THE BIODYNAMICS OF THE IMMUNE SYSTEM

"Michael J. Shea offers a potential bible for anyone wanting to support or improve their health. He generously provides specific scientific details about the physiology underlying the pandemic of metabolic syndrome and also the guidance to heal, incorporating more than 25 years of experience in the field. Beyond that, what brings the book to heart for me is Michael's personal stories. He candidly writes of his journey with fat and fasting, effects of military service–related PTSD, and his own prenatal and ancestral/ epigenetic history. His story invites us to also investigate our own lives with more curiosity. In the process, like Michael, we might find our embryo, the biodynamic fluid body of our origins, and its cosmological connectedness with all that is. This discovery is facilitated by a beautiful collection of embryo art as an additional bonus to explore in the book. *The Biodynamics of the Immune System* reminds us of the essential continuity of mind, body, spirit, and nature and how the splitting of these generates suffering and dis-ease. This is no ordinary book about metabolic syndrome! It offers paths to deep healing you have probably been craving."

CHERIONNA MENZAM-SILLS, PH.D., AUTHOR OF
THE BREATH OF LIFE: AN INTRODUCTION TO CRANIOSACRAL BIODYNAMICS

"*The Biodynamics of the Immune System* is like a tall glass of cool, clear water. Page after page, this book soothes and nourishes my mind, body, and spirit. Whether you are a health care provider, a bodyworker, or 'just' a regular human trying to make it through these challenging times, this book offers respite and incredible information. More importantly, it offers ways to incorporate many of the 'thousand faces of Health' into your daily practice."

K. MICHELLE DOYLE, BIODYNAMIC CRANIOSACRAL THERAPIST AND
FOUNDER OF LOCAL CARE MIDWIFERY

"Michael Shea brings together the ancient history of separation from nature and from each other and provides a beautiful, practical guide to bring healing and health to us as individuals and as a collective. His poetic metaphors and scientific research show us that health on every level is possible and how to live from a place of wholeness and love. The specific therapeutic applications and collaborative somatic learning experiences will benefit all humans and sentient beings on the planet. While this book was originally intended for manual therapists, all of us in the helping professions can greatly benefit both personally and professionally from the philosophy, information, and practices found here. If everyone read and applied this wisdom, we as a planet and a people could move more quickly into sustained health and happiness! I found myself inspired and my heart opened as I traveled through the pages of this incredible gift to all of us. Highly recommended!

MARTI GLENN, PH.D., CLINICAL DIRECTOR AND
CHIEF EXPERIENCE OFFICER OF RYZIO INSTITUTE

"In this paradigm-shifting book Michael Shea shares his biodynamic embryology, anatomy, and spiritual expertise so we too may clearly see. This book is about the pursuit of truth through compassion and critical thinking, giving us the insight and inspiration to see and heal the elephant in the room. In these times of COVID and a worldwide plague of heart disease, anxiety, depression, dementia, and obesity, this is the one book to read . . . and share!"

MARY BOLINGBROKE,
OSTEOPATH AND LECTURER AT THE DAISY CLINIC TRUST

"I am familiar with the beauty and biodynamic nature of this book because I've had the good fortune to have a collegial relationship with Michael for many years. We regularly treat each other, supervise each other, and share clinical experiences. This book represents an advance in biodynamic thinking to include a sense of origin and connection to the universe so necessary for the contemporary client."

BRIAN SHEA, D.O., A 30-YEAR CLINICAL BIODYNAMIC OSTEOPATHIC
PRACTITIONER IN BOULDER, COLORADO

THE
BIODYNAMICS
OF THE
IMMUNE SYSTEM

BALANCING THE ENERGIES
OF THE BODY WITH THE COSMOS

A Sacred Planet Book

MICHAEL J. SHEA, Ph.D.

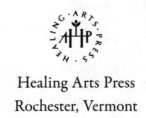

Healing Arts Press
Rochester, Vermont

Healing Arts Press
One Park Street
Rochester, Vermont 05767
www.HealingArtsPress.com

Healing Arts Press is a division of Inner Traditions International

Sacred Planet Books are curated by Richard Grossinger, Inner Traditions editorial board member and cofounder and former publisher of North Atlantic Books. The Sacred Planet collection, published under the umbrella of the Inner Traditions family of imprints, includes works on the themes of consciousness, cosmology, alternative medicine, dreams, climate, permaculture, alchemy, shamanic studies, oracles, astrology, crystals, hyperobjects, locutions, and subtle bodies.

Note to the reader: *This book is intended as an informational guide. The remedies, approaches, and techniques described herein are meant to supplement, and not to be a substitute for, professional medical care or treatment. They should not be used to treat a serious ailment without prior consultation with a qualified health care professional.*

Cataloging-in-Publication Data for this title is available from the Library of Congress

ISBN 978-1-64411-525-1 (print)
ISBN 978-1-64411-526-8 (ebook)

Printed and bound in India by Replika Press Pvt. Ltd.

10 9 8 7 6 5 4 3 2 1

Text design and layout by Debbie Glogover
This book was typeset in Garamond Premier Pro with Acherus Grotesque, Gill Sans MT Pro, and Source Sans Pro used as display typefaces
Artwork in color insert plates 1–24 by Friedrich Wolf
Photographs in chapter 25 by Almut Althaus and Beatrice Fischer
Photographs in chapters 26, 30, and 31 by Evelyn Stetzer
Photographs in chapters 28, 29, and 35 by Evelyn Stetzer and Beatrice Fischer
Photographs in chapter 32 by Beatrice Fischer

To send correspondence to the author of this book, mail a first-class letter to the author c/o Inner Traditions • Bear & Company, One Park Street, Rochester, VT 05767, and we will forward the communication, or contact the author directly at **SheaHeart.com**.

*To my mom and dad for pure love
and the support to get me this far in life.*

*To His Holiness the Dalai Lama for pure love
and the support to get me this far in life.
Please turn the Wheel of Dharma for world happiness.*

And to all life and death, the greatest teachers.

Contents

PART 1

The Current State of Ill Health and Natural Healing Antidotes

Metabolic Syndrome and Gut Health

PART 2

The Fluid Body

Biodynamics and Embryonic Healing

PART 3

Biodynamic Spiritual Healing

*Death, Distance, the Soul, and
the Influence of Covid-19*

Foreword

By Bill Harvey

For four decades Michael Shea has been learning, explicating, and evolving the field of biodynamics for the manual therapist. Through eight books and countless workshops around the world and his range and endless curiosity of how various worlds of learning interrelate, Michael has moved the field forward in numerous ways, including: greater depth of understanding of embryology; the importance of attachment theory for the practitioner's self-awareness; ways of conceptualizing and working with what is known as the fluid body; and the consequences for manual therapists of the entire culture's devolution into metabolic distress (to name just a few).

Yet before this book, I would have said that Michael's most lasting contribution to the world of biodynamics would have been his introduction of working with the cardiovascular system into the context of craniosacral therapy. This practical approach to practicing biodynamic craniosacral therapy brought the focus of the work back to the original vision of the founder of osteopathy, A. T. Still, the first D.O. Dr. Sutherland, in creating cranial osteopathy and working in a more contemplative and spiritually grounded time, moved osteopathy away from the bone and blood focus of Dr. Still and concentrated on working through the potency of the Tide. Such stillness that accompanied Dr. Sutherland's work became more and more rare as the pace of the twentieth century sped up and osteopaths changed their focus away from perceiving the patients' conditions to more pharmacological approaches to medicine. Michael Shea's realization—that working with the arteries is inherently slower, safer, and ultimately more powerfully effective when working through the potency of the Tide—will inevitably become the gold-standard approach for biodynamic craniosacral therapists.

It is always humbling to remember that the originator of craniosacral therapy, Dr. Sutherland, worked on the cranial concept for over fifty years before he made the discoveries and realizations that led to the development of biodynamic craniosacral therapy. There is certainly something to be said for putting the time in. His primary realization, that the healing impulse that accounts for the self-healing process comes from both inside and outside the body, upended the scientific materialism that was overtaking the practice of medicine during the midtwentieth century. Yet his certainty was so powerful and profound that he risked being thought of as a kook as he presented it. Ultimately his teachings were forced underground by the American Osteopathy Association.

These are times of unprecedented urgency with multiple existence-ending catastrophes looming. In considering the magnitude of the issues that we as manual therapists are now facing with our clients/patients, the tools of the trade need the possibility of a vastly more profound approach. It's not enough to tinker around the edges of our discipline, or even to upgrade the components of the field.

In a precisely similar way to the grounded spirituality of Dr. Sutherland when he presented what became known as biodynamics, in this book Dr. Shea has brought forth the necessary and critical audacity to force the issue that as a healing culture we have danced around since the advent of penicillin and the polio vaccine. That is simply to locate our existence and our actions in an acknowledged spiritual context. This potentially scary proposition is presented in the gentlest way by Michael and his superb collaborators, laying out each step of the way without even the slightest hint of proselytizing (breaking down the fourth wall of our existence). In a coherent vision of where we fit into existence, every action has a meaning: from how we eat to how we poop, how we give reverence to forces beyond ourselves, and how these actions give meaning to our lives. The presentations herein offer a level of coherence that undermine the lassitude and defeatism that we face in our extremely uncertain future. Beyond these consolations, embracing spiritual disciplines that have meaning for us in turn suggest specific ways that our healing practices can deepen and become more effective on any level that our clients are available for healing. How this is done practically is simply and comprehensively laid out for the reader with the extended examples of Tibetan Buddhism and Tantrism. Such clarity can only encourage each of us to mine the possibilities of how our own spiritual traditions can support our healing work, because the truth is, all illness is spiritual.

The Biodynamics of the Immune System is a massively generous book from a dedicated elder who is also the leading innovator in the field of manual therapy. Its generosity includes patient, accessible explanations of vast fields of research around digestion and metabolism, mature insights into the fruits of a life of dedication to a contemplative meditative path, and unvarnished autobiographical stories (with pictures!) that ground Dr. Shea's evolution as a manual therapist and spiritual seeker. Because of this generosity this book also will serve as a fundamental reference for a plethora of topics surrounding the effects of our metabolism upon our immune systems, the subtleties of the field of biodynamics, and (by the way) shockingly powerful protocols for all practitioners.

The realized vision, herein grounded in both the latest scientific inquiry and spiritual dedication, continues to evolve the field of biodynamics for nonosteopaths beyond its underground past into a coherent path to health that confers meaning and healing to the lives of all who are blessed enough to be touched by it.

BILL HARVEY has had a full-time career in manual therapies for nearly four decades. He has been a Certified Rolfer since 1984, Certified Advanced Rolfer since 1990, Rolf Movement Practitioner since 1999, and Biodynamic Craniosacral practitioner since 1984. His interest in combining these three approaches while working with clients led to the development of his trainings in Biodynamic Structural Integration, which began in 2005. He is the author of *Breathing, Mudras, and Meridians* and has an active practice in Wayne, PA. He can be reached through his website **billharvey.org**.

Preface

"The volcano of ill health has erupted." This statement was made to the European Economic Union Health Congress in the spring of 2018 by the noted cardiologist from London Aseem Malhotra, M.D. It seems like a harbinger to what would become the COVID situation. Since then, the planet earth has seen the continuous eruption of *ill health* from the emotional to the viral and the physical to the spiritual. In addition, in that same year the Institute for Functional Medicine in the United States made a call for noninvasive and nonpharmacological methods in dealing with this unprecedented eruption. This book is the evolution of a noninvasive and nonpharmacological approach to the manual therapeutic arts based on compassion and kindness. I am an expert in this field and have found methods for healing a significant part of this eruption with Real Food, associated with the work of Robert Lustig, M.D. And to heal the body one must heal the mind and the spirit. This is the work of transitioning to a compassionate approach demanded by the contemporary client and their dilemma. We are at the end of health (in this case defined by the end of disease) as we know it. It is over. Ill health does not happen in a vacuum. Antidotes, cures, and healing methods evolve and co-emerge with every new diagnosis and every angle of the numerous plagues circling the planet earth. Our work is now palliative.

To understand the situation we are in as a planet requires a language different from what we now have describing the volcano. Dr. Malhotra uses an apt metaphor for metabolic syndrome. Metaphor is an essential component of bridging from one system of thought and therapy to another, from the old to the new. In this book, whether it is science, nutrition, spirituality, eastern philosophy, or meditation, language will be critically important to incorporate a new, upgraded, wisdom-version description of the body and the mind. The update is being installed already. Our minds and bodies are being rebooted as we speak. And rather than bringing forward and dusting off some ancient therapeutic thinking and action, these beautiful streams find their way into an integrated sense of nowness. This book is full of rich and wondrous metaphors describing the integration of body, speech, and mind for the contemporary client. Every attempt is made to explain the language of metaphor either as it appears or through the glossary. And any statement made in this book and any term or metaphor used can be placed into a search engine. For example, the use of terms *pandemic, syndemic,* and *epidemic* can also mean plague, which I prefer. Just Google to deepen your understanding or to look up a reference. I have minimized the number of references for this reason. I learn more when I Google a statement or term I do not understand while reading a book. I frequently Googled numerous terms while writing this book. Use this book as a bridge to the internet.

Social media and information streams are polarized into good and bad. The essential message of this book is to reconnect with somatic empathy by investigating one's own body and slowly removing oneself from the mainstream of such polarization. The truth of any discussion can be found in one's body, and it will be the individual's truth rather than some universal truth that becomes weaponized to create separation (tribalization) and antagonize others with venomous hatred.

A major language called human anatomy is also necessary when visiting some sections of this book especially associated with the manual therapeutic arts at the end. I chose to focus on where the hands belong topically on the client without providing images of anatomy and physiology. I refer the reader to any number of anatomy texts that are available explaining the immune system and the function of the lymphatic system. Once again, the internet will provide thousands of images with a single keystroke or two on your computer.

I teach and practice slowness and stillness. This is the essence of biodynamics. Throughout this book there will be numerous terms used for slowness such as *Primary Respiration* (PR), *the Tide, the Long Tide, the Breath of Life,* and the *wind element.* Terms for stillness will include *stillpoint, the dynamic stillness, the void, quiescence,* and *the element of space.* The term *biodynamic* also has different meanings. It originally came from the work of Rudolph Steiner in Europe at the turn the last century and referred to blessing and sacralizing the earth for optimizing nutrient and spiritual value in food that is grown from it. And biodynamics means the study of the morphological development of a human embryo, which will be a theme throughout the book. More precisely biodynamics means the growth of the whole over time and the interrelationship with biokinetics, the unique development of its parts within that whole. Biodynamics implies the fluid body, which precedes differentiation in the hierarchy of growth and development yet is capable of guiding it. This leads to a discovery of an entire universe with trillions of molecules and related movements that live and die, surge and recede inside of the human body. It matches the hundreds of billions of galaxies that exist outside of our body in the totality of the universe we live in. In addition to biodynamic movement of the fluid body, every molecule in the universe must go through a phase of stillness for transformation. The universe both inside and out is moving and in a stillpoint simultaneously. Consequently, healing is explored biodynamically for the contemporary client that includes all these meanings and metaphors in one therapeutic intention and motivation; slowness and stillness are the foundation of healing.

Throughout the book I place a series of infographics that give a sense of flow to the biodynamic model of spirituality. And at the same time, they provide a glossary of terms to bridge the various models and methods demonstrated in this book into an emerging viable therapy to treat the contemporary world with kindness and compassion. I think of them as roadmaps in a traditional sense. In biodynamic embryology, the map gets unfolded first before locating one's self on the map. If the reader gets lost along the road of reading and comprehending what is written, the infographics are convenient maps to relocate oneself without Google Maps. They are linked to the glossary at the end of the book.

It is through the use of metaphor that as a culture we will transition to a higher level of functioning. The transition is upon us, and for many people it is uncomfortable. This time on the planet demands the discovery of our own personal origin story, through which the meaning of pain and suffering can be explored and incorporated spiritually. As we spiritually self-regulate, we enter the domain of coregulation and empathetic responses rather than reactivity. I believe this book is a collaborative somatic learning experience to benefit all humans and sentient beings on the planet. The reader can begin to self-regulate based on my words, practices, and metaphors and those of the contributors. I invite the reader to go inside and find their own metaphor and experience for any of the terms, ideas, and concepts I use in this book. I believe the healing process on this planet and of this planet and all its inhabitants begins with spiritual self-regulation rooted in the body and mind, culture, and nature. Self-regulation includes the notion of the exploration of these layers of the whole without unnecessary restriction but rather with direct and immediate contact with the divine, our conception right.

Acknowledgments

What an incredible network of friends, colleagues, family, and professional help-ers to get this book launched. My wife Cathy has supported every aspect of get-ting this book to print, including her contributions in the first part of the book and appendix. We know and live every part of this book through our clinical practice, our home self-care life, and seeing it all in our spiritual practice.

Bill Harvey and Ann Weinstein gave regular support as I walked the tight rope of thirty-five chapters and almost three hundred figures put together by Jeanie Burns, a fantastic friend and graphic artist. I take photographs for the sake of healing the planet and chose to keep many of the original photographs taken for classroom purposes in order to honor all of those students and assistants who willingly volunteered to be photographed: Fritz Lang, Beatrice Fischer, and my niece Erica Stetzer. Thank you to my niece, Evelyn Stetzer, for her photography prowess and to my incredible course manager and dear friend, Almut Althaus, who single-handedly manages hundreds of students every year in our classroom in Germany.

Joshua Horowitz inspired me to move toward the immune system for my teaching at the beginning of the COVID pandemic; Jörg Schürpf lent his exper-tise in many things, especially about Chi Nei Tsang in chapter 31. I am grateful to Jullian Gustavson for not only ten years of discussion but also the editing of chapter 7 on character structure. Chapter 15 was thoroughly edited by Tim Shafer, who labored over it for quite some time. I am most grateful for the time and attention Tim gave to it to improve everyone's biodynamic perception.

I have great gratitude for Michelle Doyle's editorial assistance in chapters 5 and 32. Michelle is perhaps one of the most brilliant midwives I have ever met; she gives and radiates pure love, having helped birth over 4,000 babies. I love teaching with her.

Behind the scenes is our most wonderful office manager, Lisa Fay. With her constant support editing and checking the text to make sure everything was synchronized and aligned properly, she has been a spiritual rock in my life.

While in creation, many pieces of this book were vetted, edited, looked at, discussed, and taught to my students by colleagues, teaching teams, and translators internationally. I am indebted to so many people, including Bettina Ravanelli, Ursula Walke, Joachim Lichtenberg, Carlos Rodeiro, Beata Kirscher, Claudia Oliveri, Luisa Brancolini, Javier de Maria, Ellen Grösser, Mary Bolingbroke, Renata Ritzman and her husband Barry Williams, and Dale Alexander for his encouragement in educating the manual therapy community on the meaning of metabolism.

Stephen Porges, a brilliant scientist who developed the polyvagal theory, has contributed to the book and to my life since I first studied his work in 1990 and later got to know him while on the same dais at several conferences. Stephen walks his talk regarding compassion and spirituality.

Jim Jealous, D.O., the founder of biodynamic osteopathy, died in February of 2021—a great loss to the biodynamic community worldwide. I am indebted to him for his mentorship and turning my mind and heart toward my embryo, a deep exploration of love.

Throughout this project I received spiritual support from Catherine Vitte, one of the deepest rivers and most compassionate human beings I have ever met. With her help some sharp edges were softened and my heart opened. Thank you, Catherine. I am blessed by our friendship. Annalis Prendina, my dharma sister and coauthor of chapter 23, is my spiritual mentor and a clear river of compassion. Another clear river of compassion who contributes to my life and this book is Annette Saager, a Dharmacharya with Thich Nhat Hanh.

The contributing authors are amazing and helped me with this book in more ways than contributing chapters. Thank you to Samantha Lotti, Mary Monro, and my beautiful wife Cathy again and again for our many conversations about Health, healing, and the role of spirituality in the manual therapeutic arts. Additionally, the assistant managing editor at Healing Arts Press, Patricia Rydle, was constantly available for my innumerable questions and patiently pointed out my mistakes with kindness, clarity, and precision.

Finally, I would like to give a shout out to my sister, Sheila Shea. Sheila runs the Intestinal Health Institute in Tucson, Arizona. She was the first person to alert me to the scourge of metabolic syndrome over a decade ago. She gave me my first training and understanding of the human body from a metabolic point of view. For that and many other things she has gifted me with over our lifetime,

I am eternally grateful. This sentiment includes all of my siblings. My younger brother, Brian Shea, is a biodynamic cranial osteopath practicing in Boulder, Colorado, and all of our lives we have shared our hearts, our hands, and our minds around clinical biodynamic practice. My older brother, Dan Shea, is a retired attorney who has contributed to my life in innumerable ways especially spiritually. I have the greatest siblings. How fortunate!

Abbreviations

ANS	autonomic nervous system
BCVT	biodynamic cardiovascular therapy
D.O.	doctor of osteopathy
PR	Primary Respiration
SNS	sympathetic nervous system

Biodynamics and the Mind-Body-Spirit

> *Spirituality is the aspect of humanity that refers to the way individuals seek and express meaning and purpose and the way they experience their connectedness to the moment, to self, to others, to nature, and to the significant or sacred.*
>
> PUCHALSKI ET AL.,
> "IMPROVING THE QUALITY OF SPIRITUAL CARE
> AS A DIMENSION OF PALLIATIVE CARE"

I began studying and working within the alternative health care field in 1975. I attended the Lindsey-Hopkins School of Massage in Miami, Florida, for a thousand-hour training to become a massage and colon hydrotherapist. The alternative field was still in its infancy, born from the ashes of European naturopathy with remnants remaining in the United States but soon to be forgotten. The health-food stores of the 1970s were a radically different critter than the health-food stores (or what are called health-food stores) nowadays—stacked with *natural* foods and sugar disguised a thousand different ways. The philosophy underpinning the alternative field at that time was called Cartesian duality. While in school, I was first introduced to the famous statement of seventeenth-century French philosopher, René Descartes, "I think, therefore I am." It became the foundation of the *mind-body split* philosophy. To be in this new emerging field of an alternative health care practice required healing the historical split between mind and body and returning it to a unified whole that is phenomenologically inseparable. This book explores that separation with the premise that the split happened much earlier in recorded history. This became the first pillar of the emerging field of alternative health care that was gradually co-opted by Western medicine to become the complementary medical field. The co-opting of the alternative field by the medical community coalesced at Harvard with David Eisenberg in the 1980s.

This new alignment with allopathic medicine created a philosophical dilemma for the alternative community. And it gave birth to the second pillar of alternative ethics for overcoming the *body-spirit split*. An agreement was made between the church and the emerging Western medical community around the same time that René Descartes made his famous statement in the 1600s. The body was always considered sacred from the beginning of time. But the medical community in Renaissance Europe began the practice of cadaver dissections as part of modern medical training. Initially they were illegal according to church authorities. The body as sacred became an issue with medical authorities of the time because dissection was considered sacrilegious. Cadaver dissection labs at medical schools had specially constructed tables to hide the dead bodies being dissected in case church authorities showed up to inspect. I do not know how church authorities could avoid the odor while inspecting for dead bodies. And a political deal was cut between the church and the medical community giving the right to dissect cadavers in exchange for giving up the belief in the sacredness and spirituality of the body. That was given over totally to the church. Thus the body-spirit split became deeply engrained in the practice of Western medicine.

A third pillar of the alternative community includes "The Doctrine of Discovery" written by Pope Alexander VI in 1493. It declared "that any land not inhabited by Christians was available to be 'discovered,' claimed, and exploited: 'The Catholic faith and the Christian religion be exalted and be everywhere increased and spread, that the health of souls be cared for and that barbarous nations be overthrown and brought to the faith itself'" (Khomina 2017). This act solidified the philosophy of domination over nature by man resulting in the extraction economy we have now. Furthermore it justified the enslavement of native aboriginal people resulting in numerous genocides perpetrated worldwide. It is still going on especially now in the name of communism in China. North America was home to over twelve thousand tribes of Native Americans when Christopher Columbus landed, and now it is down to 593 that are officially registered with the U.S. government.

"The Doctrine of Discovery" gave us both the *human-nature split* and the *human-human split*. Thus the third and fourth pillars of the alternative community are the reintegration of mind, body, spirit, community, and nature. Aggression and antispirituality gestated for thousands of years and was birthed around the time of the Renaissance. This book attempts to undo this history by invoking a spiritual engagement in reclaiming dominion with one's body through common sense practices and Real Food. It can hardly be called an alternative field anymore but rather an original field of being in harmony with the planet. To reclaim the body is to awaken the body's ability to know the truth of immediate experience. It begins with interoceptive awareness, the felt sense of how our organs, muscles, and fluids have a language that we can understand about what to accept and what to reject in the present moment.

- Mind-Body Split
- Body-Spirit Split
- Human-Nature Split
- Human-Human Split

A central premise of this book is that all disease is spiritual disease (see fig. I.1). That is one basic working model I use in this book and live as best as possible. The overlapping plagues consuming this planet find a common antidote in the spiritual domain. There is suffering, and it seems meaningless. There is compassion, and how do we manifest empathy for those who are suffering? How do we serve those who are suffering greatly? Contemporary forms of suffering are linked to the function of the immune system. The body is a good starting place to reclaim ownership. We live in the time of the immune system, that exquisite filter between the natural world outside of us and the natural world inside of us. That part-time barrier and part-time filter knows every cell in the body. It attempts to protect and care for every cell in the body. The immune system connects us to the moment with its benevolence. This is a major contributor to a spirituality of the body. As Alexander Lowen, M.D, said in *The Spirituality of the Body,* "in the wise individual the divine spirit is experienced as the natural gracefulness of the body and is reflected in the person's behavior." The divine spirit in this book is equated with Primary Respiration (PR), the wind element as we will see in the biodynamic practices in this book. The immune system clears the path for PR to function as grace. The divine spirit is equated with stillness that is dynamic and alive. All transformation in the body at a molecular level requires a stillpoint to function properly. Stillness is equated with the element of space in Tibetan medicine, which I have studied for forty-five years.

We will deeply explore these possibilities to overcome the basic splitting from nature, community, mind, and body. Spiritual disease begins with a gradual alienation and withdrawal from the natural world. We live in an extraction economy, and the extraction of resources and stripping of the earth for consumerism and

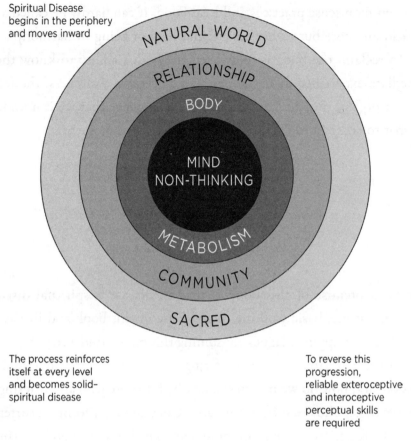

Spiritual Disease
begins in the periphery
and moves inward

The process reinforces
itself at every level
and becomes solid-
spiritual disease

To reverse this
progression,
reliable exteroceptive
and interoceptive
perceptual skills
are required

Fig. I.1. Four quadrants of spiritual disease

materialism is the outer level of spiritual disease based on European politics during the Renaissance. The great loss of the sacred begins here. And how many research reports, books, and blogs on the value of reconnecting with nature do we need before we are motivated to take a walk in the woods or a swim in the ocean or to pull weeds in the backyard? I read someone quoting Thoreau several times a month and I live by the ocean. I visit often and make my own poetry of nature. Reconnecting with nature is a spiritual process in which we begin to heal the split for ourselves and the planet. It is a central premise of the biodynamic model to reconnect with nature. Nature teaches us unfocused attention and extraordinary perception, key elements of understanding shamanism, the original healing tradition of our planet, which this book addresses. And planting an herb garden on your windowsill, in your backyard, or in a community garden is a good start.

Mainstream media promotes the separation of humans from humans in our collective social community. It breaks down our interconnectedness. Friendships lost; families broken by virtue of whom someone voted for and whether or not someone got vaccinated. The alienation from a wider social community, demonstrated by the polarization and tribalization with the emotional attitudes of hatred and anger, buries compassion in a garbage heap. We live in the charnel ground of strong emotions without civility. Digital pollution is waterboarding common sense. It also upregulates the body's immune system with unsafe stress levels and makes it prone to "cytokine storms," when your immune system releases too many inflammatory protein molecules into the bloodstream. It is a storm because almost every cell in the body has a cytokine receptor and thus the whole body is in a dangerous hurricane. Unnecessary fear captures the mind and takes it hostage, preventing a compassionate or even a balanced response to life.

PART I INTENTION

Describe Current State of Ill Health and Natural Healing Antidotes

Part 1 is subtitled "Metabolic Syndrome and Gut Health." It is what Robert Lustig, M.D., calls "the corporate takeover of the human body" with processed food that is intentionally engineered to be highly addictive. It creates the substrate of massive physiological and metabolic illness on the planet. The processed food eaten by most people biohacks our metabolism. It is like eating ransomware that shuts down critical self-healing mechanisms, especially the immune system. Food corporations make six hundred billion dollars in profit every year from this hack job, and it costs the health care system a trillion dollars to remove the ransomware without a large degree of success. We are so split off from our body that we have assigned major parts of it to various doctors and of course the belief in faulty and biased food science paid for by the food corporations. This preempts the body's ability to know the truth of experience clearly. We need a scientific mind, sometimes called a critical mind, that can weigh different arguments to differentiate good from bad science. There is such a large amount of illness that it is common to hear how overwhelmed the medical system is no matter what country. A half billion people are obese, and another half billion people have type 2 diabetes on the planet. There will be some overlap in those communities. In chapter 6 I tell my story of being morbidly obese following my discharge from the Army in 1973 and then how I lost the weight with fasting, a theme running throughout the first part. The COVID pandemic has clearly shown that those most vulnerable and likely to die have underlying metabolic conditions. This means contemporary illness is being driven by inflammation, primarily from eating processed food. The new inflammation volcano erupting everywhere in numerous organs and throughout the vascular system is the preexisting condition for mortality from COVID and other diseases.

Mary Monro contributes a detailed explanation of the cardiovascular system and its relationship with immune function. My beautiful wife, Cathy, contributes a chapter giving a general understanding of how digestion affects well-being. There is also information based on the model of Swiss Biological Medicine created by Thomas Rau, M.D. Cathy invites us to look at Grandmother's wisdom for home healing and offers simple ways to reclaim dominion over our bodies with Real Food and common sense.

PART 2 INTENTION

Describe the Fluid Body

Part 2 is subtitled "Biodynamics and Embryonic Healing" as it is found both inside of the human body and outside. Using the metaphor of the *fluid body,* an exploration of the human embryo for healing is undertaken. The fluid body is a biodynamic term coined by the late Jim Jealous, D.O. He was the founder of biodynamic osteopathy and mentored me in the mid-1990s with the proviso that I only teach the perception of love with Primary Respiration and the perception of grace with the dynamic stillness. It is important to acknowledge the shoulders I stand on and the gift that he gave me early in my career. He kept asking me every time we met, "Did you find your embryo?" The embryo is a metaphor for wholeness and love, and we will see it is the beginning of the development of the immune system. I did find my embryo, and the section on the fluid body will explore a variety of guided meditations to help you find your embryo. I have written many articles about the human embryo. I taught human embryology at the former Santa Barbara Graduate Institute in the pre- and perinatal psychology and somatic psychology doctoral programs. Just to see an image of a human embryo can change your perspective on life. I am so grateful that my friend Friedrich Wolf, who is an experienced teacher of biodynamic practice and artist, drew a series of twenty-four images with watercolors to demonstrate that the embryo is a fluid body. When you look at an embryo you are looking at yourself. This is important for healing, because in medical anthropology and biodynamic practice as I teach and practice it, illness is cured by a sacred ritual involving a return to origins, whether that is the beginning of the human embryo or the beginning of the universe. Thus, the book begins with the origin of the human body as embryo and finishes with the origin of the human body as universe. At the same time this part of the book invites the reader to begin to develop a metabolic sense of their body, a precursor to healing metabolic syndrome. Numerous practices are taught to feel the original metabolic body with its various metaphors starting with the fluid body.

PART 3 INTENTION

Describe Biodynamic Spiritual Healing

Part 3, subtitled "Death, Distance, the Soul, and the Influence of COVID-19," will begin addressing the deeper nature of recovering from spiritual disease from both Eastern and Western perspectives. The mind of altruism, compassion, and kindness is deeply buried in overconceptualization, compulsivity, wrong perceptions, and fantasy states of mind. The metaphors of fake news and conspiracy theories have become embodied in the contemporary world.

Part 3 supports the evolving paradigm I teach of biodynamic cardiovascular therapy (BCVT) by infusing it with a formal spiritual dimension. This dimension includes remote healing, distance healing, or nonlocal healing. These are terms used for healing at a distance whether it is through intercessory prayer, formal compassion meditations, and any number of perceptual processes, as the reader will see. I feel especially fortunate to have a contribution by Samantha Lotti in this section, which will provide deeper insights into healing our contemporary spiritual confusion and act as an important bridge to biodynamic shamanic healing discussed in the remaining parts. To practice biodynamically in the contemporary world requires a shift from ordinary perception to extraordinary perception, a hallmark of shamanic practice discussed in parts 4 and 5. The term "shamanic" is used to represent the original, traditional health care systems on the planet when mind, body, and spirit were treated as an integrated whole.

PART 4 INTENTION

Describe the Stillness

Part 4 is subtitled "Inner Healing Arts and Cosmology." In this section an investigation of the meditative and contemplative mind is offered. Extraordinary perception requires a calm mind for clarity and wisdom to arise. At the same time different metaphors for Health will help us bridge from a Western understanding to an Eastern understanding of the body and mind from the point of view of the five elements in Tibetan medicine. That is my primary influence both as a Buddhist therapist for forty-five years and a licensed manual therapist in the state of Florida since 1976, as well as an international educator in the field of biodynamic craniosacral therapy since 1986. However, in this book I am applying the principles of biodynamic craniosacral therapy to the cardiovascular system. I prefer to call my work biodynamic cardiovascular therapy. This is the healing necessary for the human body, mind, and spirit with the contemporary client. It is consistent with the consciousness of the osteopathic community started by Dr. Still who said "The rule of the artery is supreme" back in the late 1800s. He also said, "I love my fellow man, because I see God in his face and in his form." This part finishes with chapter 23, which creates a bridge to cosmological healing detailed in part 5. It is based on Buddhist cosmology and coauthored by Annalis Prendina, a brilliant dharma therapist.

PART 5 INTENTION

Describe Therapeutic Applications

Part 5, subtitled "Biodynamic Cardiovascular Therapy as a Healing Cosmology," takes us into a very deep investigation and exploration of manual and perceptual skills. Dr. Jealous said that biodynamics is the study of perception and wholeness. A variety of perceptual skills and hands-on skills are offered. Shamanic perception will be explored in the context of acupuncture points associated with different arteries, veins, and states of consciousness. It is in this section that we continue the formal exploration of the cosmological imperative for healing that began with chapter 23. The embryo takes us to our personal origins, while the protocols shown in part 5 are designed to reconnect the client with the cosmos as it was at the origin of the universe and the end of the previous universe, the void. This is accessible through the perception of slowness and stillness via Primary Respiration and the dynamic stillness. That is still the bread and butter of biodynamic practice and the interchange of elemental energy for harmony and balance. And Primary Respiration and the dynamic stillness function differently at different levels within the human body from an Eastern perspective. The three levels of ordinary body, subtle body, and very subtle body will be discussed and skills offered to integrate that holistic triad that exists as one thing underneath the skin of our body.

At the same time there are preliminary skills necessary to understand and experience the biodynamic session as a sacred, three-step rite of passage. This begins with the perception of a Neutral and the establishment of safety in the therapeutic relationship discussed in parts 4 and 5. Once the Neutral has been achieved and the autonomic nervous systems of both the client and therapist are coregulated and attuned to safety, the second part of the sacred process takes place. This is Ignition as shown in figure I.2 on page 12. The spark of the Breath of Life described by Dr. Sutherland initiates a quantum leap from one level of Primary Respiration and stillness to another level. Bridging to these levels requires different skills enumerated and elaborated upon throughout this book. In addition, there is a cardiometabolic protocol for babies in part 5. In this way the entire cosmos is covered from origin of the universe, conception of a human being, birth of a human being into adulthood, and death and dying. The marrow described in part 5 is the deepest part of our immune system as it exists in the body. It represents the continuity of the originality of our embryo, and at the same time throughout our life span, it is the constant creator of the blood, lymph, and cellular elements of the immune system.

The vagus nerve is a major consideration as described in chapter 25. It plays an important role in the immune response and gut pain. The vagus nerve perceives the inflammation in the gut and can regulate an anti-inflammatory response by influencing the hypothalamic-pituitary-adrenal gland axis. It modulates the autonomic nervous system in coregulating the key immune organs of the spleen, adrenal glands, and probably the bone marrow. The vagus has deep spiritual connections to the Hindu yoga of kundalini, a spiritual life force in the pelvis that can transform pain into bliss. At the very least, biodynamic practices shown in chapter 25 will stimulate the vagus for its more modest healing effects. The autonomic nervous system has been studied for a hundred years. Stress and trauma are greatly understood but a mystery when it comes to repairing them despite marketing suggesting otherwise. This is because we now live in the age of the immune system. Starting with the 1990s, every decade offered major learning about the big systems of the body starting with the brain and central nervous system. Then we had an intensive decade of cardiovascular system study and research. Now, as a culture and society, we are deep into a study and understanding of the intestines and their relationship with the immune system. The innate immune system that we are born with, which lives primarily in the lining of the intestines, is greatly damaged in most Westernized people. Compounding this problem is the fact that a critical bridge to the adaptive immune system is also found in the lining of the intestines. Its function is consequently damaged. How do we accomplish the repair? What is the antidote?

The immune system protects us from distinct forms of harm. It protects us from certain forms of death and dying. I use it as a metaphor for a spiritual system of care and nurturing of the whole experience of being human. We must learn to nurture the whole of human experience rooted in the human body. Complex trauma also compromises the immune system in the gut. This book attempts to move toward a clearer understanding of Health and healing in this new era of the immune system—and not from an eclectic point of view or cherry-picking parts of older, complex healing systems into a hodgepodge of techniques. Biodynamic cardiovascular therapy is an integrative approach that explores the complexity of the contemporary draught of well-being.

Another basic working model in this book is the biodynamic term Ignition as first coined by Dr. Jim Jealous (see fig. I.2 on page 12). The core problem in the body and mind of the contemporary client is the inflammatory process as described physiologically, metabolically, emotionally, and spiritually throughout this book. This inflammation is an Ignition of the immune system that leads to initiation in the sense of the sacred. The plague of our time has the signature of the gods. According to an ancient Asian proverb, "your illness is wasted unless you are spiritually transformed by it." The number of deaths due to the overlapping plagues on our planet lends itself to the metaphor of shamanic initiation. Ignition as initiation involves the recognition of death and dying that we have experienced already. It is a three-step process in which someone who finds themselves ill at any level described above is led to a doorway or portal that opens to the possibility of healing by sacrificing a false self for a spiritual self. And in the third step, through the choice of the individual, he or she crosses the threshold and becomes initiated and thus incorporated as a spiritual being. Incorporation means embodiment, a direct connection to the body as spiritual. The therapist is a witness and not a pill pusher. There are not any quick fixes, which is why a conscious allegiance to slowness and stillness is vital.

IGNITION, INITIATION, AND RITES OF PASSAGE

During all stages of the life journey there are required ceremonies, rituals, prayers, conversations, and rites of passage that normalize and integrate complex stages of life into becoming a progressive, differentiated, whole human being. The intention is to incorporate as a spiritual being with or without religion. Krishna said, "If you want to follow the spiritual path, I will give you the tools to follow the spiritual path; if you do not want to follow the spiritual path, I will also give you the tools to not follow the spiritual path."

Sacred rituals called *rites of passage* with accompanying prayers and ceremonies are also necessary to mitigate the effects of traumatic, pandemic, syndemic, epidemic, and cataclysmic experiences engulfing our planet. This is absolutely necessary to maintain the coherence and cohesion within a community and its members. Metabolic syndrome is a large-scale wildfire on the planet, in the planet, and filling its atmosphere. It is consuming major tracts of valuable land in our bodies and minds. It is a wildfire of systemic inflammation that will be explained throughout this book. The human organism is very combustible when its fuel is highly processed food. Processed food becomes cheap kindling inside the body. It interferes with the internal weather pattern producing lightning (cytokine) storms that continually ignite the kindling.

To snuff out the wildfire of inflammation, the element of water is needed and the repair of the container and its natural barriers, such as the epithelium of the intestines and the endothelium of the vascular system, and the perception of life as it extends out to the natural world and beyond to the origin of the universe. Such repair can happen when we stop eating for periods of time rather than following a diet that does not work such as those recommended by government and corporate agencies. For Health to flourish like a phoenix rising out of the ashes, an Ignition that incorporates slowness and stillness will transmute into a sacred initiation. This initiation requires a set of skills and practices for the scorched earth to return to its natural state to flourish and requires a period of the ground laying fallow. The herbs, the flowers, and the fruits and vegetables all return with their intrinsic, robust nature when the earth is restored after the wildfire. It restores itself with the appropriate and correct care. Such care is taught in this book for any person willing to incorporate a biodynamic perspective as a *rite of passage*.

A rite of passage comes from the study of cultural anthropology. It contains forms to assist communities with life transitions that are innate and instinctual ways in which societies remain coherent in the face of tragedy. In general such rites follow a three-step process mentioned above. This book explores those three steps in clinical practice from a biodynamic perspective as *first* achieving a *Neutral* associated with stability and the perception of safety in the autonomic nervous system, internally and externally. *Second* is an Ignition of spiritual incorporation arising from the interchange of Primary Respiration (slowness) and dynamic stillness. Some clients refer to this sensation as "grace flowing." *Third* is resting in the Health, the potency of Primary Respiration and stillness as full spiritual incorporation and the felt sense of vitality and well-being. More will be revealed throughout this book, as it is critical to understand that such rites of passage must occur in the therapist first.

The application of a therapeutically relevant antidote as used in the biodynamic practices of Primary Respiration (a metaphor for the wind element) and stillness (a metaphor for the element of space) is what ignites the possibility of Health to be remembered and restored from its hibernation in the deepest recesses of our body and mind. The capital "H" in the word "Health" comes from the osteopathic tradition. As the founder of osteopathy in the nineteenth century, Dr. Still, said in his book *Philosophy of Osteopathy,* "To find health should be the object of the doctor. Anyone can find disease." This Health is unconditional, a preexisting condition in the human body, and it will be gradually described throughout the book with numerous methods and metaphors to reincorporate it, especially in part 5 discussing manual therapeutics. Health is directly associated with the experience of well-being and thus the activity of the immune system—a well-being that is undiminished by pain and suffering and holds the equality of

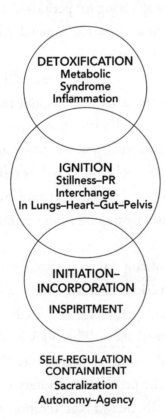

Fig. I.2. The biodynamics of Ignition. Ignition of the spiritual is a function of the heart. The spiritual at the most practical level involves self-regulation and agency. Agency is the ability to accurately perceive and change one's environment.

all experience free from judgment and duality. Some clients report feeling the movement of love in their body or the flow of grace in their body after a session. These are two of the thousand faces of Health.

Each of the sections of this book bridges to the next one until the book becomes an interrelated whole (see fig. I.3). Part 1 covers the underlying reality of a medical condition manifesting on the planet now called metabolic syndrome (MetS). It is vitally important to understand the human body now from a metabolic point of view. Metabolism refers to the incredibly complex systems that manage self-regulation of the organism and especially the immune system. It means the exchange of substances called molecules across and through barriers. In the hierarchy of embryonic development, the fluid body with its fluid forces precedes the bidirectional pathways of nutrition delivery and waste removal that molecules regulate. The metaphor of metabolism invites the reader to observe the complexities of the universe we live in, as those same complexities are duplicated inside the human body. I have attempted to simplify biochemistry and cell biology to give the reader a foothold in the inner unseen territory of the human body. It is like astrogeophysics or astronomy of the body. It is at the metabolic level, the smallest yet most global level where the human body is now most ill. That is the core of Health discussed throughout this book and the methods to reclaim it by oneself or with another. New bridges need to be built to the pre-existing intelligence of Health (see fig. I.3).

Once the process of stitching together the four domains of spiritual disease is undertaken, it is then possible upon this platform of wholeness to discern the deeper therapeutic forces binding together the quadrants in the first place. They never disappeared. These are the five elements in Tibetan medicine. The structure and function of all biological molecules are scaled across the universe as we know it now. This means that we are deeply interconnected with the whole world in a much greater and more accurate way than we can imagine because of what weaves all molecules together into similar function. This begins with the elements of space (stillness) and wind (Primary Respiration) followed by fire, water, and earth detailed throughout this book. It is possible to have an experience of the elements and the connection they provide through the practices described and shown throughout this book. It is possible to have a felt sense of our biology as a shared universal biology without unnecessary fear. Stitching together the four quadrants and beginning to access the five elements in their interconnectedness via the smallest of biological molecules is the foundation for empathy and compassion to naturally arise as the glue that binds us together. To do that we must begin to build new bridges in our mind and body with slowness and stillness. We must begin to remove the rubble of the old bridges that are in disrepair. We must rebuild the appropriate human infrastructure without interference from tribalization and talking heads. We must learn to discern the truth that already germinates forever in our body. This book is a primer on getting that seed to sprout and take root. It is up to you to water new life and claim dominion with your body.

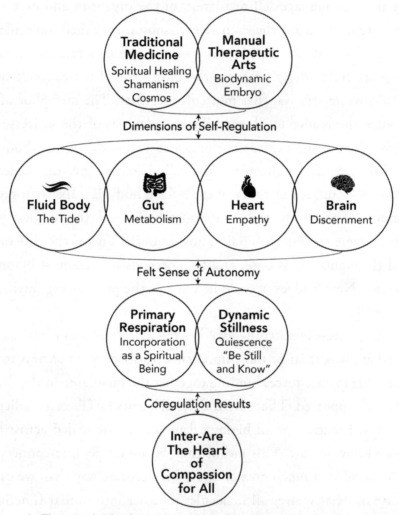

1. There is a bridge between traditional medicine and manual medicine.
2. There is a bridge between all body systems.
3. There is a bridge between Primary Respiration and dynamic stillness.
4. There is a bridge between our body and mind.
5. There is a bridge between life and death.
6. There is a bridge between our heart and our hands.
7. Thich Nhat Hanh coined the term "Inter-Are".

Fig. I.3. Bridging to self-regulation and coregulation. The neurological basis of the therapeutic relationship is based on millions of years of survival and self-regulation. The seeds of altruism and compassion are equally old. It begins with building accurate empathy.

The incorporation of spirit is an ongoing developmental phase until we die and most likely even beyond death. It is directly associated with bringing deeper, connected meaning to our existence through the soma, our biological organism as it is without negative cultural imprinting. Bringing meaning to the soma means engaging in the simple and complex repairs and maintenance of our own body via the principles shown in this book. Self-regulation then unfolds accurate coregulation by serving others. We serve others to find meaning with knowing what to accept and what to reject regarding the ownership and human right to reclaim our own body and mind. Self-regulation and coregulation, the prevailing neurological paradigm for the therapeutic relationship, is retrofitted to become spiritual self-regulation and spiritual coregulation. Everyone is empowered to have a direct connection to the divine without the middle person interpreting our sovereign connection.

Furthermore, incorporation of spirit is political. This book is the foundation of a pro soma movement. The core politics of pro soma includes a declaration of human rights associated with the sovereignty, dominion, and ownership of one's own body by each individual person. We must become the host of our sensory experience rather than a continual guest in a for-profit medical waiting room. Pro soma is about accessing the Health, the osteopathic notion of incorporation of spirit and discussed throughout this book. Thus there are numerous self-regulation and coregulation practices in this book that are tried and true. They have been vetted by the many thousands of people over thousands of years.

Incorporation is creating bridges between aspects of our body and mind with the soma being of equal priority if not more so, the temporary house of Rumi's guest in "The Guest House." So serving others at any level involves these basic principles of the incorporation of spirit. *All Sickness Is Homesickness,* as Dianne Connelly aptly named her famous acupuncture book. Or charity begins at home in the house of spirit. Spirit as metaphor includes a sense of vitality and wellbeing. It is sometimes called Buddha-nature.

It is a bridge that we cross every day and every moment with all of our senses. And in many ways the bridge seems circular with the repetition of pain and suffering that is addictive, and thus relapse is part of the terrain like hazards on a Masters-level golf course. These bridges are all self-regulated on the inside of the body based on our embryonic morphology first, then metabolism, which becomes physiology and finally a biospirituality. The body in this view is a mirror of the known and unknown universe and its hundred billion galaxies and dark energy. We are reported to have seventy trillion cells in our body. The next supercomputer modeling may double or triple that. We are destroying these somatic bridges in our body with the plague of metabolic ill health. Time to wake them up and incorporate as intrepid somatic explorers. Courage and fearlessness must be incorporated as spirit.

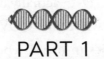

PART 1

THE CURRENT STATE OF ILL HEALTH AND NATURAL HEALING ANTIDOTES

Metabolic Syndrome and Gut Health

1

What Is Metabolic Syndrome?

Most people that die from COVID-19 actually die from the underlying preexisting condition called metabolic syndrome. COVID-19 is defined as a *syndemic* because it involves two epidemics in one. I repeat several key concepts as I go along, so forgive me if this repetition seems tedious or boring. Read with a beginner's mind. I gave it my best effort with the help of several editors to keep it at a beginner's level and not the "dummy" level as is so popular these days. Figure 1.1 gives an overview that will gradually be explained over the following chapters.

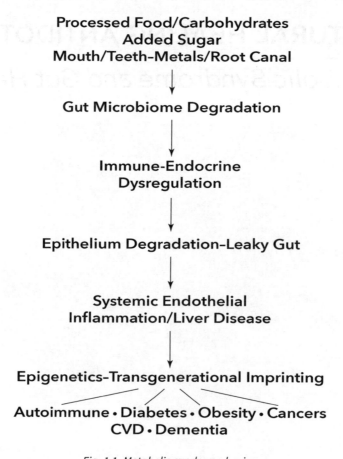

Fig. 1.1. Metabolic syndrome basics

First, metabolic syndrome is a pandemic. It has been a pandemic for the past decade. This means that over 50 percent of the population in Westernized countries on the planet have it. It is worse in the United States. Eighty-eight percent of Americans are metabolically dysregulated, and the British have 80 percent. Only one in twelve Americans are metabolically well regulated. It is shocking to me that 94 percent of people that die from COVID-19 have metabolic syndrome as a preexisting condition and consequently die from multiple organ failure brought on by a weakened innate immune system. How did we get like this? Read on.

Second, it is important to understand the word *metabolism* basically means *the conversion and exchange of substances*—from food to energy to waste—in the body. These very small substances are called molecules or metabolites and are found in all biological organisms on the planet. These substances are converted, reabsorbed, and exchanged, and waste is removed at *four basic levels* (and many intermediate and advanced levels, only some of which I mention in this chapter).

The first type of metabolic activity is *gastrointestinal,* where fat is converted into fatty acids, carbohydrates are converted into glucose, and proteins are converted into amino acids. There is also some processing of toxins and pathogens, with transportation via the blood to the liver (for conversion, storage, distribution, and elimination). The second area of metabolic activity involves the *vascular endothelium.* This is the lining of the blood vessels where the interchange of molecules between the fluid compartments of the body is managed. The third area of metabolic activity is the *surface of the cell membrane,* both internally and externally. What goes in must come out chemically altered. And finally, *internal cell structures (organelles) suspended in cytoplasm* generate energy out of the metabolites, divide and repair cells, and remove the resulting waste products out of the cells.

Trillions of such interactions and exchanges of these substances are taking place every moment in our body. It is a lot of work. These interactions are like musical notes in a larger symphony being played by the body's tissues and organs.

Molecules, these tiniest components of body metabolism, come in two basic types. One is a key and one is a lock in their appearance from scientific drawings regarding their ability or inability to connect. The two or more coming together is called *bonding* in biochemistry. Just think of oxygen and hydrogen coming together into water. Multiple bonds create a chain, and chains create groups. One such chain is called a polysaccharide (carbohydrate) like in pasta or bread, the most common and ubiquitous processed food. But a molecule can also approach the cell membrane looking for the keyhole for entrance into or out of the cell and then bond.

When the key enters the lock, a stillpoint takes place in their combined vibratory movement. The tumblers in the lock align. This allows for a transformation to take place. This is like when a sperm cell enters the egg cell, and a pause takes place in the alignment of the two genomes, which may last up to twenty-four hours before the first cell division. A brand-new molecule (water) and a brand-new human being (cell) are created. Thus, a stillpoint is the basis of all human transformation. It is the foundation for bodily life: all movement in the body at every level, from micro to macromolecular, is oriented around and toward such stillness for Health, stability, and growth.

For example, eating processed food with added sugars and unpronounceable additives makes a lot of work for breaking down the polysaccharides. This creates more free radicals than the body can use and recycle for natural metabolism. These extra-hungry free radicals interfere with the homeostatic function of the blood vessels' endothelium. This leads to chronic inflammatory problems and metabolic syndrome. Processed food is basically pollution like hydrocarbons from cars, planes, and buses that we breathe in all the time, which also create more free radicals to break pollution down and excrete it out of the body.

It is easy to see why O_2 is a foundation for life on this planet. Our metabolism is always working and always playing music whether awake or asleep. When it gets rusty the music sounds out of tune. If it is out of tune long enough, the physiological systems of the body become disordered and diseased via metabolic syndrome. How is this music tuned and organized?

Third, metabolism is organized around *anabolism and catabolism*. Anabolism means the buildup of tissues and supporting functions in the body. Catabolism means the breakdown of tissues, cells, and metabolites. Food is broken down metabolically to build up living energy such as glucose (mostly from monosaccharide carbohydrates) and ketones (mostly from good fat) for feeding the mitochondria inside the cell. The mitochondria then converts (the ATP cycle) glucose and/or ketones into the energy necessary to live and grow. There is always a lot of work going on at this tiny level. This is anabolism. Anabolism includes a simultaneous breaking down or *catabolic* effect of the anabolic waste products.

Catabolism also describes the way in which tissues such as muscle and fascia break down from cell death (*apoptosis*) and the conversion of some dead cells via a molecular system called *autophagy* into excretable waste products. (More on autophagy below.) Thus, catabolism describes the journey of these waste products in their complicated lock and key conversion into molecules that can be excreted out of the body via the lymph, kidneys, skin, or large intestine.

Polysaccharides from the ultraprocessed food mentioned above are a good example. A polysaccharide must be broken down into a disaccharide and then into a monosaccharide and finally into glucose for the mitochondria inside the cells to use it for energy production. That is a lot of metabolic work to break down a complex macronutrient (carbohydrate) into a single molecule for building up cellular energy! And an emerging body of science suggests the human body does not need carbohydrates at all since the small amounts of glucose that are needed can be derived from fat and protein in quantities enough to sustain full body energy, including some elite athletic performance. Ketones are quite enough for most of the body's cells, especially the brain, which are also derived from protein and fat. The brain prefers ketones for optimal functioning.

In each stage of digestion and elimination (anabolism and catabolism) the music being played by our metabolism organizes itself into different functional cycles most often depending on our last meal. Think of these cycles as playing musical octaves, where the musical notes (molecules) are organized (bonded) into octaves called *cycles*. The *Krebs cycle* is a series of chemical reactions used by all aerobic organisms to release stored energy through oxidation, which is how our muscles move. The octaves are organized into major and minor tonal systems like the renin-angiotensin-aldosterone system, a molecular hormone system that regulates blood pressure and water (fluid) balance. There are many metabolic cycles and systems operating constantly in the body, divided into anabolic or catabolic cycles and systems.

So one of the basic problems with carbohydrates in general is the amount of work (cycles and systems) necessary to get to the simple glucose molecule distributed for energy in most every cell in the body. On the one hand there are too many free radicals hungry to dissolve inappropriate chains and systems. And on the other hand, there is usually *too much glucose* created from this process of breaking down *too many complex processed carbohydrates*. All of the metabolic processes, such as the one for the carbohydrate macronutrient, must also take place for the other two macronutrients of fat and protein. There is a whole lot of activity going on in what seems like simple digestion, absorption, and elimination.

This activity requires long breaks from all the action. Intermittent fasting for at least twelve to sixteen hours overnight, with no snacks between meals, keeps anabolism and catabolism balanced, reduces free radicals, supports autophagy, and allows for excess insulin to be processed out of the blood, thus reducing inflammation.

WASTE REMOVAL AND RECYCLING

From the moment of conception, the human body builds two waste processing systems. Recycling happens for cells that are dying or cells that have waste products that are positioned in a place in the body with no obvious pathway out of the body. The skeletal system is a recycling center par excellence. It can take certain waste products during both anabolism and catabolism and use them to make bones. Bones, of course, require other metabolites and micronutrients (the *fourth category* of the basic components of Real Food along with carbs, fats, and proteins). The inside of the heart is partially built embryonically from recycled cells.

When the body has obvious pathways for waste removal, then natural elimination can happen. When it does not, then it recycles. The recycling systems are also sensitive to excess free radicals, and a blocked recycling system can lead to sepsis or high levels of metabolic dysfunction and consequently excess physiological toxicity and decreased internal safety. The organ systems of the body become overwhelmed in their physiological functions with garbage, especially the liver. The spectrum of dementia disorders are like this. Amyloid plaque and related waste product proteins are metabolic waste products that build up around brain cells, since they are not being eliminated via their natural cycling. Such recycling requires good quality and quantity of sleep for a balanced metabolism.

But waste removal also has a series of metabolic cycles and systems depending on the bonds, chains, and size of the waste, like a dying (senescence cycle) cell or dead (apoptosis cycle) cell. One such intermediate-advanced metabolic system is called *autophagy,* in which dead and dying cells are broken down into easily eliminated byproducts. *Cytokines* are immune factors that every cell in the body can read to alert the immune system to help remove the waste products, especially during senescence. (I call cytokines the internet of the body.) While waste removal takes place at a cellular level, it leads to the macro level of sweating, urinating, and defecating. Thus, anabolism and catabolism together contain multiple musical notes (molecules) with multiple octaves and major and minor tones (types of cycles and systems) signifying stages in each phase or movement in the symphony.

Opening and clearing the detoxification pathways in the body therefore becomes a critical factor in managing metabolic syndrome as does the critical necessity of eating Real Food. The different macro and micro detoxification pathways are blocked from eating excess processed and ultraprocessed food. Eating such food especially blocks the liver, which I will address below.

By way of review at this point in our story, there is a balance of body energy buildup and storage for a period and then the different levels of breakdown mentioned above. This breakdown takes longer to accomplish and is why the embryo sets up this waste removal system first (endoblast). All the associated cycles and systems of anabolism and catabolism need time to successfully complete their work.

Good sleep (which is different for many people) is critical to catabolism, and really there are simple solutions to what appears to be a very complex chemical soup that lives in our body, such as not eating for at least twelve to sixteen hours between dinner and breakfast the following morning. These elimination processes are highly contextual based on a person's lifestyle and epigenetics (changes in our body caused by modification of gene expression, which are usually reversible such as through diet, behavior, attitude, and emotions) rather than alteration of the genetic code itself. For example, type 2 diabetes in some people can be reversed in less than a month. When either the buildup or breakdown is interfered with through pollution, trauma, and especially a poor diet, various disease processes and disorders can arise in an individual based on changes to their epigenetic pattern. This gets back to oxidative stress and endothelial inflammation.

Think of epigenetics as sheet music and that each human being, although having similar genes, plays different symphonies and at different times with different instruments. Every human has a repertoire of their own melodies that their metabolism plays. No two embryos differentiate their organ systems and thus their related metabolic pathways at the same time. Different timing creates different melodies. *One size does not fit all* (or there is no universal symphony) but everyone has the same basic instruments (metabolic cycles and systems) in a symphony orchestra. And the instruments need to be tuned properly and know when to play and what notes to play while looking at the sheet music in front of them.

THE EPITHELIUM

Due to the collision of our contemporary society and its consumerism—especially of processed foods, added sugars, poor hydration, inherited traits, and myriad activities that generate pollution internally and externally—our body metabolism becomes dysregulated. We get out of tune with the whole of the natural world. We lose our molecular bonding with the earth and the ocean and the sky externally as we lose our connection with our organs and tissues internally. This dysregulation is organized by oxidative stress interfering with molecular bonding.

This sequence breaks down the epithelium of the intestinal lining (leaky gut). This leads to systemic inflammation via the endothelium of the cardiovascular system and lymphatic systems (leaky blood vessels). Inflammation arises from overstuffed insulin-resistant fat cells starting in the liver. The endothelium is the gate keeper for nutrition delivery via arterial blood to all levels of the body. The lymphatic system is a toxin recognition and removal system. Anything that leaks through the gut, because the innate immune system in the gut does not recognize it, creates cytokines to alert the global body immune system of a problem, and the lymph tries to process these oversized and irregular molecules that create free radicals. Then the endothelium breaks down and loses its quiescence or stillness. This is the essence of metabolic syndrome.

The conductor of the metabolic orchestra is the *endocrine system,* and the principal instrument in the symphony is the liver. Together they regulate glucose metabolism, especially when too much insulin is created, for example from excess processed carbohydrates (polysaccharides). This creates hyperinsulinemia in the liver, which I think of as an out-of-tune violin. Inflammation arises from overstuffed insulin-resistant fat cells starting in the liver. Fat cells are inflamed cells and make obesity a critical problem for most people metabolically, especially with fatty liver disease. All tunes in the gut go to the liver. The liver is a *master metabolic regulating organ.* Its sound is extraordinary.

The entire orchestra and conductor is tuned to its harmony, as is our body, like the first violin in a symphony giving the proper tone at the beginning of the symphony. It is the field commander directing the metabolites from the food we eat and their processing for delivery to the cells of our body via the blood. And at the same time the liver manages waste products such as food additives that the body does not recognize. It also must manage excess glucose and thus hyperinsulinemia.

At this point with hyperinsulinemia in the liver, one's epigenetics choose which disease/disorder to accelerate or express in one's body (or which out of tune, atonal, discordant symphony to play). This could be inherited family traits or personal expression. Identical twins do not express the same metabolic disorders even with similar diets and lifestyles! The timing of each of their embryonic organ differentiations is different. And each differentiation requires a nutrient level at its critical time of differentiation. If that nutrient level is not available in utero, a potential disease expression can take place later in life or right after birth. The most common postnatal expressions are cardiovascular disease and obesity, but there are many, many others. The lining of the gut (epithelium) has already alerted the innate immune system to trouble with its barrier function. It happens in seconds, whereas the adaptive immune system may take days or weeks to shift. Then, since the cardiovascular system is already badly out of tune systemically, the endothelium is always an underlying problem because of the breakdown in its barrier function of keeping pathogens sequestered or quarantined, and likewise with the epithelium. Together these systems and organs choose whatever metabolic syndrome to express in one's body.

Metabolic syndrome is a catchall term for a variety of disordered states resulting from this continued dysfunction of anabolism and catabolism. If left unchecked for too long, genetic damage of one's sperm cells and egg cells takes place, affecting the Health of future generations. Some researchers have said that it may take up to fourteen generations to repair the genetic damage and cease inheriting metabolic disorders. Others have suggested that insulin resistance is passed on to the developing fetus through the placenta and cannot be reversed.

Even though the word *syndrome* is singular, it refers to the plural including a variety of conditions such as obesity, type 2 diabetes, dementia disorders, cancer, autoimmune diseases, and the wide prevalence of cardiovascular diseases. There are primary markers for metabolic syndrome used in biomedicine to determine its severity, which we have all heard of, such as waist circumference, blood sugar, triglycerides, inflammatory cytokine levels, and others.

RECLAMATION

There are also numerous secondary symptoms such as constipation, diarrhea, skin problems, and so forth. But it is most important to understand the source of the problem and natural solutions first (cleansing and Real Food) before pharmaceutical considerations are employed, in my opinion. Metabolic syndrome is a huge wake-up call for taking charge of one's body and reclaiming its ownership. Since *one size does not fit all* again, but this time in terms of natural or medical solutions, reclaiming our body becomes a *trial-and-error* process that requires patience and good coaching from appropriate and qualified helpers. This also depends on our age and stage of life, because metabolic syndrome can incubate for seven years or more. Each stage of life changes the body's anabolic and catabolic competence. I feel shopping for a doctor is wise. I believe there is a doctor for every condition in every phase of life.

Besides the chemical free radicals, key/lock-disturbances, liver overload, and leaky gut/leaky blood vessels, the fluidity and water quality in the interstitium is also essential. After all, we are over 90 percent water. The metabolic body as described here is a system of chemical and biokinetic (morphological) communications. Cell membranes need to stay intact and whole as they also interact with our moods and emotions that also create metabolism. Water carries cytokines wherever they need to go, especially in the lymph. Metabolism and related endocrine-immune cycles and systems are based on feedback loops and cycles of communication and flow, like an orchestra playing at an outdoor amphitheater in the summer. As the orchestra members need to exchange information internally, they need Real Food from nature externally (listen to Beethoven's *Pastoral* Symphony). The natural world is a major player in rebalancing from metabolic syndrome.

Metabolic syndrome occurs when a person has three or more of the following measurements:

1. Abdominal obesity (waist circumference greater than forty inches in men and greater than thirty-five inches in women)
2. Triglyceride level of 150 milligrams per deciliter of blood (mg/dL) or greater
3. HDL cholesterol of less than 40 mg/dL in men or less than 50 mg/dL in women (I disregard this recommendation because cholesterol is a nonissue in heart care according to new research)
4. Systolic blood pressure (top number) of 130 or greater, and diastolic blood pressure (bottom number) of 85 or greater without medication
5. Fasting glucose of 100 mg/dL or greater

Doctors most familiar with metabolic syndrome now recommend these tests:

1. Insulin (fasting and particularly postprandial)
2. Inflammation
3. Coronary artery calcium
4. Carotid ultrasound
5. Triglyceride/HDL ratio

Metabolic syndrome is the backdrop of this book. It is the doorway to understanding and feeling our body in our contemporary culture. The following chapters in this section will detail the depth of the challenge for healing.

RECOMMENDED READING

A Statin-Free Life: A Revolutionary Life Plan for Tackling Heart Disease—without the Use of Statins by Aseem Malhotra (Yellow Kite Books, 2021).

Fat Chance: Beating the Odds Against Sugar, Processed Food, Obesity, and Disease by Robert Lustig (Avery, 2013).

Metabolical: The Lure and the Lies of Processed Food, Nutrition, and Modern Medicine by Robert Lustig (Harper Collins, 2021).

The 21-Day Immunity Plan by Aseem Malhotra (Yellow Kite Books, 2020).

The Big Fat Surprise: Why Butter, Meat and Cheese Belong in a Healthy Diet by Nina Teicholz (Simon & Shuster, 2015).

The Hacking of the American Mind: The Science Behind the Corporate Takeover of Our Bodies and Brains by Robert Lustig (Avery, 2018).

The Immunity Fix: Strengthen Your Immune System, Fight Off Infections, Reverse Chronic Disease and Live a Healthier Life by James DiNicolantonio and Siim Land (self-published, 2020).

The Obesity Code: Unlocking the Secrets of Weight Loss by Jason Fung (Greystone Books, 2016).

2

Autoimmune Disorders
in the Intestines

By Cathy Shea

CATHY SHEA has been a licensed massage and colon hydrotherapist in the state of Florida since 1992. She also holds full certification in Swiss Biological Medicine from Thomas Rau, M.D. Additionally, she is a certified instructor with the International Association of Colon Therapy and holds the highest credential in her profession as a nationally board certified colon hydrotherapy instructor. Her passion for health education is shared with her husband Michael J. Shea, Ph.D. as they have collaborated on teaching and writing since 1990. Cathy has personally instructed health care providers in thirty-four countries who share knowledge and experience as they continue to expand upon the value of gentle, routine cleansing practices and positive health outcomes.

Metabolic syndrome now exists in the majority of the world's population, especially in Westernized countries eating a diet rich in processed food and under constant stressors. Depending on an individual's epigenetics (the genetic imprinting from a person's family lineage as well as prenatal imprinting), an individual can express metabolic syndrome quite differently on a scale of cancer, dementia, type 2 diabetes, cardiovascular disease, obesity, and autoimmune disorders such as irritable bowel disease (IBD).

IBD begins/incubates with IBS (irritable bowel syndrome). It has mechanical contributors, metabolic contributors, and emotional/sexual abuse contributors. The metabolic issues cause low-grade inflammation, primarily from eating processed food. Most people don't know the difference from a food sensitivity, which is more insidious. Food sensitivities show up three to five days after eating a certain food. Full-blown allergies give immediate conscious feedback, discomfort, and/or pain from distension either in the gut or any place in the body via the vagus nerve's role in the neurological inflammatory reflex cycle.

There are three categories of IBS: constipation related, diarrhea dominant, and the combination of intermittent diarrhea and constipation. Therefore it is very difficult for most medical doctors to diagnose it without also knowing abuse history. Functional medicine doctors tend to understand it better. When the inflammatory condition persists over a period of time, which again is different for each person based on their genetic predisposition from prenatal imprinting and/or abuse history, it leads to IBD: inflammatory bowel disease. The most common forms of IBD are Crohn's disease and colitis.

The main symptoms of IBD are blood and mucus in the stool. The typical medical intervention is steroid medication. Some complementary medicine therapists find that rectal insufflation of ozone is much more effective and safer. There is a German protocol by the name of Koch that outlines the frequency of ozone and the concentration needed in the progressive stages of a treatment plan for IBD.

However, what initiates all metabolic syndrome disorders is the very common "leaky gut syndrome." The barrier function called tight junctions between the cells of the epithelium of the small intestine and its villi become weak. They become progressively more damaged by inflammatory cytokines from an upregulated innate immune system initially and the adaptive immune system over time. The weakened barrier function of the epithelium allows inflammation-causing bacteria (and other molecules) to pass through to the gut, lymph, and vascular systems, then directly to the liver and from there to the entire cardiovascular system, especially the endothelium. The vascular endothelium also has different levels of tight junctions, which then lose their integrity. Leaky gut becomes leaky heart and vascular system, which then becomes leaky brain. Since 80 percent of the immune system is in the epithelium of the intestines (Peyer's patches form most of the innate immune system and create the bridge to the adaptive immune system), complex inflammatory conditions become systemic in the body via the endothelium of the arteries and veins. The lining of the gut is an integrated circuit involving barrier function, the innate immune system, and the microbiome. This integrated circuit sends regulatory metabolic signals throughout the body and is further integrated neurologically by the anti-inflammatory function of the vagus nerve as well as the enteric nervous system, which registers pain in the gut. It consists of two layers of the intestines.

Kolacz and Porges (2018) say this about IBS:

Rates of gastrointestinal problems such as irritable bowel syndrome are similarly elevated in survivors of abuse. Meta-analytic evidence supports this with childhood sexual abuse being associated with higher risk of gastrointestinal problems. It is estimated that individuals with a history of sexual abuse are about twice as likely to develop abdominal pain and gastrointestinal problems than those without an abuse history. As seen with fibromyalgia, rape survivors are among those with the highest risk, with meta-analytic methods suggesting their odds of having a functional gastrointestinal disorder are about four times greater than those without an abuse history. Those with an abuse history also have higher severity and quantity of gastrointestinal symptoms and seek medical help more often. Overall, these robust associations suggest that abuse and trauma experiences may be key to understanding the pathogenesis of fibromyalgia and irritable bowel syndrome.

Finally, in the most recent psychiatric research (Norwitz and Naidoo 2021), inflammatory processes are linked to anxiety. The authors suggest that solutions could be nutritional rather than pharmaceutical. It is important to know all these side effects from metabolic syndrome and inflammation. We must understand that the kitchen in everyone's home is the new emergency room, and the goal is to put out the fire in the intestines and vascular systems for optimal innate and adaptive immune flexibility, inner safety, and well-being.

3
Nonalcoholic Fatty Liver Disease

As the global epidemic of obesity fuels metabolic conditions, the clinical and economic burden of nonalcoholic fatty liver disease will become enormous.

YOUNOSSI ET AL.

Nonalcoholic fatty liver disease (NAFLD) is a metabolic syndrome. A principal element in MetS is hyperinsulinemia, which is linked to chronic inflammatory conditions in the epithelium of the gut and endothelium of the cardiovascular systems. MetS is otherwise known as "leaky gut" and "hardening of the arteries." Processed food and added sugars are the main drivers of MetS and destroy the protective lining of the gut including its innate immune system layer, which comprises 80 percent of the entire immune system as mentioned earlier. When the liver is overloaded from trying to digest processed food loaded with preservatives (some of which are unrecognizable), excess complex carbohydrates, and added sugars, the liver works overtime (hyperinsulinemia) converting much of the excess sugar and molecular waste into adipocytes. These are fat cells that are also inflamed cells now encased in dense insulated fat.

This type of fat is so dangerous in obesity because it is an inflammatory cell and has a unique ecology with its own functioning immune system linked to the inflammatory conditions. At a simple level, the innate immune system generates inflammation to alert the whole body, including the adaptive immune system, to potential trouble. The trouble becomes chronic, and the cycle of nonstop inflammation becomes challenging to reverse. The obese immune system upregulates the entire immune system to generate more inflammation and even cytokine storms popularized in the literature from COVID. Cytokines are the internet of the immune system, as these immune cells have receptors on almost every type of cell in the human body. Cytokines constantly communicate with the whole. If a

31

person has an underlying metabolic condition (syndrome) in which the immune system is already upregulated with inflammation, then catching the flu bug or COVID would set off an intense cytokine storm in the whole body, especially the vascular endothelium that is already dysregulated and trying to mediate the underlying or preexisting cytokine weather. Concurrently, the lymphatic system is overloaded because it must manage the waste products from systemic inflammation and obesity.

This cascade not only generates excessive fat cells blocking critical cellular functions in the whole body, but the inflammatory process shuts down half of the function of the endothelium of the arteries in the body by stopping vasodilation so that only vasoconstriction can happen as a protective mechanism. The artery cannot breathe. This is the start of cardiovascular disease, which is usually comorbid with NAFLD. This patient profile usually includes type 2 diabetes.

Once the normal storage areas of the liver and muscles are full of fat cells, the fat heads to the mesentery, which distributes the fat by surrounding all the other organs, including the heart. This suffocates their normal intracellular and extracellular metabolic activity. Since the liver can normally handle some storage deposits of fat cells, that liver storage system gets easily overwhelmed resulting in hyperinsulinemia. Due to the epigenetic constitution of the individual, some people will be prone to get NAFLD and others will be headed for autoimmune disorders, cardiovascular disease, or cancer. Obese patients have a much higher incidence of cancer. But it is not just the liver that is overloaded with fat. It is simply a major marker systemically of a variety of metabolic dysfunctions associated with NAFLD coming mainly from processed food and added sugars. Liver function is greatly diminished. There are, of course, other mitigating factors that could cause fatty liver disease, but the main one is the diet-insulin-inflammation-endothelia cycle.

4

Obesity and Metabolic Syndrome

Every year, three million people die of causes related to being overweight, including from COVID. The distribution of overweight people in the United States is not limited to gender or ethnicity. Recent studies estimate seventy million Americans over the age of twenty-five are considered obese, and an additional sixty-five million Americans are overweight. These numbers show that more Americans are now obese than overweight. Despite numerous calls for nutrition standards (Real Food versus processed food), exercise, common sense, and medical care, obesity remains a metabolic syndrome with complex origins and most certainly a complicated cure (Yang and Colditz 2015; Skinner, Perrin, and Skelton 2016). Obesity is also on the rise worldwide (Zhang et al. 2016). Every year, nearly three million people die of causes related to being overweight. From a metabolic point of view, heart disease, stroke, and diabetes are the main disease processes resulting from the effects of obesity. This chapter touches upon medical issues, defining terms, and the psychospiritual dimensions of obesity.

Three terms apply to the structure of obesity: body fat, adipose tissue, and visceral fat. These terms refer to empirical evidence gathered through three common measurements. The first and most reliable is by simply measuring the circumference of an individual waist (Dimitriadis et al. 2018). Guidelines generally define abdominal obesity as a waist size of thirty-five inches or higher for women and a waist size of forty inches or higher for men. Waist circumference measurements are best obtained at the level of the iliac crest or midway between the last rib and the iliac crest. Whatever location is chosen, it should be used consistently. The measurement of waist circumference improves patient management and affords medical therapists with an important opportunity to improve their care and the Health of their patients.

The second measurement is called the body mass index (BMI). BMI uses a simple calculation based on ratio of a person's height and weight. BMI is a less reliable indicator of metabolic syndrome and not necessarily definitive. It is an indicator. It was originally noticed in the literature that approximately 20 percent of obese people do not have metabolic syndrome (Phillips 2016). But this is no longer the case as there are clear cardiovascular markers, meaning inflammatory molecules, that are expressed in most if not all people who suffer with obesity. BMI is a simple tool to discover information about one's body and its potential for metabolic syndrome (Padwal et al. 2016). It has been used however, to predict a woman's possibility for heart attack (Schmiegelow et al. 2012). Numerous smartphone apps can be downloaded to help determine an individual's BMI, or a quick search of Google will provide the formula.

The third and most accurate way to measure someone's visceral fat would be to use medical technology such as an MRI, especially in NAFLD (an accumulation of excess fat in the liver caused by obesity that can lead to liver failure) mentioned in the previous chapter. At least five million Americans have NAFLD. It is now estimated that a half a billion people worldwide have diabetes, and 650 million people worldwide are obese.

The premise of this chapter is to attend to this pandemic of obesity that has reached catastrophic proportions worldwide. It is the most significant factor in the morbidity of COVID, and there is a need to sort out the plethora of seemingly conflicting information and address the difficulty of being kind to one's body. This information becomes increasingly important with the rise in awareness of the side effects of obesity. One in three Americans and one in four adults worldwide have at least three conditions associated with obesity such as type 2 diabetes, high triglycerides, and high blood pressure. At the same time there is a lack of nonpharmacological remedies that are effective in exploring the problem even considering constant antidotes being offered in the media and literally thousands of diet books and health-food cookbooks. The argument runs that the traditional government-supported diet of foods low in fat and high in carbohydrates needs to be replaced by its opposite: low carbohydrates and high fat. Recent research is clear that there is not one diet that fits everyone because of one's genetics (Goni et al. 2015). This means that any diet should be approached as simply trial and error. Gradually I will dissect the problem with these opposite diets, their context (the human body), and ways to explore the obese body through kindness to oneself with or without commensurate weight loss.

CENTRAL OBESITY

The most difficult type of obesity regarding medical outcomes is what is called central obesity. Central obesity is visceral fat that is stored in the abdomen surrounding the organs and filling the mesentery, the big net that holds all of our abdominal organs in place and is a communication pathway between all the organs. The highest mortality risk for being overweight and obese is for those people who carry the visceral fat centrally (Sahakyan et al. 2015). Complex inflammatory conditions go together with obesity because a visceral fat cell is functionally considered an inflamed cell. Inflammation causes a significant disruption in heart, intestine, and brain function.

The biggest challenge with central obesity is the relationship to cardiovascular disease and endothelial dysfunction. The epithelium is the surface lining of the gut, and right underneath that is the vascular endothelium and capillary beds receiving and distributing the metabolic breakdown of nutrients coming through the epithelium. The endothelium is the innermost lining of the blood vessels of the gut and all the arteries and veins of the body. The rule of thumb is that once one endothelial area of the body is disrupted with inflammation, such as the lining of the gut blood vessels, then many other endothelia are disrupted throughout the body. This especially includes the endothelium of the heart, arteries, and veins just mentioned. As discussed earlier, obesity creates cellular changes in the cardiovascular endothelium because the immune system is already upregulated from gut inflammation, which causes a disruption in blood flow and compromises localized passage of nutrient molecules to their end organs such as brain tissue and a dysregulated nervous system in general.

The apple, pear, and olive-on-a-toothpick body-shape metaphors are used as simple descriptors of central obesity (apple and olive on a toothpick) or noncentral obesity (pear). Some people with metabolic syndrome will have an apple-shaped or olive-on-a-toothpick-shaped body, meaning they have larger waists and carry a lot of weight around their abdomen. Some researchers feel that having a pear-shaped body, carrying more of your weight around your hips and having a narrower waist, will not increase the risk of type 2 diabetes, heart disease, and other complications of metabolic syndrome, although that research is being challenged (Jialal et al. 2013). Remember that science frequently is polarized in its results depending on who funded it, the author's corporate affiliations, and so forth. This is the day and age we live in, where science is constantly being challenged.

VISCERAL FAT AS
AN ENDOCRINE ORGAN

Some definitions to consider:

Adipokine is in the family of cytokines (cell-signaling proteins with receptor sites on almost every cell in the body, but mainly associated with immune system reactivity). Cytokines are secreted by visceral fat and alert the body to inflammation.

Adipocytokine is the same as adipokine. It is a general term for a bioactive product produced by visceral fat. Adipocytokines include inflammatory mediators, angiogenic proteins, and metabolic regulators (adiponectin, leptin). Angiogenesis is the process of new blood vessels forming from other ones, which in this case is to supply the visceral fat.

Adiponectin is a hormone. It is involved in regulating glucose levels (carbohydrate) as well as fatty acid (fat) breakdown.

Resistin, also known as adipose tissue-specific secretory factor, is a visceral fat-derived hormone. It plays a critical role in the maintenance of intestinal barrier function (epithelium) and gastrointestinal innate immunity. Epithelial function breaks down in the inflammatory process creating what is called leaky gut discussed earlier in this book.

Leptin is a hormone secreted by visceral fat that acts on a receptor site in the hypothalamus. It is designed to curb appetite and increase energy expenditure as body fat reserves increase. Levels are lowered by fasting and increased by inflammation in the gut lining and endothelium of the vascular system.

Visceral fat is a dynamically active endocrine organ system. It is traditionally considered to be the primary site of energy storage when food supplies are sparse. Now, however, excess sugar consumption, ultraprocessed food, and subsequent changes in sugar metabolism are the principal causes of excess visceral fat. It serves as an endocrine organ capable of synthesizing several biologically active molecules that regulate metabolic homeostasis (Coelho, Oliveira, and Fernandes 2013). The most basic cell of visceral fat is called an adipocyte. Visceral fat, a type of adipose tissue, makes different bioactive peptides called adipokines, which influence adipocyte-endocrine function and affect more than one metabolic pathway primarily through the bloodstream. One notable metabolic pathway is the renin-angiotensin-aldosterone system. It is a hormone system that regulates blood pressure and water (fluid) balance in an exchange of molecules between the kidneys, liver, lungs, and heart. When the water molecule reduces its natural flow in the body, trouble may incubate for years before manifesting as a specific metabolic syndrome.

Increased production of many adipokines impacts multiple bodily and metabolic functions such as appetite and energy balance, immunity, insulin sensitivity, angiogenesis, blood pressure, lipid metabolism, and blood formation. All of these influences are linked with cardiovascular disease (Ronti, Lupattelli, and Mannarino 2006). This again is because the endothelium is the coregulator of homeostasis in the body. It is dramatically impacted by obesity and its associated inflammation that affects and changes the function of the endothelium, thus contributing to and increasing atherosclerosis. This is discussed in detail in chapter 11 by Mary Monro.

Atherosclerosis is now considered an inflammatory process of the arterial endothelium. Monocytes adhere to the endothelium and then migrate into the subendothelial space, where they become plaque. This leads to a potential rupture of the atherosclerotic plaque's fibrous cap and then to rupture of the plaque itself into the artery. The possible consequences of such a rupture is blockage of the artery leading to a heart attack or stroke. Thus, an inflammatory process in the gut accounts both for the development and evolution of atherosclerosis. The inflammatory process of the arterial endothelium starts with the inflammation of the intestinal lining, goes to the liver, and then the endothelium systemically. Once the epithelial lining of the intestines is inflamed, the endothelial lining in the cardiovascular system becomes inflamed. The artery responds by losing vasodilation and stiffening. Thus, visceral fat represents a complex organ system with numerous functions that link the gastrointestinal, cardiovascular, central nervous, endocrine, and immune systems (Batra and Siegmund 2012).

Obesity is associated with these unfavorable changes in hormone expression, such as increased levels of resistin and leptin as well as reduced levels of adiponectin, all of which affect glycemic homeostasis from consuming too many carbohydrates. Vascular endothelial function is compromised, especially in the brain, and even blood coagulation can become dysfunctional. Visceral fat-related hormones, a proinflammatory state in the endothelium of the arteries and in the epithelial lining of the intestines, are most likely the links between metabolic syndrome and its cluster of obesity, type 2 diabetes, hyperinsulinemia in the liver, and cardiovascular disease.

Now loaded with this basic information on obesity, we can turn our attention to other issues associated with obesity and possible antidotes.

5

Origins of Obesity

The origins of obesity are deep and wide, beginning at conception and even earlier. To consider an individual with obesity, we need to view that person as a biological, emotional, and spiritual being in a historical and social context. I was that person. I was overweight as a child and very aware of these aspects yet had no idea how to lose weight or find spiritual ground until I became an adult. My mom smoked and drank every day of her pregnancy with me. I sometimes say that I gestated in a barroom and was born looking and sounding just like Baby Herman (a cartoon character from the movie *Who Framed Roger Rabbit* who wore diapers, smoked a cigar, and had a gangster's gravelly voice). I know my mother struggled with her own issues around weight for her whole life, as she frequently quoted Wallis Simpson, the Duchess of Windsor (whom she resembled), "you can never be too rich or too thin." It is most likely that I experienced nutritional deficits in the womb as my mother concurrently smoked a pack of cigarettes a day (this was 1948 when 75 percent of pregnant woman smoked) and drank two or three scotch and waters every evening. During my younger brother's pregnancy, my mom was told she was too thin and needed to gain weight, so the doctor put her on drinking an extra six-pack of beer every day! Yes, it was a medical prescription in 1951.

Factors included in the known influences on the development of obesity are:

- Epigenetics: transgenerational imprinting
- Nutrition (both inadequate and excessive calories)
- Chemical exposure
- Microbiome
- Stress

EPIGENETICS:
TRANSGENERATIONAL IMPRINTING

The ovum that became you resided inside your mother as she gestated in your grandmother. Quite literally, your physical beginning was once encased within three female generations at the same time. This reality has lasting and profound effects as the environment on one generation enfolds the next. The ovum that originates in a time of scarcity is overprepared (imprinted) if the resulting individual is subsequently raised in a time of excess. A dear friend of mine is an active, lovely woman with Class III obesity (high-risk). Nutritionists have been baffled with her obesity since her calorie intake, type of nutrition, and activity level would predict a much smaller body habitus. But epigenetics can give a clue. She "existed" as an egg in her midwestern grandmother in the dust bowl during the Great Depression. This same egg then basked in the nutritional wealth of postwar Southern California. After conception, this egg was gestated inside a woman encouraged to minimize weight gain by taking appetite suppressants (a.k.a. speed or amphetamines). As an ovum, then an embryo, and then a fetus, her cells were programmed to maximize nutrition, and now as an adult being, her cells do that exceedingly well. When viewed through the lens of epigenetics, my friend's obesity is not baffling but a result of cellular and genetic programing over three generations. A serious impact of the problem is the transgenerational imprinting on the genes of the parents and child, which in turn influences how the genes are expressed and how they are carried forward across generations (Saben et al. 2016). It is not just the current mother and child who are affected by suboptimal diets and/or obesity, but future generations can wind up carrying this stress imprinting. Since I am of Irish descent (Shea is a shortened version of O'Shea), many Irish people have told me that my obesity and my mom's anorexia (her maiden name was Murphy) was imprinted from the Irish Potato Famine, a period of mass starvation and disease in Ireland from 1845 to 1852. The biggest cause of the famine was not a plant disease, but England's long-running political hegemony over Ireland and a blockade of their ports to prevent food coming into the starving country. One million Irish people died during the Potato Famine. Millions more, like myself, carry the imprint of this historical horror in our very genes.

NUTRITION

Ideally, every being would have good, clean, Real Food and water in the right amounts, at just the right times, and be able to dine in safety, comfort, and with good company. However, in the contemporary reality, people (including pregnant ones) distractedly consume large amounts of poor quality, highly processed foods. Thirty-three percent of Americans reportedly do not know how to cook, and many Americans have three meals a day of take out or fast food from drive-throughs. The type and amount of nutrient and the timing of nutrition matters, especially to a developing fetus. The context of eating well-prepared meals at home and sitting with a family to eat is the tradition I grew up with. We always said a blessing before we ate, and I still do. With every meal my wife and I eat at home or out a restaurant, we take a quiet moment and bless our food before eating. I consider the kitchen to be the new ER because the kitchen is the hearth, the place where love is placed into food during preparation, and love is the original, most important medicine.

Both low and high maternal weight gain during pregnancy create the potential for negative effects on the fetus and the child after birth. According to one study, barely a third of pregnant woman have appropriate weight gain during pregnancy: "Overall, 20.9%, 32.0%, and 47.2% of women gained inadequate, adequate, and excessive gestational weight, respectively" (Deputy, Sharma, Kim, and Hinkle 2015). The Institute of Medicine guidelines recommend gaining twenty-five to thirty-five pounds if normal weight at the start of pregnancy; twenty-eight to forty pounds if underweight; fifteen to twenty-five pounds if overweight; and eleven to twenty pounds if obese at the start of pregnancy.

A diet that provides inadequate maternal nutrition modifies the physiology and metabolism of the pregnant woman, her unborn child, and her postpartum self and imprints the fetus for heart disease later in life (Saad et al. 2016). The Dutch famine affected 4.5 million people and resulted in over eighteen thousand deaths. This was a famine that took place in the German-occupied Netherlands, especially in the densely populated western provinces, during the winter of 1944–45 near the end of World War II. It was caused by several factors: in addition to an exceptionally harsh winter, bad crops, and four years of brutal war, the Nazis imposed an embargo on food transport to the western Netherlands in September 1944 in retaliation for the exiled Dutch government supporting the Allies. Thousands of pregnant women starved, which in turn stressed their developing babies. The Dutch Famine Birth Cohort Study showed that babies who gestated during the Dutch famine had increased risk of obesity, cardiovascular disease, renal disease, and a variety of other chronic physical and mental care problems.

Just as undernutrition is detrimental, consuming too many calories also has serious consequences for the preborn. Excessive weight gain during pregnancy is more common now than several decades ago (Deputy et al. 2015). Children of women who gain an excessive amount of weight during pregnancy have more than four times the risk of being overweight at age three (Oken et al. 2007). By age four, almost 25 percent of children are obese if their mothers had been obese in the first trimester of pregnancy compared with 9 percent of children whose mothers had been normal weight. Mothers' excess pregnancy weight gain and elevated blood sugar imprint obesity onto their children (Leddy, Power, and Schulkin 2008). Elevated blood sugar in pregnancy increases the childhood obesity rate by 30 percent, incidence of weight gain during the life span more than 40 percent, and a risk for increased obesity by 15 percent in the life span.

The effects of sugar consumption carry significant risk factors for not only obesity but other metabolic syndromes for the child's life span (Asghar et al. 2016; Azad et al. 2016; Fowler, Williams, and Hazuda 2015; Howie et al. 2009; Karachaliou et al. 2015; Sovio, Murphy, and Smith 2016). The effect on the baby's metabolism from prenatal exposure to excessive maternal weight gain and excess sugar consumption may be as important as what happens after the child is born.

CHEMICAL EXPOSURE

Pregnancy is a minefield of dos and don'ts, such as: Do take prenatal vitamins. Don't drink coffee. Many of the common dictates are not based on fact, but on concern and recognition that the maternal environment affects the developing fetus. For decades, Western medicine considered the placenta to be an effective barrier between maternal body and fetal body, filtering out chemicals and pathogens. Then came the thalidomide scandal. In the late 1950s and early 1960s, babies who had been exposed prenatally to thalidomide were born with a variety of defects, most notably missing and deformed limbs. These "thalidomide babies" opened our collective eyes to how the "filter" of the placenta is very porous.

Cigarette smoking and exposure to secondhand smoke are also stressful to the embryo and fetus and are linked to childhood obesity, anxiety, and cardiovascular disease. Nicotine binds to receptors in the fetal brain that are the same receptors for oxygen. My mother smoked a pack of cigarettes a day while pregnant with me, and my father also smoked in the house, magnifying her exposure to secondhand smoke. The atrial fibrillation I experience is sometimes caused by holding my breath for no known reason. (Maybe my Inner Embryo is recreating the prenatal experience?) I link this breath holding and some of the symptoms

I have from a 100 percent service-related posttraumatic stress disorder (PTSD) disability to my fetal nicotine exposure.

MICROBIOME

It is currently well accepted that an individual's microbiome affects their inner well-being, including metabolism and weight. Human genes only regulate 30 percent of gut function in adults. The other 70 percent is regulated by the microbiome. Once thought to be sterile, we now know that the fetus and placenta have small amounts of bacteria and viruses acquired during gestation entirely from the maternal system. At the moment of birth, this baseline microbiome is inoculated with millions of microbes from the birth canal with a vaginal delivery or with different and fewer species after a surgical birth (C-section). A mother's breast milk contains prebiotics that provide a seeding of the intestinal microbiome of the baby. Commercially made infant formulas are chemical concoctions that strive to imitate human-made milk. While crucial for some babies' survival, they are detrimental to the intestinal tract of an infant for short- and long-term well-being outcomes. Skin-to-skin contact between a caregiver and a newborn baby also seeds the baby's body with the caregiver's microbiome. Optimal time for skin-to-skin contact is four to five hours a day in the first days after birth. Skin-to-skin contact is not only building a beneficial microbiome but also enhancing the infant's thermal regulation and appropriate appetite while also increasing the emotional and physical bond between caregiver and child.

STRESS

Recent research has identified prenatal stress as a serious detriment to the immediate and long-term well-being of the embryo, fetus, infant, and adult (Danese and McEwen 2012; Lupien et al. 2009; Sandman and Davis 2012; Shonkoff, Boyce, and McEwen 2009; Van den Bergh et al. 2005; Wadhwa et al. 2002; Wadhwa 2005; Wadhwa et al. 2011). Many women and girls who are pregnant report experiencing high levels of stress in their lives and feel they have little time and limited resources to fulfill their needs in appropriate ways.

Researchers Wadwha, Entringer, Buss, and Lu (2011) explain that stress is a "person-environment interaction, in which there is a perceived discrepancy between environmental demands and the individual's psychological, social or biological resources." This is frequently the core of posttraumatic stress disorder, another contemporary pandemic. There are direct links between prenatal maternal mood and fetal behavior as well as significant genetic adaptations in the human placenta from different types of stress (Monk, Spicer, and Champagne 2012; Myatt 2006; Wadhwa et al. 2002).

Some pregnant women and girls have experienced severe stress and trauma. This stress may be past, recent, or chronic. Robert Scaer, an expert in the field of trauma, notes that during a traumatic experience, severe stress escalates to the point where an individual feels her life is threatened. A feeling of helplessness is a key component of traumatic experience (Scaer 2007, 2012). These pregnant women and girls may experience traumatic stress symptoms and PTSD during pregnancy, which may be associated with pregnancy complications that impact the well-being and development of their offspring (Yehuda et al. 2005), including their birth weight and length of gestation (Seng et al. 2011). Some women who have experienced rape, a particularly severe and overwhelming stress event, may choose overeating to protect themselves, what I call Obesity Safety Insulation. One explanation for weight gain in those with a history of childhood sexual abuse is binge eating disorder. Binge eating disorder is at least six times more common in people with obesity and three to four times more common in people with obesity who report a history of childhood sexual abuse. The effects of childhood sexual abuse (poor self-esteem, poor body image, impulsive behavior, and drug abuse) are common predictors of binge eating and obesity. Compulsive eating may be an attempt to manage the mental care issues resulting from childhood sexual abuse.

Fetuses can become obese along with their obese mother. Fetal programming for obesity may cause a newborn baby within weeks after birth to become obese. Researchers have found a larger proportion of children were overweight or obese when they had higher than average fat mass as newborns. For example, when neonatal adiposity was one standard deviation below the mean, about 3 percent of five- to six-year-olds were overweight or obese. Among children born with adiposity one standard deviation above the mean, 23 percent were overweight or obese. Consequently, the onset of cardiovascular disease now occurs during childhood, much earlier in the life span of our society than ever before.

CHILDHOOD OBESITY

Childhood overweight and obesity has increased dramatically during the past several decades in both developing and developed countries (Zhang et al. 2016).

This presents a significant challenge to health care systems in developing countries, which are poorly equipped to deal with such problems.

FACTORS PLAYING A ROLE IN CHILDHOOD OBESITY

- Epigenetic factors
- Family history (especially parents or siblings that are obese or overweight)
- Gestation and early infant feeding
- Early childhood trauma
- Lifestyle and activity level
- Excessive screen time (TV, iPads, video games, smartphones . . .)
- Role models for diet, exercise, self-image

Major contributors to the development of childhood obesity are overeating processed food, not enough exercise, and excessive screen time. A poor diet, what is commonly called Standard American Diet (SAD), containing high levels of processed food and sugar, can cause children to gain weight quickly. Highly processed foods such as fast food, prepackaged foods, candy bars, protein bars, smoothies, "pouches," and soda are common challenges for contemporary children. Too many parents and their children eat most of their meals from drive-in fast-food chains. Some people eat all their daily meals from such places. Children who only stop drinking soda can lose significant weight (Lustig et al. 2016). Lustig, at the University of California San Francisco, has started the Real Food movement to improve childhood and adult nutrition. The United States Department of Health and Human Services reports that 32 percent of adolescent girls and 52 percent of adolescent boys in the United States drink twenty-four ounces of soda or more per day. Sugar is now known to be addictive. It is a dose-dependent chemical toxin. Sugar activates the dopamine addiction pathways in the brain and reduces serotonin well-being pathways in both the brain and the gut.

Even one ten- or twelve-ounce can of soda activates the addiction centers in the brain that are run by dopamine. Over time, as the dopamine system takes over, the serotonin system in the gut is severely compromised. The receptor sites in the brain for sugar are the same receptor sites for addictive drugs like cocaine. With SAD, we are creating a generation of addicts. These obese (and sugar addicted) children become obese adults. Research has shown that, unfortunately, less than 10 percent of obese adults are ever able to lose their excess weight, keep it off, and sustain a normal weight (Fildes et al. 2015). Childhood obesity can cause body dysmorphia, a mental challenge like a body image problem on steroids. It is a mental disorder in which a person cannot stop thinking about defects or flaws in their appearance. It is a flaw that appears minor and cannot be seen by others. A person suffering from body dysmorphia may feel so embarrassed, ashamed, and anxious that they may avoid many social situations. The misperceived flaw and resulting obsessional behaviors cause significant distress and impact one's ability to function in daily life.

COMMON PROBLEMS IN CHILDHOOD OBESITY

- onset of type 2 diabetes
- heart disease
- asthma
- sleep disorders
- orthopedic problems such as chronic pain because of too much pressure on the joints

BODY IMAGE

Body image is important at all ages. There are five aspects to body image:

1. Perceptual: The way you see or conceive of yourself
2. Emotional: The way you feel (sad, mad, glad, afraid) about the way you look
3. Cognitive: The thoughts and beliefs you have about your body
4. Behavioral: The actions you take in relation to the way you look
5. Interoception: The way you sense your body

Body image is strong during childhood, adolescence, and young adulthood. Children imitate the posture and body mannerisms of their caregivers, which may become habitual patterns. It is problematic at a metabolic and psychological level to carry a negative body image, and the effect is compounded with time. It takes much effort to unwind a negative body image, and more the longer it exists. Given the body image issues women face during pregnancy and the anorexic appearance many young women aspire to, issues around weight before a pregnancy can remain in place during pregnancy. Health care providers must be sensitive to body image issues and any history of trauma and PTSD as well as potential medical issues regarding weight.

There is a risk that therapists who read this may begin to advise a woman to focus on the number on the scale rather than on the quality of nutrition she is providing for herself and her fetus. Gaining the right amount of weight, which differs for each woman, still does not tell you whether her baby has received adequate nutrients. It is not just how many pounds a pregnant person gains but finding out what they are eating and how they are eating and where they are eating. If they are carrying more than one fetus, what are their nutritional needs in that situation? Weight gain or loss during pregnancy involves many issues that must be explored without scaring the mother or her unborn child. Kindness must be the priority when approaching the subject of weight gain, nutrition, and body image, especially with a pregnant individual.

When looking at this information on prenatal and childhood obesity, the enormity of the problem at a social, cultural, and individual level is seen. Major commitments are necessary at the level of government policy regarding food and nutrition, but that is difficult since the USDA will not lower the recommended amount of sugar in a child's diet nor are they willing to recommend a reduction in processed carbohydrates. It is through the individual that change must happen. I recently saw this aphorism on the internet: "Stop asking why the government isn't doing what's in your best interest. Save your own life!" Eat Real Food. Disorders caused by diet need to heal by diet. Pregnant people and the next generation they are carrying need community gardens, kindness, and love, not more junk food.

RECOMMENDED READING

"Substance Abuse During Pregnancy," CDC (website).
"Thalidomide Scandal," Wikipedia (website).

6

Fat Shaming and Me

One of the more curious aspects of our contemporary culture is a phenomenon called "fat shaming" (Wann 1998). Fat shaming occurs in many segments of society, whether it's children making fun of each other's bodies (or worse, parents shaming children) all the way to public figures denigrating some other person's body, especially if that person is overweight. In our contemporary culture, the line between fat and thin is constantly shifting. A person with the same body can get very different responses to that body in different situations, especially in adolescence. When I was a teenager, I was called "fatso." In the military, my nickname was "whale" (see fig. 6.1 on page 50).

The words "tubby," "fat," "fatso," or "fatty" are pejorative adjectives in our society and have been used for most likely a century or more to tease and shame other people, especially in family systems. I have heard them all personally. So visceral fat carries a double bind with it: medically because medical professionals frequently have contempt for obese patients and psychologically because of shame. Thus, a person who is obese can see their doctor and be told they have too much visceral fat and feel shamed by that statement because of the attitude of the doctor. Even the term *adipose tissue,* a synonym for visceral fat, will still be held as shameful.

However, acceptance of overweight and obesity is being taken on by our society via glamour magazines with the addition of plus-size models wearing clothes that show off with some pride their extra weight wherever it might be found on the model's body. In the spring of 2016, *Sports Illustrated*'s annual swimsuit issue featured a plus-size model on its cover for the first time. So the fat-thin border is constantly shifting in society. The propensity for giving people of any weight or size a nickname will likely continue. Pejorative nicknames and teasing are shaming and destructive to one's emotional well-being. It depends on the inner growth and spiritual strength of an individual to become mindful of their body, develop self-compassion, and recognize the suffering of the person giving the insult.

We also live in the day and age of reality TV with weight-loss competition shows like *The Biggest Loser,* whose participants regain a substantial portion of their lost weight within six years after the competition. Nevertheless, participants were deemed "quite successful" at long-term weight loss when compared with other commercial weight loss programs. Quite successful is corporate hype, a joke when compared to eating Real Food. It was concluded that long-term weight loss requires "vigilant combat against persistent metabolic adaptation that acts to proportionally counter ongoing efforts to reduce body weight" (Fothergill et al. 2016, 7).

UP CLOSE AND PERSONAL

Upon leaving the Army in 1973 with a 100 percent service-related PTSD disability, I was a hundred pounds overweight after the terrorist bombing attack I experienced. I was morbidly obese with a forty-four-inch waist size (see fig. 6.1 on page 50). As I was finishing my doctoral work in 1995, I wrote an essay about my body image from the experience of being obese. I called it "Every Ugly Man." Here it is:

> I remember my first bad acid trip. It was in my midtwenties. I had just experienced a terrorist bombing attack in the military. I felt the fullness of the impact of the explosion on my body and mind for the first time. I touched my fat, my lumps, my parts. I had begun to overeat after the bombing and blew up to 275 pounds. It all felt like excess baggage, a densely insulated sack. Nothing short of a monster, a cadaver coming to life. It scared and fascinated me at the same time. I felt fragmented not knowing anything about PTSD at the time. Each part had a different shape, a different feel. Some were sticky and sweaty, unconnected. Some were heavy, some hurt, some cried out, some were angry. Every part was confused. My head ached relentlessly for days. I was scared, but I found my body on LSD. I got a foothold back in.
>
> I wanted to dismember myself, strip myself, lay bare my flesh and bones in my fascination. I had to get out of the Army as much as I enjoyed it. I was driven. I stopped eating and lost one hundred pounds in six months. I felt a false vitality return to my body. I learned control and excitement with food, a first for me. I obsessed. I fasted on water for weeks and months. I became

celibate. I became uncelibate. I stopped doing drugs. I started again.

I was raw meat, exposed and shivering, but in contact with my interior, morbid thing that I was. PTSD is so damaging to one's body image, like being in a permanent state of fear and anxiety, never feeling safe inwardly or outwardly. I started gestalt therapy and found my body contained even more and more feelings! I quit therapy. I started another. I cried a lot. I mourned for the unknown soldier.

I sobbed for the loss of a soul blown away never to return. I wanted to scratch and claw at a something inside my body. I keep picking the PTSD scab over and over again. I further dismembered myself ritualistically with laxatives, marathon running, and anything that could excavate the intensity of the feelings from my body. Purge them out. I became bulimic for years after getting out of the Army trying to flush out the memories. Flush them down the toilet. Puke them out. How I hated those feelings. Jesus, did I hate myself.

I went back to school for more training to outthink myself. I wanted to learn more techniques to apply to myself and my client. It was the great quest of "more is always better." I converted to Buddhism to make friends with my mind. Impossible. I converted to the culture of bodywork to make friends with my body. Another group of narcissists looking for a spiritual bypass. I accomplished nothing except two divorces.

I am the new Terminator, the new Frankenstein, my new hero. I wanted a body impervious to the inner daily pain and nightmares. Disfiguration is no big deal. I am already there. Salvation will come through a cauldron of molten metal that I must swim in to save myself. I am a steelworker: Local 295 South Chicago. I shoveled iron ore off the decks of Great Lakes ore boats for two years. I am homeless, nowhere. Who the hell can save me anyway? I hate it. I can't even save myself.

I contract with each new feeling rather than open. I am hostile toward each sensation rather than friendly. I ignore emotions, rationalize, project, deny, and kill my feelings. I'll do anything to avoid the reality of my body. Laxatives, pills, dope, alcohol, speed, overwork, undersleep, exercise, no exercise, relax, no relaxation, friendliness, no friendliness, hatred—no damn end to hatred of the body. Thanks, PTSD.

This is a stunning indictment written three decades ago when nothing much was known about PTSD and how to work with it. My memories of this time included

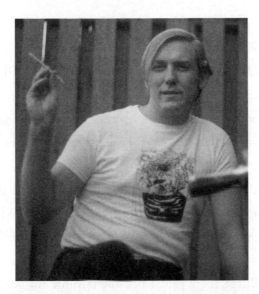

Fig. 6.1. Michael at discharge from the Army in 1973

experiences of fat shaming. I am sensitive to fat shaming and its prevalence in everyday life. I have learned to observe bodies with utmost neutrality because I can never know what a person's inner experience is. But if that person's inner experience was anything like mine, I am humbled every time.

When I landed back in the United States in September 1973, I slept on my parent's living room floor with no mattress and photographed the Watergate hearings from the television screen. I was a mess. I knew it. I knew I had to lose the hundred pounds as the residue of ingesting recreational drugs in the military after the bombing gave me the felt sense and cognition of a deep suffering rooted in my body. I woke up to my body with its extra weight.

In the spring of 1974 I shipped out as a merchant seaman, registered as a deckhand with the U.S. Coast Guard on the *SS Samuel Mather* (see fig. 6.2). The *Mather* was a 1920s-style, Great Lakes coal-fired bulk ore carrier. I bunked in an eight-by-five-foot room with two other deckhands. We each had one drawer in a triple-decker chest of drawers. It was cramped and sweaty. The ship had six-foot-tall, all-steel bulkheads, which I constantly banged my head on (being six feet four inches tall). I brought with me a supply of Shaklee protein powder and Shaklee lecithin tablets to clear out my arteries. As I began to lose weight and feel more energy, I noticed I was constipated and had not had a bowel movement in several days. I talked to my sister from a pay phone at the next port. She sent me several boxes of Arnold Ehret's Innerclean herbal laxative pills. She recommended I take twenty tablets. The main ingredient is the herb senna, which is a bowel irritant. Knowing my sister's recommendations were likely on the extreme side given her personality, I decided to take half that dose even though the box said only two or three. I had never taken a laxative before and gobbled down ten tablets. In a short time I was on the toilet, and as my father-in-law was fond of saying, "I shit a pile." The volume of feces that came out of me not only filled the toilet bowl but came above the waterline pressing into my buttocks. When I was done and wiped myself there was a large object hanging from my anus. It was a massive double thrombosed hemorrhoid the size of a quarter in diameter that was blocking my anal canal. It had been freed and was now hanging out of my anus and was damned uncomfortable.

While overcoming tremendous embarrassment, I had to request a medical appointment at the next port of call through a ship's officer. I got an appointment with a public health doctor in Buffalo, New York, while we were in the process of offloading grain at the General Mills Cheerios factory on Lake Erie. And the doctor gave me my diagnosis of a double thrombosed hemorrhoid after looking at it. He then made two recommendations that changed my life. First, he handed me a tube of KY Jelly (no gloves). He said I needed to lubricate my anus several times a day and make circular motions inside the anal canal to stretch and tonify the tissue around the hemorrhoid. I learned my first massage routine from a public health doctor in Buffalo, New York! He then said that I needed hot sitz baths and to use as hot a water as possible. I told him there were only shower stalls on the boat. He said to let the water run down my back as hot as

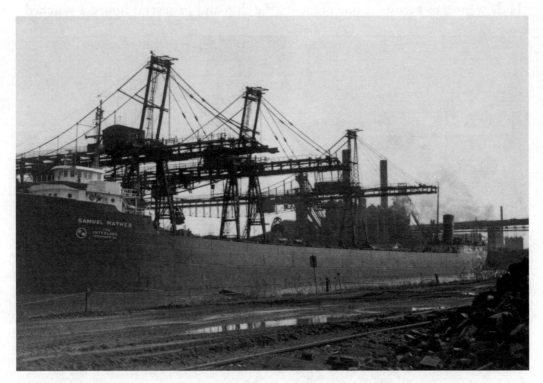

Fig. 6.2. Michael's first ship, SS Samuel Mather, *unloading iron ore at a port on the Great Lakes*

possible and cup my fingers into the perineum between my anus and genitals so the water could pool around the hemorrhoid for as long as I could take it.

What I found out is that on a coal-fired boat, if you turn the hot water in the shower on full with no cold water turned on, only steam will come out. I could do my standing sitz bath and then a steam bath. This was usually late at night when everyone was either sleeping or up in the pilot house. I turned the head on the ship into a spa sauna! Within several weeks the hemorrhoid had diminished significantly, and over the years it periodically returned in the form of a bleeding hemorrhoid from way too much travel, sitting on planes, trains, buses, and automobiles and occasionally drinking too much wine. I learned that hemorrhoids were a direct reflection of the condition of the liver, and that it would be several years before my history of obesity could metabolically normalize.

I continued to fast on Shaklee protein powder. By the end of my first season on the Great Lakes, I had lost one hundred pounds while also taking the Innerclean tablets in a much more limited fashion. Since constipation was rampant on the boat, I was distributing boxes of Innerclean to most of the crew. I was given several endearing nicknames. It was a very mixed crew, and we all worked well together and even had picnics on deck in the summer (see fig. 6.3).

I was also reading my first book about diet called *Arnold Ehret's Mucusless Diet Healing System*. It fortified me in trusting my body. This is critical as my body went into ketosis at one point on the ship and in several hours, I watched

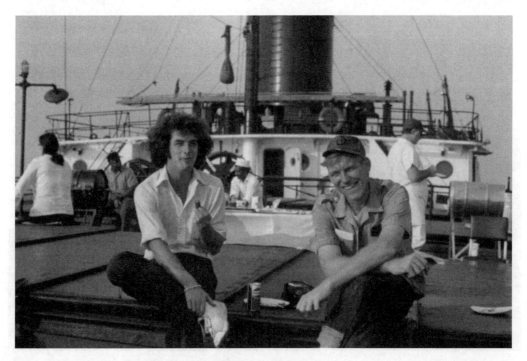

Fig. 6.3. Michael with his roommate and crew on board the Mather in 1974

with curiosity at the loss of my buttocks muscles. My urine and whole body smelled like the ten thousand hotdogs I ate growing up. I then remembered going through a polio vaccine detox on the boat as well while losing the hundred pounds. I was getting a cluster of symptoms, and when I cross-referenced them in a medical dictionary while on leave from the boat one day, I found out those symptoms were exactly the symptoms of having polio, and that's when I knew it was the vaccine that was being detoxed. This was the beginning of deobesifying me. I completely trusted my body and the enormous energy I had with the heavy manual labor performed every day on the ship. It began with senna tablets, Shaklee protein powder, anal massage, and steam baths while on an old coal-fired boat delivering iron ore, grain, and coal to and from various ports of call on Lake Superior, Lake Huron, Lake Erie, and Lake Michigan. However, the greatest healing aspect associated with the weight loss while on the Great Lakes for two full seasons was watching almost every sunset and sunrise over the water. I made a deep connection with the Great Mother and her water. She has been very generous with me for my whole life.

And all good things come to an end. In my second season I was in the storm that sank the *SS Edmund Fitzgerald*. It was a nasty gale, and on November 10, 1975, she went down with all hands (twenty-nine) in Lake Superior. We were about two hours behind her, and of course the radio traffic informed us of the tragedy, about which Gordon Lightfoot later created the famous song. I still get chills up and down my body when I hum those lyrics or even think about that time and that song. We were headed to Burns Ditch, Indiana, with a load of iron ore. We tied up to the steel mill, and I jumped ship and quit my job. I walked through several steel mills and found my way to a Greyhound bus station in Gary, Indiana. I went straight to New York City to set up the next phase of my life. I had just repaid all my college loans and, with a decent grubstake, took up residence in a raw food commune with my sister and her business partner, Betty Dodson, a famous sex educator who mentored me the rest of her life until her death in late 2020. I also began receiving colon hydrotherapy treatments and studied the naturopathic traditions of Ann Wigmore in Boston at her original Hippocrates Institute. My new life was ignited.

7

Character Structure

Obesity as character structure is an integrated body-mind-cultural-spiritual process. Awareness of how human bodies are shaped via cultural and political influences is important to understand and contemplate. As mentioned earlier, body image and body dysmorphia are contributing factors to the psychophysical aspects of obesity. Character structure is both a psychophysical and psychospiritual shaping process according to Wilhelm Reich (2000) in the sense of how political systems and social media affect emotional development and the embodiment of emotions. The human body responds differently to each phase of human development because of different environmental stressors. This relates to the different typologies observed since World War I. Thus, the psychophysical dimensions of character structure are constantly evolving. However, the premise of this chapter is that there is a common psychospiritual core of all character structures according to Reich.

Obesity is a type of character structure because of government-sponsored dietary advice promoted by Big Food corporations and followed by the medical community. This corporate takeover of the human body as described by Robert Lustig (2018, 2021) generates obesity and is reinforced by corporate messaging from social media regarding well-being, body shape, and fitness. Consequently, character structure involves habitual and unconscious musculoskeletal holding patterns based on emotional and spiritual development. The classical definition almost a hundred years ago—the source, so to speak, of character structure—was that it was generated from a sexual neurosis (Reich 1986). That is not accurate anymore and perhaps never was, given the statistics on sexual trauma and the prenatal origins of obesity that I will address more thoroughly in this chapter. Reich did evolve his observations about sexual neurosis over the years and focused on pleasure, especially sexual pleasure, as curative for many problems because the corporate takeover of the human body specifically reduces pleasure through food addiction and emotional addiction. There are far too many influences on character structure, especially considering the evolution of the concept showing changes in body types being more a direct reflection of both epigenetics and culture at any given time. However, this interpretation points to the psychophysical dimensions of obesity from eating processed foods rather than sexual neurosis.

In the original literature on character structure, Wilhelm Reich essentially said two things about the psychophysical dimensions of character structure, the first of which was his view on sexual neurosis above, which is inaccurate as mentioned. But importantly, the second thing he said was that our character structure is also a political form. The human body is shaped by the political environment of the country and region a person lives in. He was living in a fascist culture in 1930s Germany and Austria. He observed that his clients' bodies were being shaped by fascism and thus by fear. Thus, the political environment is a prime source of the psychophysical shaping of the body.

Reich continued to develop his thoughts about a type of universal fascist character structure after World War II. This is the psychospiritual dimension of character structure that is more universal and less adaptable than the psychophysical dimension. He felt that all character structures had a foundation of three layers:

1. Ordinary everyday social consciousness at the surface
2. An inner layer of irrational hatred
3. A third layer that requires deep personal inner work to access, the layer of rational hatred balanced by and with love

One's deeply held irrational emotions must be transformed spiritually to access the third layer. This is a viable message in today's world. The messaging we receive from the outside reinforces the second layer of irrational hatred, and people are stuck in that innate consciousness of survival and separation into protected tribes of like-minded people. This is a spiritual dilemma. Now couple this dilemma with the food being eaten as metabolically unsafe. It interferes with psychological function and creates the perfect storm for irrational hatred. How can inner transformation occur to reach the deep layer of love and the transformation of hatred without the support of Real Food? How can we as a species detoxify from overexposure to negative messaging by the media or what used to be called propaganda?

When talking about its evolution and the roots of character structure in *The Mass Psychology of Fascism* (1980), Reich said it was not in the best interest of political systems to have body freedom, pleasure, and creativity nor a population that has the capacity to sense their bodies from the inside. He said that people stay stuck in their own unique adaptive character structure through government/political/media propaganda filled with fear mongering, militarism, and divisiveness. The political messages of today are like the past; however, today's body responds differently to abusive messaging because of the sophistication of the delivery method—electronically, verbally, and visually combined with gratuitous violence, junk food, and prescription drugs advertising. The character structure of this day and age is a metabolic syndrome type that is associated with the prevalence of corporate processed food and a political environment of fear and anger fed with prescription drugs (such as the opioid epidemic in which 85 percent of the world's prescriptions for opioids are written in the United States). Medications are constantly being advertised in the media, especially during televised sporting events. "Better Living Through Chemistry" was a sixties TV commercial slogan by Dupont. I saw that ad a thousand times.

The stages of Western body psychophysical adaptations via malnutrition and emotional imbalance leading to changing forms of character structure continued with Lowen (1994). He proposed five different character structures in the early 1950s that still persist in some body-centered therapy communities. Likewise, Sheldon (1970) proposed three "somatotypes" after World War II, which evolved into constitutional psychology in the 1950s. Clearly, with each generation, these thinkers looked at the shaping of human bodies through the lens of contemporary culture and saw how the human body became shaped in those eras. The post–World War II era ushered in the age of speed from amphetamines but also transportation systems and body conditioning.

Fear is a significant contributor to a contemporary character structure, especially the way in which the autonomic nervous system is constantly cycling through fight/flight and then withdrawal and collapse (Porges 2011). It is extremely difficult to access the deep layer of love in a character structure without an environment of both inner and outer safety. Fear and despair are major well-being factors in America because of domestic terrorism, gun violence, COVID, drug addiction, overdoses, suicide, and eating corporate processed (junk) food, among other things. This all relates to obesity as a character structure being shaped by these contemporary psychophysical and psychospiritual factors. Obesity in this context is driven by inner metabolic fears resulting from processed food and from an outer fear based on contemporary messaging and family systems. Fear, whether it is necessary or unnecessary, is linked to physical and spiritual stress. The point is that diet is metabolically linked to stress-related fear. Appropriate choices around food are virtually impossible when consumed with fear.

A major factor that influences the metabolic syndrome character structure is the pervasive use of prescription drugs that are designed to be metabolic balancers yet are equally metabolic imbalancers. Just read the side effects of any prescription drug for a lesson in fear. Just listen to a client describe his or her medications and how many of them are to treat the side effects of the others. It is a vicious circle. There is a continual shaping of the body's metabolism, especially when medications and prescription drugs are ingested with processed food that persistently inflames the gut and cardiovascular system, along with a television constantly running in the background or foreground. Keep a person fearful, and they are easier to control as they lose touch with their body. This was Reich's central message. People become ill mentally and emotionally and then come under the control of allopathic medicine and prescription drugs, some of which are necessary and lifesaving. Modern people, however, have abdicated responsibility for their own bodies. Sad. As one example, this metabolic syndrome pandemic, as it is known medically, preceded COVID and is the basis of mortality with COVID. The suppression of the sensual and the loss of kindness coupled with the diminishment of common sense is manifested in American culture and every other developed country. Inciting fear triggers hatred and aggression toward other humans. But at the core is self-hatred and self-aggression. This is deep suffering underneath an obese frame.

The degradation of the gut with contemporary lifestyle and processed food are major contributing factors to the metabolic syndrome character structure because of their influence on the brain, the changes in physiology of the cardiovascular system, the changes in the hormone metabolism of the immune system, and the way this shapes the body from inside to out. So the person with the beer belly or excess visceral fat or inhabiting an apple or pear shape is maintaining a character structure constantly being formed from a host of complex factors internally and externally. The character structure is centered internally around a loss of self-respect and a diet that causes epigenetic switching from optimal expression to suboptimal expression of the body's immune and vascular systems. Then cultural and societal factors build the contemporary character structure of metabolic syndrome. Genes rarely cause disease. Instead, genes influence disease susceptibility. It is not any longer nature versus nurture. It is nature and nurture. The environment and the food we eat profoundly influence how genes behave. The last meal eaten by someone has the biggest influence on gene expression.

We now live in the age of mainly one character structure: a metabolic syndrome character type such as obesity. When 88 percent of Americans are metabolically dysregulated, then the remaining 12 percent is the only control group in this experiment of metabolic overload. We have now reached the end of our health as we know it. Although there is some attempt to describe a metabolically healthy character type by the Weston A. Price Foundation, this research was done on traditional cultures almost one hundred years ago. All we must do is look around and see misshapen bodies, whether obese or not, struggling with well-being, emotions, and spiritual formation.

As Victor Frankl once said, the only freedom we have as human beings is the freedom to choose how we respond to life circumstances. This includes what we put in our mouth and into our minds. Once anger is elicited, the creative spark of innate well-being and the control of our body, agency over our body, is forgotten. This anger is fueled by too much media, too much processed food, and too much hatred. The sociology of hatred and despair involves depression and suicide, which are both increasing in the United States. Fear, anger, and hatred is the diet that many people consume in the contemporary political and social landscape. By turning off the television and reducing smartphone consumption, it might be possible to lose emotional weight so as not to be exposed to propaganda of all sorts, especially to the prevalence of junk food and sugar that dominates both adult and children's television. Essentially, many forms of bodywork as they evolved in our society over the past one hundred years attempt to undo the character structure, either directly or indirectly, and to become more mindful. Numerous systems such as massage therapy are promoted for relaxation, but relaxation is not enough to transform the layer of hate to one of love. Even relaxation and mindfulness have become more corporate hype. Appropriate body-centered therapy can be seen as anarchistic because it is a resistance against the political and corporate takeover of the body in contemporary society.

The more times someone eats at chain or franchise restaurants, the more that person allows the corporate ownership of the restaurant to shape their body. It is virtually impossible to know all the additives that chain restaurants put in their food. Body-centered therapists are the new anarchists. Therefore, Reich was such a renegade (and saw it early on) for espousing body-centered therapy, especially breathing techniques and sexual pleasure as a type of silent, nonviolent revolution.

He was the Gandhi of the Western world resisting the corporate industrialization of the body just as Robert Lustig, M.D., is today with his book *Metabolical* (2021). Even the spa and massage industry worldwide is owned mostly by large corporations. Is this about well-being? How do we start to reclaim our body and form a resistance to its corporate takeover?

Seventy percent of American bodies are overweight, 30 percent are morbidly obese, and a whopping 88 percent of Americans are metabolically unhealthy. The rotund shape of the American body could be seen as having a prenatal origin as mentioned earlier. Now we know another link to prenatal stress from obstetrical violence (especially against women of color and minorities) that contributes to obesity and all other forms of metabolic syndrome. Fetuses can become obese from a variety of different circumstances, even transgenerational imprinting or a mother's history of trauma. Stress and trauma at any time in a person's life interferes with the metabolism of both the gut and the brain. This sends a message to the hypothalamus in the brain that the body is in survival mode and must eat as much as possible. It also activates the deep, evolutionary urges of survival before we are even out of the womb. Prenatal metabolism is much more active proportionally than at any other time in our life. Without adequate and proper nutrition and low stress, the body of a prenate can become toxic, leading to metabolic syndrome for both mom and her baby.

The first principle of metabolic healing is to reduce the toxic load at any level possible. This is because the majority of the human embryo's period of growth is about the metabolic development of nutrition delivery systems and waste removal and recycling systems. Since much of the food people eat is not Real Food (fresh or any portion of it from a home garden), the waste removal systems are backed up, creating a huge toxic load in the body. At one level, the obese body is also a malfunctioning waste removal system. However, there is another way to view the problem. The solution co-emerges with the dilemma.

METABOLIC ANTHROPOLOGY

Rotundity, portliness, fecundity, and roundness from being obese are synonymous with the original female form from the perspective of depth psychology (Neumann 1963). In the anthropology of matrilineal or goddess cultures, the first cultures to appear in recorded history, rotundity was the vital and most sacred feature in the iconography and symbolism of the feminine. Neumann called this "the elementary character." The body itself was considered feminine.

Woman = body = vessel = world. How often do we see someone who is obese and think that the person looks pregnant? Obesity represented fecundity, a fullness of life, such as being pregnant. From this perspective, the symbol of a contemporary overweight body contains both a positive (anthropologically) and a negative (medically) image or connotation.

In the trauma literature mentioned above, the term *survival resource* is used to indicate that a person with PTSD from whatever source is fixated on survival and rightly so. It is a type of survival that includes a broad spectrum of possible resources to simply get by in life, especially with comfort food usually of the processed, sugary variety. Obesity is also a survival resource from that point of view, and thus the lifestyle patterns underlying the survival resource may be difficult to change without relating to one's origins—in other words, to relate to the preexisting condition in the whole evolutionary pattern of mankind. Thus, the metabolic syndrome character type is in survival mode at its prenatal core, and healing requires going back symbolically to one's origins, to "the elementary character" as Neumann called it.

This is a basic principle of healing in cross-cultural medical anthropology. It is a return to the body as feminine, not as gender but to its original shape. This is our origin and paradoxically the double bind of healing. The problem contains the solution or antidote. The healing event in traditional cultures is to focus on the Health that is preexisting and available in the present moment. It was also present at the origin of the universe or conception when each person was originally whole—fresh from the factory, so to speak. Cultural healing also involves reconnecting to the natural world that lives inside the body and supports the body as well as the natural world outside. How?

The patient needs to symbolically return to the moment of origin and begin again in their original wholeness. This may involve retrieving it from that place as a remembering but integrated in this present moment. Or maybe it is simply entering a profound state of transformation by fasting without eating as was part of many cultural rituals. From the standpoint of depth psychology, one must return to the original state, that moment of conception of one's original wholeness to be reconceived into right relationship with their body in its perfection at the moment of creation. The return to origin may involve a symbolic return to the beginning of the universe. The ritual return to wholeness is interconnected from the body outward to the mind, the community they are in, and finally the world of nature (Eliade 1958, 1963, 1964). We need a different image and metaphor of obesity given its complexity, and since much of obesity begins prenatally or in preconception, the obese person is already going in the right direction but without the sacred container for transformation. An appropriate biodynamic practice can provide such a container.

I see the obese abdomen as a placenta rather than representing pregnancy. Both visceral fat and the placenta are endocrine organs, and both are attached to the body as if from the outside, much like air tanks worn by divers or babies wrapped in a sling close to their mother's body after birth. The placenta is a fetal organ derived from the father's genes. If the body is feminine, then obesity is its masculine component. Sometime obesity regresses further toward embryonic origin by displaying a yolk sac structure from the second week postfertilization. This is the giant abdomen with multiple overlapping rolls of visceral fat. The yolk sac is an embryonic structure attached to the umbilicus like a huge beach ball hanging from the front of the body. This to me is a healing phase of obesity going back to one's origin with a bigger and bigger belly. Obesity represents a return to origins whether prenatally or preculturally. Either way it is a spiritual journey requiring a sacred container for transformation.

This is the healing direction, but it needs sacredization in a spiritual container provided by a knowledgeable biodynamic or other appropriate therapist. If most metabolic syndromes start prenatally, then it is logical that the body returns to that state for healing. So it is invaluable to look at it symbolically and as a potential source of healing for psychological wounds. A healing container needs to hold the totality of the person in all their wholeness like a tapestry being woven together. That means being held with compassion and loving kindness as it was in the beginning of the universe, because there is immense suffering at the core of obesity.

A child being wounded is unavoidable. Such wounding happens on such a broad spectrum. However that wounding occurs, it may include obesity being its expression or its survival resource. Parenting is never perfect, but parents do need to get involved when their children are obese (Wolfson et al. 2015). The critical part is how the parents form a receptive container to help children become well differentiated, free of body shaming and body teasing. Parents need the greatest amount of support, particularly in the prenatal period. It is vital that parents do not shame their children's bodies, as the metabolic syndrome character structure is very complicated. This is especially the case if the child has had preverbal attachment problems in the first two years after birth

(Schore 2005). About 75 percent of children have some variation of an insecure attachment. Becoming overweight and obese can also be a compensation for an insecure attachment.

Looking at my own service-related PTSD disability, I can say genuinely that I needed to experience my own obesity after my discharge from the Army to be who I am right now. I deal with my symptoms much better now with one hundred fewer pounds, which is the psychophysical component. I avoid overeating or being emotionally unavailable (well, most of the time). Back then I did not know I was unhappy, even after two divorces. For almost a decade after the military, I expressed it through my body in a preverbal, not-knowing state of obesity. At the same time, I am 100 percent of Irish descent, and numerous therapists have told me that my obesity most likely came from the Irish Potato Famine right through my mom and dad. It is essential to understand that all developmental pieces in a life decade after decade, especially those involving the body, contribute to the possibility of becoming more and more whole and sometimes unfortunately less and less whole. It is possible to gradually see the importance of obesity in one's life and how it is a constant shaping of mind-body-spirit, without rejecting it or oneself. It is a constant shaping and renewal from the energy of origin. That origin may or may not have a fixed point or specific triggering event. It is possible to change the past layer by layer, through trial and error and deep listening with the utmost self-compassion and loving kindness. That is the psychospiritual component.

The metabolic syndrome character type (of which obesity is just one variation of a single character type) is the prevalent contemporary character structure. It requires becoming deeply mindful of the body and emotions without judgment or interpretation. It is about one's ability to see through the character structure; not give it up initially nor transform it, but just to see that it is a mask or part of a false persona. It may be held for a reason historically—such as preconception or prenatal or childhood stress—and reinforced by trauma and PTSD. Trauma is also a part of the planetary diet plan. Obesity may also be a necessary resource to get us through certain situations and circumstances in life, especially if it is associated with shock and trauma. It is crucial to understand and to sense character structure as being translucent or semisolid. This is a lifelong process and a gentle holding of the body with self-compassion. Self-compassion, a deep self-respect, is critical for self-regulation of the body-mind internally. Self-regulation in this sense is the ability to contemplate, contain, and transform emotions, cognitions, and perception quickly, without prolonged activation of the nervous system. This is also called resilience. Mindfulness is the foundation for a continual exploration of one's body-mind.

Mindfulness is the innate radar system detecting when our attention has been captured in an unwholesome way; in other words, when we are obsessing mentally and emotionally. To be mindful of this shaping and holding process and to see how it arises in certain circumstances in life and wakes up a healing instinct—the return to origins. Mindfulness is invaluable in bringing attention to one's holding patterns and character structure. Sometimes it is noticing a breathing pattern that is restrictively holding the trunk and abdomen up or pushing it down in defiance or resignation. Every cell in the body can be recruited to adopt a shape that may become long lasting and diminish body function and the experience of nonaddictive sensual pleasure. With such attention, the journey to healing begins. We will continue to explore such healing throughout this book.

8

Ultraprocessed Foods

Sugar inhibits three mitochondrial enzymes—AMP kinase, ACADL and CPT-1, all necessary for neurons to burn energy. No surprise that sugar is linked to Alzheimer's—it's a chronic dose-dependent neurotoxin.
ROBERT LUSTIG, M.D., TWITTER, AUGUST 2, 2021, 5:26 A.M.

More so than any other Western country, Americans are being bombarded with food products that are high in sugar, saturated fat, salt, and calories. More specifically, after analyzing over two hundred thousand food products packaged in the United States—including bread, snacks, salad dressings, sugary sweets, and sugary drinks—researchers found that a whopping 71 percent were classified as ultraprocessed. Furthermore, 86 percent of the packaged foods sold by the twenty-five top food corporations were found to be ultraprocessed. According to Robert Lustig, M.D., food corporations earn a yearly profit of $600 million while it costs the health care system a trillion dollars to attempt to repair the damage.

The term "ultraprocessed" means *foods that are industrial formulations made entirely or mostly from substances extracted from foods (oils, fats, sugar, starch, and proteins).* These foods are usually created in laboratories and derived from hydrogenated fats and modified starch that are indigestible and ultimately wreak havoc on the body's metabolism. They may also contain additives like artificial colors and flavors or stabilizers.

Examples of these foods are frozen meals, soft drinks, hot dogs, cold cuts, fast food, packaged cookies, cakes, and salty snacks. According to one study, bread products seemed to be especially bad. "Bread and bakery products" was the only studied food category that ranked high (negatively) in all four nutrient categories: calories, saturated fat, sodium, and total sugars. Ultraprocessed foods are the main source (nearly 60 percent) of calories eaten in the United States and contribute almost 90 percent of the energy we get from added sugars. It is no wonder so many are so metabolically dysregulated.

While foods packaged in the United States are similar in overall negative qualities to those of other Western countries such as Australia, American food products were found to be significantly more processed and contain larger amounts of sugar and sodium. For example, U.S. bread products contain 12 percent higher sodium levels than bread made in the United Kingdom. The United Kingdom has made a concentrated effort to lower sodium levels in their packaged foods. This is one reason 88 percent of Americans are metabolically dysregulated. It is difficult to paint an accurate picture of the processed food industry because it is constantly changing, with about 20 percent of packaged foods in the United States being replaced or modified each year. Better information is necessary about this constantly changing food supply to improve its authenticity as Real Food. That is not likely going to happen because of the successful lobbying efforts against it by food corporations.

With the prevalence of ultraprocessed snack food advertising on television, it is best to consider fasting from the media, which numerous experts have recommended. I accomplished numerous water and juice fasts up to sixty days in length without a problem when I was younger. I did not own a television or even a radio at the time. I know it is possible to stop eating for short periods of time without overeating when breaking the fast. I have lived without a television for most of my adult life. Consider the following chronic disease triggers:

1. Sugar
2. Processed denatured grains
3. Industrial seed oils

Cheapest processed ingredients:

1. Sugar
2. Processed denatured grains
3. Industrial seed oils

Highest profit for food corporations:

1. Sugar
2. Processed denatured grains
3. Industrial seed oils

DIABETIC STARTER KITS

Energy gels and granola bars are diabetic starter kits. All they do is damage teeth, promote hunger, excite abnormal behaviors, inhibit fat metabolism, promote fat deposition, increase hyperinsulinemia, and delay recovery from exercise. I ate them for years when the fad started—especially those bars found in health-food stores. But they are all the same. It is not Real Food.

HIGH GLYCEMIC INDEX

The glycemic index is a scale that ranks the number of carbohydrates in foods from zero to one hundred. This indicates how quickly such food causes a person's blood sugar to rise. Foods high on the glycemic index can cause harmful blood sugar spikes in people with diabetes. High glycemic index foods also make it more difficult for a person to maintain an appropriate weight. Therefore, some people with diabetes use glycemic index to plan their meals.

In a recent study it was found that a diet with a high glycemic index was associated with an increased risk of a major cardiovascular event or death, both among participants with preexisting cardiovascular disease and among those without such disease. Among the components of the primary outcome of the study, a high glycemic index was also associated with an increased risk of death from cardiovascular causes. In a meta-analysis of glycemic index research in 2021, a diet with a low glycemic index reduced metabolic syndrome.

It is very easy these days to go online and find the glycemic index for most foods. However, once again, processed foods, especially grains, are very high on the glycemic index. Death by carbs could be another interpretation of this study. Carbs (triglycerides and diglycerides) break down into sugar (monoglycerides) and when coupled with added sugars, the body's metabolism is overwhelmed. This leads to any number of metabolic syndromes depending on one's epigenetics and family history. Whether it is processed food or high glycemic index food, these two are major troublemakers for the body's metabolism.

In this first part of the book a rather big problem is defined and some solutions pointed toward. What follows in the next chapter and the rest of the book are a wide variety of solutions from the physical to the spiritual. It is important to have as many tools in our toolkit or medicine pouch as possible in this day and age. What is clear is that all of us are different in terms of how we respond to food sensitivities and stress levels. We must be able to explore with an attitude of trial and error in which the error part of the equation is normal rather than a threat to our self-esteem. We must be able to experiment with how we nurture and care for ourselves, knowing the ups and downs of our self are waves that we learn how to surf. We all wipe out when the wave is too big and we all come back to the surface and get back on the board looking for a wave to catch that can take us all the way in, close to the shore of sanity. And even that wave comes to an end. We keep repeating that pattern over and over until we get the hang of it and enjoy both the wipeout and the long fun ride.

Above all we must learn self-compassion.

9

Intermittent Fasting

The probability of attaining normal weight or maintaining weight loss is low (less than 10 percent) as mentioned previously. Obesity treatment programs, such as Weight Watchers and Jenny Craig, may also be ineffective (Fothergill et al. 2016). Such research calls into question not only weight loss programs but exercise programs in general. Some studies suggest that walking is the best exercise regardless of one's weight, but that requires motivation. Motivation is lacking in many people who are obese because of feelings of shame about being seen in public. Other evidence suggests that combining aerobic and resistance training has better outcomes for the cardiovascular system in general for both overweight and obese people. *Fat Yoga* is now becoming popular in the United States as yoga classes are being offered exclusively for overweight and obese people. It is mostly done sitting on a chair, as mobility on a floor is difficult.

The conflicting research on the capacity to lose weight is not connected to simple mindfulness of the body. In this case mindfulness refers to being non-judgmental about the body one inhabits. Obese people have a deep, personal experience of their body, usually negative or judgmental. This is not mindfulness; it is obsessive and shame-based. To become mindful of the body is an act of kindness toward oneself. In becoming mindful, judgments and interpretations of one's body and behavior are welcomed and viewed with kindness. Mindfulness is unbiased without judgment or interpretation. Neutrality allows for deeper healing instincts to become active, such as the kindness of self-compassion. Then appropriate choices can be made that are gentle and use the right effort and discipline. This includes choosing a lifestyle of mindfulness and dietary coaching to repair the damage from metabolic syndrome.

Ludwig (2016) suggests that the old "calories in, calories out" method of diet and nutrition needs to change as an approach to treating obesity and weight gain in general. In *Always Hungry?*, he writes that weight gain occurs because fat cells are stimulated by insulin and other metabolic signals such as leptin to take in and store excessive calories. Because of this, blood concentration of available calories is lowered, leaving too few for the rest of the body. When the brain perceives this problem, it increases hunger and lowers the metabolic rate to store the energy from the food that is eaten. In this sense, the conventional low-calorie diet can make the problem worse and contribute to obesity.

The fat cell model of body weight control is an alternative to the "calories in, calories out" model for obesity treatment. The fat cell model says that the high glycemic diet (grains and processed grains) drives hyperinsulinemia and consequently more interference with the body's metabolism, including weight gain. When people have insulin resistance, glucose builds up in the bloodstream instead of being absorbed by the cells. Why is glucose not being accepted into the cells? High levels of insulin remain in the bloodstream and especially in the liver. The high levels of insulin have reduced the number of receptors on cell walls leaving fewer doors and entrances into the cell, especially for leptin to use and regulate insulin. The bloodstream is saturated. The liver is saturated, and this liver saturation is called hyperinsulinemia. A high glycemic diet in which sugar is rapidly released into the bloodstream or a diet of predominantly processed carbohydrates is the culprit driving this condition of hyperinsulinemia. The "calories in, calories out" model says that if you exercise more and eat less, you will lose weight. The calorie restriction model is false and debunked in countless studies.

The brain responds by increasing hunger and lowering metabolic rate—akin to a state of starvation—undermining long-term weight loss. Starvation physiology manifests as increased hunger, decreased metabolic rate, and rising stress hormone production. Hyperinsulinemia also heightens the palatability of artificial sweeteners (because by taste, the brain thinks it is actual sugar) and increases greater food intake. These metabolic changes occur before overeating and obesity occur.

Ludwig states that a calorie restriction strategy makes the body-mind disconnect worse for biological and biochemical reasons. The idea is to connect the body and mind through our dietary behaviors. "The Almost Hungry Solution is designed to work from the inside out, creating the internal conditions for weight loss to occur naturally" (Ludwig 2016, 13). People focus on the quality of food, not the calories.

Ludwig reports on research that indicates there is less weight loss on conventional low-fat diets compared to all higher-fat diets, low-carbohydrate diets, very low-carbohydrate diets, or Mediterranean diets. He encourages whole plant foods, while limiting the highly processed carbohydrates that dominate the fad diet industry and remain prevalent in the current era of low-fat/high-carbohydrate dietary guidelines recommended by the USDA for the past thirty years. Those guidelines continue despite the mounting evidence against them. Nuts, olive oil, avocado, and dark chocolate are some of the natural foods derived from plants featured on Ludwig's fat cell model meal plan. The high-fat and low-carbohydrate foods recommended in the new era of ketogenic diets are not associated with weight gain in the best observational research.

INTERMITTENT FASTING

To eat or not to eat is the question in order to heal being overweight or obese. Special diets involving cultural rituals and fasting have long related to spiritual, religious, and political systems. Thus, eating and not eating or fasting is also associated with spirituality, psychological attitudes, and self-development. From a contemporary point of view, special diets and fasting are about nurturing a compassionate instinct and the realization that there is not a "one size fits all" diet. One must realize the necessity of trial and error regarding diet and nutrition. It is all an experiment that shifts from decade to decade as we age. Being overweight or obese requires as much of a spiritual commitment as a physical commitment. An instinct for healing preexists in the body. When a body is out of harmony with its internal and external environment, it is very difficult to self-regulate at any level or to maintain mindfulness and compassion. Animals, when ill, generally know which bushes and trees to eat from that contain the medicine necessary for healing. They also generally fast on water when sick. In other words, our mammalian body knows how to heal by itself.

Typically, stopping eating and beginning fasting is a spiritual time of renunciation. One is not simply renouncing food, but renouncing the world for a short period of time for a correct and right balance to manifest between one's body, mind, spirit, and connection to community. Fasting was the primary way I initially lost over one hundred pounds in the mid-1970s as mentioned in chapter 6.

During the middle and end of the last century, many *fasting farms* existed around the United States. The most famous was the Natural Hygiene Society in Texas run by Herbert Shelton who wrote almost exclusively about fasting (Shelton 1978). The health-food stores of that time had numerous books on the importance of fasting with water only or raw fruit and vegetable juices by naturopaths such as Norman Walker (1978), Bernard Jensen (2000), and Paul and Patricia Bragg (2004). That literature is hard to find in health-food stores anymore, but they are available online at Amazon. I began fasting with a traditional text by Arnold Ehret (2011, 2014) and was familiar with Shelton's work and DeVries's (1963) text on fasting. Contemporary literature on fasting is available both in the medical community (Fuhrman 1995; Carrington 2006) and is reappearing in Christian communities in America such as *The Daniel Plan* (Warren, Amen, and Hyman 2013).

Water fasting and juice fasting are still viable approaches to one's self-care, well-being, and a lifestyle that includes cleansing. Fasting is usually done under supervision or proper coaching to help manage the potential side effects. The most basic fast is from the time of the evening meal to the breakfast meal the following morning with a minimum of twelve hours between these meals. Some naturopaths recommend fasting one day a week (for twenty-four to thirty-six hours) simply to give the digestive organs a rest. Recent medical research available by searching the internet for the term "intermittent fasting" also refers to periodic food restriction. This is now called intermittent fasting.

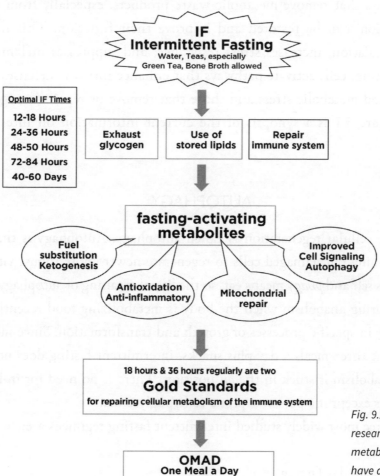

Fig. 9.1. Intermittent fasting, research and definitions. The metabolism of the body must have adequate time between meals to thoroughly digest and eliminate waste products down to the cellular level.

Fasting is a challenge to your brain, and it appears that the brain reacts by optimizing the function of the immune system, since the gut can repair itself. It restores the lining of the intestines (leaky gut) by giving the intestines a much-needed rest from constant work. The body then converts fat to ketones as a substitute for glucose to function properly. The brain prefers ketones to glucose.

Intermittent fasting in both humans and mice results in fewer circulating immune system monocytes and lowered monocyte inflammatory activity. This, of course, is a useful observation if applied to someone suffering from a chronic inflammatory condition, but how does this immune system impairment affect a balanced body's ability to heal wounds or fight off an infection?

Many of the benefits of intermittent fasting are not simply the result of reduced inflammatory molecules or weight loss. Instead, intermittent fasting elicits older metabolic and adaptive cellular responses that are integrated between and within organs. The pathways that deliver nutrition molecules and the pathways that remove metabolic waste products, especially from chronic inflammation, can be restored and improve their function. This improves glucose regulation, increases stress resistance, and suppresses inflammation. During fasting, cells activate pathways that enhance intrinsic defenses against oxidative and metabolic stress and those that remove or repair damaged molecules. Figure 9.1 is a synopsis of the current information on intermittent fasting.

AUTOPHAGY

The key to cellular regeneration is called autophagy. Autophagy is the body's way of cleaning out damaged cells to regenerate newer, more robust vital cells. *Auto* means self and *phagy* means eat, so the literal meaning of autophagy is "self-eating." During anabolism when the body is metabolizing food recently eaten, cells engage in specific processes of growth and transformation. Since most people consume three meals a day plus snacks, intermittent fasting does not occur because anabolism is stuck in the *on* position. There is no need for in-between meal snacks except if a person is prone to hypoglycemia.

The three most widely studied intermittent fasting regimens are:

1. alternate day fasting
2. 5:2 intermittent fasting (fasting 2 days each week)
3. Daily time dependent eating

Diets that attempt to reduce calories one day or more each week usually result in elevated levels of ketone bodies (from high-quality fat consumption) on those days. The metabolic switch from the use of glucose as a fuel source to the use of fatty acids and ketone bodies generates greater metabolic flexibility and efficiency of energy production from fatty acids and ketone bodies.

Ketone bodies are not just fuel used during periods of fasting; they are strong signaling molecules with major effects on cell and organ functions. Ketone bodies regulate the expression and activity of many proteins and molecules that are known to influence well-being and aging. By influencing these major cellular pathways, ketone bodies produced during fasting have profound effects on systemic metabolism. Moreover, ketone bodies stimulate expression of the gene for brain-derived neurotrophic factor, with implications for brain care and psychiatric and neurodegenerative disorders. The use of ketogenic diets for neurological disorders in children for a century is clear evidence of their value. Intermittent-fasting interventions have a positive benefit for obesity, insulin resistance, dyslipidemia, hypertension, and inflammation. The benefits of intermittent fasting are the cornerstone of contemporary fasting clinics in Europe such as the famous Buchinger Wilhelmi Clinic in Germany. The Buchinger Wilhelmi Clinic has done the world's largest study on fasting.

APOPTOSIS (CELL DEATH)

The average adult human loses between fifty and seventy billion cells (out of thirteen trillion cells) each day due to apoptosis. That is, about five out of every thousand cells die each day. For an average human child between the ages of eight to fourteen years old, approximately twenty to thirty billion cells die per day.

Autophagy and apoptosis are really elements of a critical metabolic *detoxification* necessary at the basic level—the four-phase catabolic cycle for cell/ mitochondrial waste products: recycle, rest, restore, and transform. The waste products must have time to be broken down from the cellular level to the physiological level to the structural level of urination and defecation. At the same time the breakdown of the waste products provides metabolites that can be recycled and used to build up tissues. Many cells that die burst open and spill their contents into the interstitium. Since the contents contain cytokines, which are necessary in apoptosis, naturally, the rest of the body's cells may misinterpret the presence of cytokines and react with more inflammation or a cytokine storm if there are underlying metabolic issues. It takes time for the body to sort out both recycling and waste removal without adding more fuel to the fire with snacking. Therefore, the most basic regular interval between the evening meal and the morning meal is twelve to sixteen hours (see fig. 9.1 on page 71).

KETO DIET AND ALZHEIMER'S

The prevalence of Alzheimer's disease, a devastating neurodegenerative disorder, is increasing. Although the mechanism of the underlying pathology is not fully uncovered, there has been significant progress in its understanding in recent years. This includes progressive deposition of amyloid plaques, intracellular protein tangles, neuronal loss, and impaired glucose metabolism. Some dieticians now call this *leaky brain*. Due to a lack of an effective prevention and treatment strategy, emerging evidence suggests that dietary and metabolic interventions could potentially target these issues. If Alzheimer's is a diet-caused disease, then logically it requires a dietary solution or at least making diet a major component of its management and potential healing.

The ketogenic diet is a low-carbohydrate, high-fat diet. It has a fasting-like effect that brings the body into a state of ketosis. Ketosis is a process that happens when the body does not have enough carbohydrates to burn for energy (glycolysis). Instead, it burns fat and makes nutritional molecules called ketones, which it can use for fuel. The presence of ketone bodies has a neuroprotective impact on aging brain cells. Their production may enhance mitochondrial function and reduce inflammatory and cell death (apoptotic) mediators. Thus, it has gained interest as a potential therapy for neurodegenerative disorders like Alzheimer's disease and many other metabolic syndromes, especially obesity and type 2 diabetes.

BLOOD BRAIN BARRIER DAMAGE

Metabolic syndrome damages the blood-brain barrier, which is the normally tight border that prevents harmful molecules in the bloodstream from entering the brain. The endothelial cells that make up the blood-brain barrier have many specialized proteins that help them to form tight junctions called fenestrations. These cellular structures act as a strong seal between cells. When a person has *leaky gut,* the common denominator of metabolic syndrome, then it causes *leaky heart,* in which the space between endothelial cells expands throughout most of the vascular tree, including the brain. In the brain this is called *leaky brain.* In the liver it is called hyperinsulinemia. It is one's epigenetic expression, which is unique for each person, that determines one's metabolic syndrome typology.

No matter what type of metabolic syndrome a person has, the brain will always be affected. The most common term being used is brain fog. The vagus nerve as discussed in chapter 25 is clearly a coregulator of intestinal metabolism. From food to fuel to waste products, the vagus nerve keeps track of the body's metabolism, especially inflammation. Inflammation is synonymous with the term leaky gut. One of the functions of the vagus nerve is to stimulate the metabolic processes of anti-inflammation. But it still includes shifting toward a low-carbohydrate, high-fat diet through a process of trial and error and receiving sound, compatible nutritional coaching from someone who has been on the path and knows the territory. Intermittent fasting is the major support for the metabolic cycle called catabolism (the removal of waste products and recycling of metabolites). Eating supports anabolism, the buildup of tissues and energy to run the body.

Not eating for longer periods of time during a twenty-four-hour period is vital to cellular detoxification and metabolic renewal of the body down to its subcellular components. Thus, there is a ratio of eating time/not-eating time that is unique to everyone. This ratio reflects each person's epigenetics regarding the percentage of time during a twenty-four-hour period in which one eats and digests Real Food and the percentage of time during a twenty-four-hour period where one does not eat for the purpose of cellular waste removal, cellular recycling, and metabolic repair. The removal of waste products is a critical part of embryonic development, since we were a single-celled, whole human being at conception. One diet does not really fit everyone, and as I said in the previous chapter, the trial-and-error diet is most acceptable. A low-carbohydrate, high-fat diet functions on a broad spectrum of exploration and experimentation. All diets rely on trial-and-error and will change as a person ages. Food corporations knowingly make processed food addictive. Big Pharma makes drugs that are addictive. The new lifestyle is a cleansing lifestyle to enhance the necessary repair of leaky gut, leaky heart, and leaky brain. Timeliness of intake followed by removal, recycling, and repair is a commitment to Health and ownership of one's body.

10

Human Digestion, the Microbiome, and Elder Wisdom

By Cathy Shea

CATHY SHEA has been a licensed massage and colon hydrotherapist in the state of Florida since 1992. She also holds full certification in Swiss Biological Medicine from Thomas Rau, M.D. Additionally, she is a certified instructor with the International Association of Colon Therapy and holds the highest credential in her profession as a nationally board certified colon hydrotherapy instructor. Her passion for health education is shared with her husband Michael J. Shea, Ph.D. as they have collaborated on teaching and writing since 1990. Cathy has personally instructed health care providers in thirty-four countries who share knowledge and experience as they continue to expand upon the value of gentle, routine cleansing practices and positive health outcomes.

I am an international health educator and have worked on six continents with Michael since we married in 1990. It has been a rich inquiry as we teach and learn in a lively exchange with so many gifted people from around the globe. Every day that I interact with my team, it humbles me to learn more from the professionals that I have trained in thirty-four countries. I earned my license in 1992 to practice massage and colonics in the State of Florida, instructor certification status from the International Association for Colon Therapy, and national board certification for colon hydrotherapy. Florida is the only state that licenses colonics and we are governed by the Department of Health and regulated by the Board of Massage.

SWISS BIOLOGICAL MEDICINE MODEL

I earned full certification in Swiss Biological Medicine from Thomas Rau, M.D., in 2016. So much of what I have gathered since 2009 came from my study with Dr. Rau. He was the first medical doctor I found who understood the necessity for cleansing especially through colon hydrotherapy. It is the first pillar of his Swiss Biological Medicine model (see fig. 10.1). I am truly honored to be part of his global team of gifted providers who are trained in this progressive body of knowledge and give him my sincere thanks for all he has taught me so I may share this with my clients and students. His network spans six continents, and I have the privilege of training many of his health care professionals, including medical doctors, in the art and science of colon hydrotherapy.

Dr. Rau is the originator of the Swiss Biological Medicine model, and his patient protocols follow the three pillars below (see also fig. 10.1).

The first pillar is detoxification. Biological dentistry is a cornerstone of the model. Every patient receives a full dental evaluation to begin with, and Dr. Rau measures the electricity in each patient's mouth as part of this routine evaluation. This is because he is particularly concerned with the use of metal amalgam fillings and root canals in the dental industry. The teeth are the shelf upon which the brain sits. The metals carry an electrical charge and create a neurological disturbance called the galvanic field response. Also, root canals carry hidden

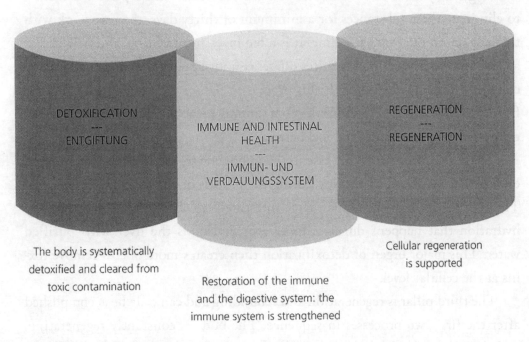

Fig. 10.1. Dr. Rau's Three Pillars of Swiss Biological Medicine. (Image adapted from Dr. Rau's original.)

infection that can enter the bloodstream and cause the infection to become systemic. Therefore, Dr. Rau insists upon the removal of any amalgam and metals in the teeth and the proper extraction of all root canals. A typical biological dentistry protocol includes extraction of the tooth, then the socket is injected with ozone (O_3). We breathe O_2, and ozone carries an extra molecule of oxygen that disarms harmful microbial activity.

The second pillar is immune and intestinal well-being. Dr. Rau believes that leaky gut syndrome is a pandemic and a root cause of the disease process. When the small intestine's lining barrier is damaged and breached, toxins enter the blood and create a full-body inflammatory response. His protocols include natural remedies and homeopathic medicine—not available in the United States—to heal the intestinal lining and curb the cytokine storm in the immune system that results from the inflammatory response. His vegan menu plan at the clinic in Switzerland supports healing at the cellular level and excludes the most common food groups that create intestinal irritation. Food sensitivities, including dairy, gluten, soy, tree nuts, sugar, alcohol, caffeine, shellfish, chicken eggs, and chemicals in food and water (see fig. 10.12) are the main cause of this irritation.

Unlike a full blown allergic reaction that creates an immediate histamine response that is sometimes life threatening, food sensitivities may take from three to seven days to present with symptoms. Since most people are used to low grade headaches, stomach discomfort, joint pain, and other chronic symptomology, they must be educated about this process. When a person is willing to eliminate these substances for a minimum of thirty days, then we work with them to reintroduce one at a time. It is a big investment of time and heightened awareness that pays off and requires diligence and support. Our coaching during colon hydrotherapy assists with this process to reduce the antigens in the body from the irritants. The person's level of commitment is directly related to the time it takes to see results and feel better.

Colon hydrotherapy is an essential component to the healing process, and each patient receives this therapy during the process of eliminating the irritants. The first function of the human large intestine is to absorb water and the deep hydration that happens during this treatment floods the liver with purified water. This major organ of detoxification then creates more bile to remove toxins at the cellular level.

The third pillar is regeneration and rebuilding and can only be accomplished after the first two processes in sequence. The body is constantly regenerating, and now that the detoxification process and intestinal lining are improved, rebuilding can be accelerated. Dr. Rau has formulated specific medicines to be given orally or injected, depending on the patient. He also implements pulsating electromagnetic field technology to accelerate rebuilding at the cellular level.

Dr. Rau believes there is a need for everyone to practice routine cleansing to counteract the toxic exposures that are unavoidable in this world. Our routine cleansing program includes rectal insufflation of ozone and has been very helpful, as it also improves the body's defenses and immune activity.

My story includes a recent injury resulting in a diagnosis of osteoarthritis. This chronic inflammatory condition is being managed well with daily exercises, systemic enzymes, routine skilled bodywork, acupuncture, and avoiding the top twelve gut irritants shown in figure 10.12 on page 95. What was fascinating is my recent discovery of how a flare-up of pain diminished by 80 percent after having my routine dental hygiene to manage periodontal disease. You can see my teeth with and without metal fillings in figure 10.2. It is clear to me that periodontal well-being relates directly to the body's systemic inflammation. Leaky gums, leaky gut, leaky heart, and leaky brain are all related. I am living testimony that Dr. Rau's guidance has allowed my well-being to soar.

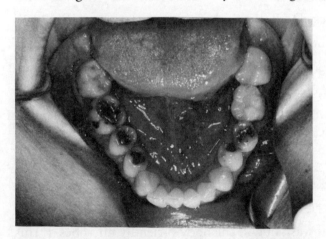

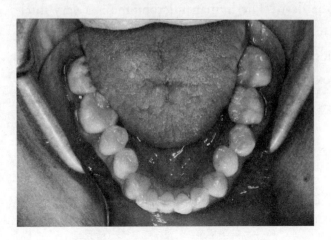

Fig. 10.2. Cathy's lower teeth before and after metals removed

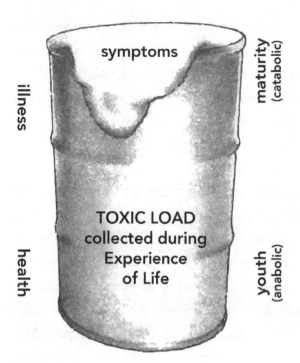

Fig. 10.3. Dr. Rau's metaphor for the overflow of the accumulated toxic load that includes the toxic residue from prescribed medications. (Image adapted from Dr. Rau's original.)

This book is full of metaphors, and there is one that is very helpful when explaining how people get so sick. Dr. Rau uses the image of a barrel (see fig. 10.3). He explains that when we are born, the toxic barrel has very little in it, unless of course it was a challenging pregnancy and birth. As we move through life eating, drinking, and breathing, we are exposed to unavoidable toxins. There comes a point when the barrel overflows and symptoms appear. Therefore his first pillar requires detoxification before the process of regeneration can occur efficiently (see fig. 10.1 on page 77).

Colon hydrotherapy (also known as colonics) is a gentle way to incorporate the therapy that Dr. Rau prescribes at his Swiss clinic for all his patients. It is a fallacy that colon cleansing will wash out all the body's friendly microbes. If this were true, many of us would be dead! The human microbiome is a very intelligent system of organisms that will self-regulate when fed the proper nutrition and purified water. We are guests in this microbial world. Dr. Rau states it very simply, "We must reduce the toxic load and weed the internal garden so the flowers can grow."

DIGESTION

Digestion is also important to gut health, so I continue with a simple overview of the structures and functions of digestion to understand how it all works from

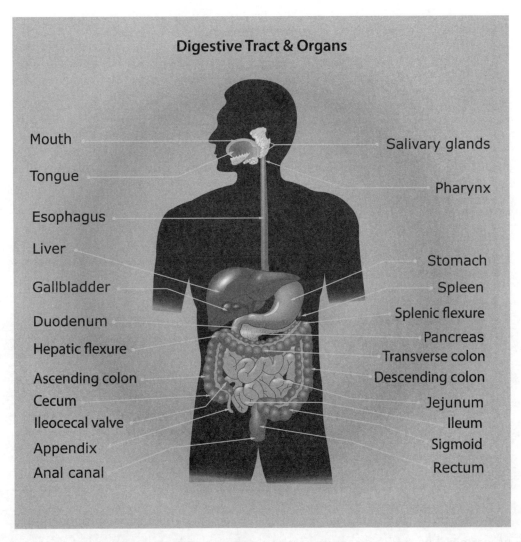

Digestive Tract & Organs

Mouth

Tongue

Esophagus

Liver

Gallbladder

Duodenum

Hepatic flexure

Ascending colon

Cecum

Ileocecal valve

Appendix

Anal canal

Salivary glands

Pharynx

Stomach

Spleen

Splenic flexure

Pancreas

Transverse colon

Descending colon

Jejunum

Ileum

Sigmoid

Rectum

Fig. 10.4. A basic view of human digestive system structures

mouth to anus (see fig. 10.4). In my clinical practice, this is what most people have questions about, since it is likely they learned very little if anything about this in early school experience.

The functions of chewing and mixing in the mouth are the most important aspects of eating along with a sense of relaxation. The gut needs to access the rest-and-digest branch of the autonomic nervous system for optimum gut activity. This branch speaks to the enteric nervous system, which is exclusive to our digestive system's electrical activity as it moves things along this long tube from mouth to anus. This movement is called peristalsis and is constantly in motion, even during sleep. The enteric nervous system is designed to function as an independent system from the central nervous system. In fact, it has many more neurons than the brain and spinal cord combined. It is also the main regulator of serotonin, the feel good hormone, and creates 90 to 95 percent of the body's supply of this essential substance in the gut as reported by Michael Gershon, M.D., in his book *The Second Brain*.

Digestion begins with a thought. Even thinking about food will stimulate the saliva to flow in preparation for eating. The mouth is responsible for breaking down the food substantially prior to swallowing, and therefore chewing mindfully until the food is completely broken down into the consistency of a smoothie is essential. Less chewing may be an indicator of rushing, stress, jaw or teeth pain, and loss of mindfulness. The adult mouth usually has thirty-two teeth managing this mechanical reduction. A simple practice is to chew each bite thirty-two times or keep liquid in the mouth for half a minute. The saliva assists in liquifying the food to make it easier to swallow. It also triggers a neurochemical signal to the stomach that food is coming down. Carbohydrates (starches and sugars) must mix with the saliva to begin metabolizing properly. A simple axiom is to remember to *drink your foods and chew your liquids*.

This is especially important for those who are following the recent trend of ingesting mostly liquid foods like juices and smoothies. These constitute a meal and need to be sipped slowly after holding them in the mouth to warm up if they are cold. If the liquids are not mixed with the saliva, there is a loss of mechanical signaling that chewing provides along with the loss of chemical signaling from the saliva. The result is typically a sense of bloating and discomfort in the belly, especially if the fluids are cold; it's advisable to drink them at room temperature or warmer. I have found that its best to sip these slowly over a period of thirty to forty-five minutes to avoid this unpleasant result.

The tube that carries the food from the back of the throat down into the stomach is called the esophagus. Gravity assists in this process along with the wave-like motions of peristalsis. When digestive acid from the stomach backs up into the esophagus, it is known as acid reflux. Major causes of acid reflux include drinking cold liquids during meals, improperly mixing food groups, and overeating, and these lead to digestive upset and metabolic syndrome. The resulting acid reflux can damage the tissue of the esophagus and lead to esophageal cancer—an entirely preventable disease. My father died of esophageal cancer and I watched him take many over-the-counter remedies for years without breaking the habit of improperly mixing food groups and overeating, two major causes of digestive upset and metabolic syndrome which may result in cancer.

The stomach sits under the ribs on the left side of the body when full. It expands when food enters from the top at the esophagus and contracts when food leaves at the bottom through the pylorus. This expansion promotes the secretion of leptin to signal a feeling of fullness (satiety) so we stop eating. When the stomach empties, there is a secretion of ghrelin to signal hunger.

Not everyone senses hunger in their stomach. My experience with my body has shown a different list of signals that may appear when I get hungry. These sensations include feeling cranky, "hangry," thirsty, spacey, loopy, dopey, sweaty, and sometimes even blurred vision.

These two hormones are major players and become skewed when obesity is present. Their presence and quantity are also influenced by the quality of food and sleep patterns. The pylorus allows three to five tablespoons of liquefied food to exit the stomach at a time. This is called chyme. If the food is not adequately chewed, it lingers until the acid and enzymes in the stomach can break it down more. Nothing leaves the stomach until it reaches a body temperature of 98.6 degrees (see fig. 10.5). That is why drinking cold liquids and eating cold foods during meals will slow down this process. It is better to have the soup first before the salad or a cup of hot water or tea with a lemon to warm up the stomach environment. In ayurvedic medicine, the digestive fire is called Agni, and we must stoke this fire with heat before eating raw foods. Personally, I have found that I digest and eliminate much better with a more macrobiotic approach that includes more cooked foods. It is also helpful to snip the raw greens into small pieces with a scissor and place them under soup or cooked foods to wilt them. In this way we still get the nutritional boost from the greens.

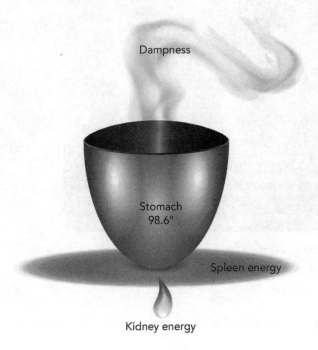

Fig. 10.5. Digestive fire needs heat like a pot on the stovetop.

Next, food exits the stomach and enters the small intestine. This is considered *small* because it is usually the diameter of the person's thumb. It is by no means small in length. It is coiled up within the belly measuring twenty to twenty-two feet long. Inside this tube are small, fingerlike projections called villi that resemble a shag rug. Each villus has even smaller structures on the surface called microvilli. If the food is sufficiently liquified, the villi will grab the microscopic nutrients and transport them into the venous blood supply within the lining of the gut. These micronutrients then travel up a tube called the portal vein and send it all off to the liver for the next round of metabolic processing. If the food particles are too large, they will move through undigested and be marked as a toxin in the body by the lymphatic system. The resulting loss of barrier in the villi, called leaky gut (see fig. 10.6), leads to many metabolic issues. Some people are diagnosed with an autoimmune disease called celiac disease and must avoid gluten-containing foods at all costs. Gluten sensitivity is also a condition where the person cannot tolerate gluten found in wheat, rye, spelt, kamut, and other grains. The amino acid L-glutamine is helpful in healing this inner wounding. A simple stool test that we provide in our clinic will determine this condition.* Until the person eliminates the top twelve gut irritants, the villi continue to deteriorate and no supplement will be effective.

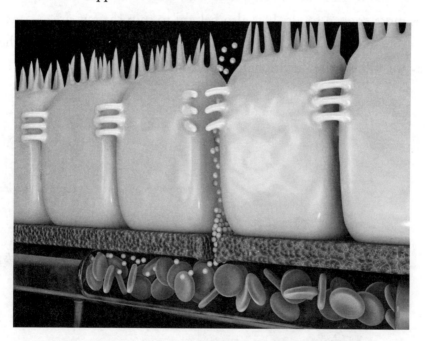

Fig. 10.6. Leaky gut and the loss of tight junctions in the small intestine, indicating a loss of barrier and proper filtration function

---

*Another valuable product for gut healing is formulated by Zach Bush, M.D., called ION Gut Support.

The villi have a configuration called *tight junctions,* meaning they are knitted close together to form a necessary barrier, an exquisite and delicate filtering system integrated with the immune system in a well-regulated small intestine. Undigested food, medications, toxins in food and water, and lack of fiber damage the junctions leading to inflammation and what is termed "leaky gut." I also learned that when my mouth was full of amalgam fillings, each time I chewed the metals leached into my saliva and I was swallowing these! If the metabolized food particles are not flowing south, they will migrate east or west through the single layer of gut lining into the bloodstream and lymphatic system depending on the size of the molecule. These villi form an integrated unit of structure and function with the immune system, the vagus nerve, and the microbiome that live in this part of the body. The small intestine is home to lymph tissue that acts as a guard at the gate of digestion. We've all experienced swollen glands in our neck when toxins enter the sinus or throat area. The same lymphoid activity is dominant in the small intestine—70 to 80 percent of our immune activity is regulated there. *Leaky gut syndrome* is inflammation at the level of the villi and creates a cascade of symptoms throughout the body as toxic molecules interfere with the lining of the arteries and veins called the endothelium. Inflammation—an adaptive mechanism of protection—is orchestrated by immune molecules called cytokines. Swelling such as lymph edema anywhere in the body is directly related to leaky gut. The proper metabolic channels for digesting food and eliminating waste products is broken. Leaky gut is also attributed to common conditions such as asthma, eczema, allergies, autoimmune disease, and autism.

Within the lining of the small intestine are several layers of tissue. One deep layer houses essential immune activity occuring within lymphatic tissue called Peyer's patches (see fig. 10.7). They are designed to assist with homeostasis—the body's ability to maintain balance within narrow operating ranges. These tiny lymphoid nodules form an important part of the immune system by monitoring intestinal bacteria populations and preventing the growth of pathogenic bacteria in the intestines. A recent phenomenon called small intestine bacterial overgrowth has emerged as a modern condition related to the weakness of this tissue. There are specialized bacteria in the small intestine that require fiber to synthesize and do their job. Lack of appropriate fiber to feed them will also create leaky gut as the bacteria begin to feed on the mucous membrane that houses the immune system cells. This is another major contributor to leaky gut syndrome. When this occurs, the immune system determines that it's being attacked by a pathogen and will begin an inflammatory process to help protect itself immediately, calling out an army of immune system cells to assist over time. Symptoms appear sooner or later depending on a person's transgenerational and prenatal epigenetics.

Trauma also plays a role in triggering leaky gut. Chronic digestive issues, swollen joints and glands, skin eruptions, allergies, and a host of other metabolic syndrome symptoms are directly linked to leaky gut syndrome and lead to serious metabolic consequences if not addressed. There are numerous small lymph nodes in the gut that assist in providing the proper drainage of toxins (see fig. 10.9). Stagnation in this flow is a major cause for cancer. By now you are beginning to understand how gut well-being influences overall Health (see fig. 10.8).

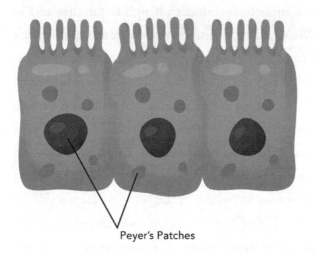

Fig. 10.7. Innate immune system tissue called Peyer's patches within the epithelium of the small intestine. Peyer's patches contain critical molecules bridging the innate and adaptive immune system.

Peyer's Patches

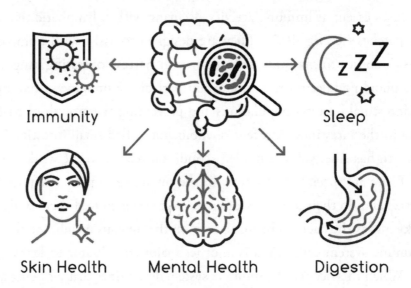

Fig. 10.8. Why gut health matters

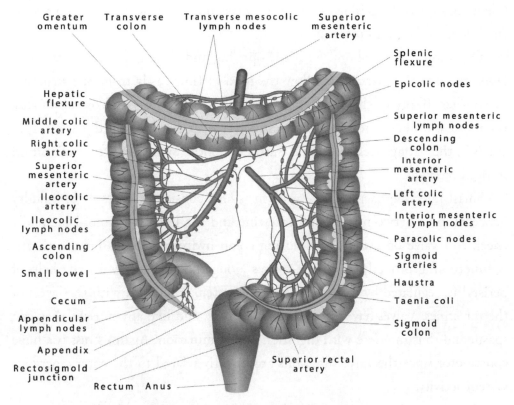

Fig. 10.9. Large intestine anatomy and lymphatic drainage pathways.
Note that the superior mesenteric artery supplies two-thirds of the colon up to
Cannon's point and is then supplied by the inferior mesenteric artery to the anus.

The Western world has a massive population of people without tonsils, adenoids, and appendix. These organs are vital to the lymphatic system's ability to protect the gut. When they are not present, the person is considered immunocompromised. All structures in the human body have a purpose. Hang on to them!

As a person smells food and chews, there are neurochemical and neuroendocrine signals that begin to stimulate the accessory organs of digestion. For example, the pancreas must adequately produce specialized enzymes and insulin to help metabolize sugars as they break down from complex to simple carbohydrates. The pancreas is also busy making protease, the enzyme that helps to digest protein. The largest internal organ, the liver, has hundreds of functions, almost two dozen different types of cells, and very likely more to be discovered in this miraculous organ. The liver cleanses itself by producing a substance called bile. Bile is mostly water based, and when dehydration is present, stagnation of the bile occurs often resulting in constipation and the risk of gall stones. The liver bile flows down to the gallbladder for storage.

Chewing signals the gallbladder that food is coming so it will prepare to release the bile into the small intestine.

Digestion is a symphony, with the opening and closing of numerous valves along the intestinal tract that allow the food to flow easily from one structure to another. If any of these valves is compromised by stress and/or substances, the music is off key. Stress is the biggest deterrent to harmonious digestion since cortisol, the strong stress hormone, shifts the entire symphony from relaxation to fight or flight.

Small intestine bacterial overgrowth is also considered a result of a faulty ileocecal valve between the small intestine and the large intestine. I manually check this valve on every client during colon hydrotherapy sessions so that it is functioning properly as chyme moves along the gut tube with the help of peristalsis, regulated by the enteric nervous system embedded with the layers of the intestines. Valves have circular muscle fibers, and like any muscle, they can spasm and thus interfere with digestion and elimination. Again, stress is a huge contributor since the valve functions are directly related to the enteric nervous system activity.

The chyme that departs from the small intestine enters the large intestine on the right side of the body at the ileocecal valve near the appendix. This is meant to be a one-way valve, allowing the contents to change from alkaline to acid as they enter the large intestine. The appendix is attached in this area and assists in this process unless it is removed, which creates another set of challenges for gut functions and overall immunity. There are unique families of bacteria that inhabit the small intestine as it absorbs nutrients versus the bacteria in the large intestine that assist with decomposition and synthesis of micronutrients. Anabolism and catabolism can occur simultaneously. The primary job of the large intestine's five- or six-foot tube is to absorb water. Since most people are dehydrated, constipation is epidemic. Pharmacies and other stores are chock-full of over-the-counter laxatives. Unfortunately, these substances only release the soft, watery stool and leave behind the dry, hard pieces. I had the distinct privilege of training a progressive gastroenterologist years ago who called this "overflow diarrhea." With continued laxative use, the bowel muscles get lazy and then stop doing their job. The rectum turns to leather, obliterating the nerve reflex to evacuate the bowel. This common diagnosis is called melanosis coli and is often a precursor to colorectal cancer. As a licensed colon hydrotherapist, I can help this condition with retraining the bowel if the client is willing and able to make certain changes in their lifestyle habits.

Routine cleansing is an ancient practice that dates from 1500 BCE and is historically part of all ancient spiritual practices. Colon hydrotherapy is the modern version where we gently infuse filtered, temperature-controlled water into the body via the rectum.

COLON HYDROTHERAPY AND CONSTIPATION

As mentioned earlier, I am a licensed colon hydrotherapist in the state of Florida. This therapy resides under the massage therapy license and has since the 1940s. Colon hydrotherapy is a much more thorough colon cleanse than an enema, which often only clears the rectum and lower bowel. I utilize an FDA-cleared, Class II medical device called a *closed system* (see fig. 10.10). This means that all the gas, water, and waste materials are contained so there is no exposure to the waste. The waste flows from the client's body through disposable tubing then through the device and may be inspected in the viewing tube before exiting the device into the sewer. It is common to see big and small mucus clots, undigested food particles, and foamy water. The tubing and the speculum that enter the anus are ergonomic and comfortable. They are well lubricated with a natural salve or KY jelly. Since the equipment is all disposable, there is no risk of contamination. The device below has numerous safety features including the control of temperature and pressure. It also has state-of-the-art filtration to guarantee the large intestine is saturated in purified water. Colon hydrotherapy has been shown to be effective as a safer alternative way to prepare for a colonoscopy procedure.

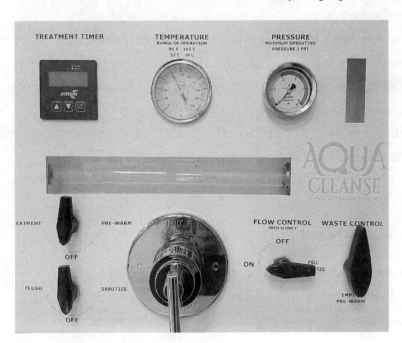

Fig. 10.10. Quality colon hydrotherapy device. It is an FDA-approved Class II medical-grade device. This is the industry standard that my school adheres to.

(The study was presented in 2006 by Joseph Fiorito, M.D., of Danbury Hospital in Connecticut.)

My experience in this cleansing field of study since 1988 shows me that colon hydrotherapy is of great value when someone is ready to stop using laxatives. People can deliberately hold the waste from exiting the body, and that is called *functional constipation*. It is a throwback to nineteenth-century Victorian manners to consciously hold back the gas and waste that the body must excrete. But halting the natural flow of feces from the body causes numerous issues including creating a serious physical and behavioral stagnation pattern and setting the body and mind up for a variety of metabolic syndromes. I hear it often from clients that they are just too busy to use the toilet.

The tube from mouth to anus is approximately thirty feet in length in the adult human. The last portion is a holding tank called the rectum, which stores the fully composted waste until the signal to defecate (called interoceptive awareness) initiates a behavior to find a toilet. There is a very sophisticated signaling system in the rectum that sends interoceptive information from the pelvic nerves to the gut brain on to the head brain to initiate a behavior to find a toilet. Unfortunately, many people ignore the urge, which is the main cause for constipation and other digestive issues. I have heard many stories of people who cannot use public restrooms, either because of a sanitary phobia or simply because they are ashamed to be heard by others. This is known as a *shy bowel* and contributes greatly to ongoing constipation. One such client told me she was on a vacation for two weeks and could not have a bowel movement. No wonder she reached out to me for colon hydrotherapy!

The entire digestive system has a unique nervous system innervation called the enteric nervous system, also known as the *gut brain*. The enteric nervous system consists of two layers of neurons sandwiched between the three muscle layers of the intestines. The enteric system registers pain from the distension caused by gas and bloating. It also is the main driver of peristalsis, which moves digested food forward through the tube and is ultimately responsible for the mechanics of a bowel movement.

HUMAN MICROBIOME

This term is everywhere on the internet now. It relates to the colonies of bacteria and other microbes that live on and in our human body. What is fascinating is that the new science confirms that our body has many more microbes than human cells. There is a plethora of unique and distinct organisms that inhabit our eyes, nose, ears, mouth, respiratory tract, reproductive system, gut lining, and even between our toes and under our arms. How marvelous that we live with them and it is impossible to sanitize them away. If we do, we die.

The microbes carry an electrical charge and messenger molecules signal the head brain that it is time to eat, drink water, use the toilet, stop eating, and other behaviors related to assisting the process. As mentioned earlier, these microbes are interacting with the vagus nerve and the immune system as a unified function. Current research from John Cryan, Ph.D., of the University of Cork in Ireland, has shown that the gut microbiome also coregulates moods and emotions, cancer risk and outcome, neurological risks like Alzheimer's, and a host of other metabolic issues. Other luminaries that I studied in this field include Emeran Meyer, M.D., and Zach Bush, M.D. The human microbiome is now a hot topic of dialogue among many progressive health-care-minded professionals, and the reader is invited to search YouTube for more information from the authorities just mentioned.

According to Zach Bush, M.D., the condition of the human microbiome is in direct relationship to the natural world's microbiome including soil, air, and water conditions. Remember that these three elements are the original source of our sustenance from the land and water supply. He shares a new perspective for humans that includes a reminder that we are guests in this microbial world. We live in their world. They do not live in our world. These colonies of microbes will live much longer than humans and will continue to inform necessary genetic upgrades along the way for future generations. He speaks eloquently about our connection to nature as a *spiritual realm*. Simply reflecting upon the unknown forces that move the stars, tides, and planets keeps all living organisms connected to the mystery of the seasons as well as light and dark. Noticing the moon phases is good for us, as there is a tide being moved by the moon inside our body fluids. This is of particular importance to women who are menstruating since that is the same cycle as the moon.

So much of the earth is polluted with toxic chemicals that leech into the food and water supply. Dr. Bush is passionate about how we must take better care of the earth and ourselves, since we have this intimate link to all life on the planet. He makes a strong recommendation for home-grown, organic foods and has launched the Farmer's Footprint website to support this effort to bring more vital vegetables into what he calls "nutritional deserts," also known as *obesity swamps*. We applaud his team, who are building gardens around prisons and the

Navajo reservation as well as other places in great need of Real Food for their populations. His words caution us to avoid the "unreal world" and spend more time in the "natural world." For me that means turning off technology as much as possible.

The gut microbiota has recently been recognized as a separate endocrine organ, which is involved, through a molecular crosstalk with the host, in the maintenance of host energy homeostasis and in the stimulation of host immunity. Shifts in gut microbial composition caused by external factors can result in a dramatic alteration of the harmonious relationship between gut bacteria and the host, which promotes the development of metabolic diseases. In particular, the gut microbiota is believed to contribute to metabolic diseases via stimulation of low-grade inflammation.

THE CHEMISTRY OF CRAVINGS

The body is a sophisticated factory of specialized substances that include numerous categories of metabolites. This section of the book is a discussion of the relationship between foods, microbes, and behaviors with obvious natural remedies. The human gut harbors a dynamic and complex microbial ecosystem consisting of approximately two pounds of microbes in the average adult, approximately the weight of the human brain. Recent investigations indicate that these organisms have a major impact on cognitive function and certain behavior patterns, such as mood regulation, social interaction, and stress management.

These microbes produce many neurochemicals. Many have heard of serotonin and its common name, *the happy hormone,* since it is vital to the regulation of many metabolic functions including moods, sleep, and appetite. Serotonin is produced in abundance in the human small intestine. In fact, Michael Gershon, M.D., has written in his book *The Second Brain* that the gut creates 90 to 95 percent of the body's serotonin from enterochromaffin gut cells. "Entero" relates to the gut, and "chromaffin" is a chromium salt reaction shared with chromaffin cells in the adrenal glands on top of the kidneys. When someone is under a lot of stress, serotonin production is reduced because of this relationship to the adrenals. Serotonin is involved as we all experience emotion, which often affects our overall mood. Upsets in the gut brain will create upsets in the head brain and vice versa. Dopamine is another metabolite produced by the body, creating a sense of reward or euphoria in the human body. This chemical messenger plays a key role in memory, learning, cognition, emotion, and addiction. Sugar interferes with proper dopamine balance and is addictive. That is why many people crave it and reach for junk foods.

An upset in this balance between dopamine and serotonin from eating processed foods and drinks and drinking water with chemicals has been implicated in ADHD, Parkinson's, depression, bipolar disorders, addiction, binge eating, and gambling.

The immune system provides a further route of communication between gut microbes and the brain (see fig. 10.15). Microbiota and probiotics have direct effects on the immune system via the Peyer's patches in the small intestine lining (see fig. 10.7 on page 86). In fact, John Cryan mapped out which organisms have the capacity to generate individual neurotransmitters traveling between the gut brain and head brain. Indeed, a specific form of *Bifidobacterium breve* protects the bacteria from acid and bile in the gut and shields the bacteria from the host immune response. As we grow older, the microbiota becomes more diverse with the emergence and dominance of Firmicutes and Bacteroidetes. It is the delicate balance between these two phyla (the taxonomic category above class and below kingdom) that sets us up for food cravings and addictive behaviors as well as our ability to extract calories from food. Many people with metabolic syndrome (especially obesity) test out with much higher colonies of Firmicutes and lower concentrations of *Bifidobacterium breve*. Science has confirmed that this essential organism is lower in cesarean born people and those not breast fed. This explains one of the big contributors to obesity. The bacteria create a craving for obesity-causing foods.

Dopamine is released from the brain when it is expecting a reward and

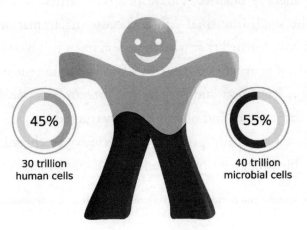

I am ~~not~~ only human after all
A complete biosphere

45%

30 trillion
human cells

55%

40 trillion
microbial cells

Fig. 10.11. Human vs. microbial cells. We live in their world. They do not live in our world. Each organ and each system of the body has its own unique and interrelated microbiome thoroughly integrated with the immune system.

associates a certain activity with pleasure, which leads to cravings. Simple sugars upset the balance of these chemicals and create a craving for more sugar as dopamine becomes dominant. Many food industry processors know this and have added hidden sugars to many processed foods. This opens the brain pathway in the same way that cocaine does, leading to addiction. According to neuroscientist Austin Mudd from the University of Illinois at Urbana-Champaign, changes in neurometabolites during infancy can have profound effects on brain development, "and it is possible that the microbiome—or collection of bacteria, fungi, and viruses inhabiting our gut—plays a role in this process."

Zach Bush, M.D., states emphatically that the "virome," a collection of viruses that thrives on bacteria, is essential to human growth and development along with fungi and other parasites. Therefore, the idea that we can sanitize against these organisms, when our body has numerous *barrier functions and immune filters* to protect us, is misinformation based on a hundred-year-old germ theory. These barriers are in our nasal passages, our gut epithelium lining, vascular endothelium lining, skin and lung tissue, and it's likely more will be discovered. These barriers are now leaking in many people and lead to the symptomology associated with metabolic syndrome. In addition, the COVID situation created a germ-phobic pandemic along with the fear. To think that we can sterilize ourselves or surfaces is unrealistic based on the science of the microbiome. We must learn to live in harmony with the microbial world, and that requires keeping a strong immune system. This process is known as symbiosis. When we are out of balance it is called dysbiosis. Current research is validating the importance of maintaining the gut's balanced terrain as the first line of defense.*

OBSERVATIONS

In thirty years of colon hydrotherapy practice, I have observed which of the most common foods irritate the small intestinal villi and cause inflammation that travels through the body. I have learned that when a person has a full-blown allergic reaction to certain foods, it is usually immediate, like swollen tongue or lips. This is caused by a histamine reaction and may lead to *anaphylactic shock* and be life-threatening as the throat closes and breathing is obstructed.

Food intolerance or sensitivity typically presents less serious yet chronic responses, including gas and/or bloating, pain in the abdomen, nausea, diarrhea,

*Learn more about Zach Bush's unique perspective and commitment to offering solid scientific information on his website.

headache, dizziness, sleep disturbances, mood swings, loss of concentration, cravings, skin eruptions, and/or joint pain. Often the person is so used to these symptoms that there is a belief this is "normal." It is not. It is metabolic syndrome gestating. The big chain drugstores are full of products that are used to self-medicate the symptoms. This will not address the root cause that lies in the gut. In fact, many of these are laboratory or chemically based. They might give short-term relief but also act as a contributor to more long-term damage to the sensitive gut lining that keep the cycle of symptoms circulating.

Most people who avoid the items in figure 10.12 will see rapid improvements in their digestive process and overall sense of well-being. This may look like all that is in your kitchen, so start with a few and gradually eliminate the others. Once you have stopped consuming all of them for at least six to eight weeks, you may explore adding one back into your diet at a time. Remember, a food sensitivity often shows up three to five days after ingesting the substance, so reintroduce one per week. This way you can note the responses you may be having over the days after eating it. Be mindful of stressors as well. If there is not a noticeable reaction, go to the next one. I first learned this "elimination process" from my physician students who have studied functional medicine at the Institute for Functional Medicine. It is wise to have three colon hydrotherapy sessions consecutively per week for three months while eliminating these twelve substances. This is the most successful protocol that I have developed with Michael over our combined seventy-plus years of exploring gentle

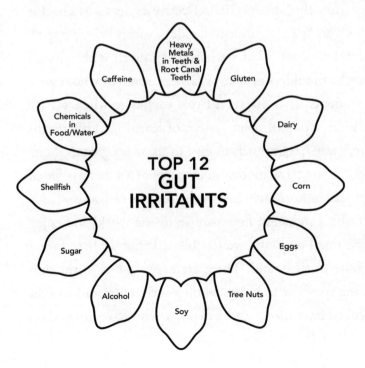

Fig. 10.12. The top twelve gut irritants. Follow the instructions given in this chapter to become your own food scientist and to discern as gently as possible how to identify and tame the cravings for foods that harm you.

cleansing. My heart aches for the people who pay us handsomely during the cleansing process and then sabotage their progress by eating at restaurants or making unwholesome food choices. This behavior is self-destructive. It is not my job to judge them but respect each person's individual choices on their journey. Often this is difficult and as therapists, we must be accepting and supportive of those who suffer.

Please learn to read labels and if it cannot be pronounced, it is not food for your body. If it is delivered through a window to your car, it is not food for your body. If it is in a package with more than three ingredients, it is likely to be too complex for your body. Eat Real Food in its most natural state and follow the seasons and your region. It is often wise to ask your grandparents or other elders in your circle about family traditions and how they managed nutrition and home remedies before the advent of modern medicine walk-in clinics so prevalent today. So much of what I have learned comes from these people that I revere. I distinctly remember my paternal grandma had a barrel of sauerkraut in the basement and insisted we eat it to "keep us regular."

ELDER WISDOM

The past thirty-plus years of a blissful marriage to Michael has been a journey of discovery as we grow deeper in love, age together, and work together on courses and book projects. This is a time of life review, and much of what I will share in this chapter comes from this age-specific reflective cycle, as Michael is seventy-four and I am sixty-eight. We are considered elder experts in our respective fields, and it is wonderful to share what we have been given with all who are interested. We stand on the shoulders of many teachers, some of whom were family members and our students. It is always a lively exchange when we are in the classroom since we teach from an open system of learning. This means that everyone who comes our way has as much to give to us as we give to them. Since our students hail from around the globe, much of what we hear is based on ancient traditions, giving us authoritative knowledge in our respective fields of expertise. We are promoting a model of how we live in the world and enjoy nature's bounty. Work is one small part, and we feel blessed that we have found meaningful ways to contribute to the world. There are many colors in the tapestry of life, and we are doing our best to create wholesome circumstances that match our values. It is joyful to have nieces and a nephew who have jumped on our train.

Eastern cultures revere their elders and reach out to them for guidance and information that is based on life experience. Very often the elders live with the children and grandchildren, and they contribute greatly to the household. Their presence provides safety and stability for the family unit. We have seen this beautiful relationship in many of the international homes that we have visited. Fortunately, we also witness this locally with several of our friends who are recent grandmothers. The time I spend with these women is always rich as they recount the changes that grandparenting has brought to them. Many do not color their hair, and their faces carry a grandmotherly glow. I call them the silver foxes! Their eyes twinkle as they tell stories about their grandchildren. One woman spoke of a newfound feeling that includes the lack of selfishness in her desire to be generous with her growing family. The other woman choked back tears as she shared of her estrangement from her grandchildren and need for group support to manage her emotional pain. Another friend is actively involved with her granddaughter every week, and their special day is Thursday. Aging brings change and, with it, the possibility for wisdom. Certainly, patience is a core requirement of wisdom as the body moves more slowly and priorities change.

My fondest memories are sharing time with both of my two grandmothers in their respective kitchens. As I recall, that is where they spent most of their time, and now I do the same most days. It is my fondest wish that the readers of our book will share time with their grandparents. Sit with them, listen to them, and write down their pearls of wisdom, memories, family history, recipes, and home remedies. This is an oral tradition for healing that *must* continue through the next generations. Follow their commonsense guidance and pass it along. Reverence for family and healing lineage is most needed these days in our complex world.

Western culture is fixated on extending the appearance of youth with drugs, injections, surgeries, and implants along with other ways of attempting to stem the tide of time. Media hype blares the promise of eternal youth, and this fallacy began to infect women's consciousness in the early 1960s with Twiggy and *Glamour* magazine. Too many elders are isolated in adult facilities/warehouses and are often neglected and abused. Michael and I have had firsthand experience with this including visits to such places with both of our parents. This strikes me as an unfortunate contrast between East and West. When I look back on my childhood, both of my grandmothers were present with me in our home at one time or another. Neither of them would have considered dyeing their hair or getting a facelift or breast implants, nor would they have spoken about trying to look younger than their actual age. It was a time of respect and reverence for the aging process as they shared their experiences and knowledge with my parents and us children. They honored the natural progression of time and how it manifested in their bodies, lives, and psyches. Slowing down was expected as part and parcel of the aging process. It is inevitable, so we must learn to embrace the changes.

My first exposure to the natural way of well-being came at a very young age in my large, loving family. My six brothers and three sisters were blessed to share time with our grandparents, who lived nearby and ultimately lived in our home. My paternal grandmother loved to drink beer and do jigsaw puzzles. She let us take a few sips now and then, and I distinctly remember the dizzy feeling from that. On the other hand, my maternal grandmother was a baker and had sacks of white flour on the floor of her kitchen along with numerous cans of Crisco shortening. This grandma always told us if we didn't feel well in our tummy, "go sit on the toilet and relax!" Very often, that was all we needed to release the discomfort of gas or waste. If we did not expel, she would administer an enema to us. I remember kneeling at the bathtub with a pillow under my head as she put water into my rectum. It was not the most pleasant experience, but I can honestly say that I always felt better afterward because it was done with care and kindness, free of abuse. This was standard procedure in our home for all of us no matter our symptom, age, or gender. I also remember my mother using a small enema ball syringe like the one shown in figure 10.13. The enema bag was a permanent fixture on the back of our bathroom door. Unfortunately, most people have no idea what this is or how valuable it can be. One of my elder friends called to thank me for telling her caregiver to give her enemas while she was ill with COVID. She told me that it likely saved her life.

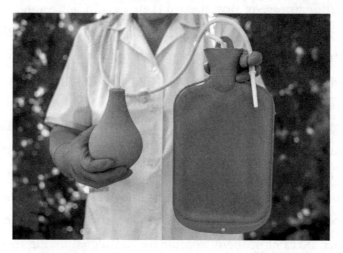

Fig. 10.13. Nurse with enema bag and baby ball syringe.
The baby ball syringe is also used to clear the rectum
when a full enema is not indicated.

Then Grandma would give me a cup of hot tea and a piece of dry toast and put me in bed. She would rub my belly and just sit with me until I dozed off. She also came from a large family, and many of her siblings never married. My dear Great Aunt Lu was the midwife as well as the death doula for many in the community. I can still remember being eight years old and stepping into her home and helping to bathe her sister, my Great Aunt Lizzie, who was dying. I had no fear, since Aunt Lu told me Great Aunt Lizzie would be meeting Jesus in heaven soon. Aunt Lizzie died that night peacefully and bathed in love. She also had her best Sunday dress on! Aunt Lu was a hoot! She had the rock-and-roll station on her radio all the time, and I remember dancing with her often.

I have also been blessed by many elder women who have brought me Grandmother's voice in their sharing. One such group is a global network called the International Council of Thirteen Indigenous Grandmothers; each woman comes from a different tribe. I have a long list of wise, healer women who have nurtured and nourished me with their knowledge of home remedies and natural healing ways. Sometimes a good, long, hot salt bath is all we need. No wonder I love swimming in the ocean and seek out thermal waters when we travel. Or perhaps application of a simple essential oil and a hot cup of herbal tea is what's called for. These simple ways are returning to us as the population seeks out more gentle ways of healing in the wake of aggressive and often failed medical interventions that do not treat causes, only symptoms. And in that vein, often a complete bowel movement is the best medicine to provide relief, and this takes time with the necessary relaxation response. The gut's enteric nervous system is governed by our ability to rest and digest.

THE THRONE ROOM

Recommended Bathroom Protocol

1. Listen to your body's signal as soon as possible and go sit down on the toilet.
2. Use the squatting position while seated on the toilet as shown in figure 10.18 on page 108.
3. Relax, belly breathe, and read daily affirmations or other spiritually uplifting literature.
4. When finished, turn and look at the feces in the toilet. Contemplate what may have contributed to the shape, density, and consistency.

5. What did I eat yesterday? How much water did I drink yesterday? Was I upset yesterday or today?

6. Reflect on what was eaten and what may have been eating at you emotionally. Remember that the shape and volume of feces is directly related to the amount of fibrous foods eaten.

7. Double wipe the anal area from front to back. One dry paper and one wet paper.*

8. Close the toilet lid before flushing to contain the fecal bacteria.

9. Inspect toilet and seat, top and underneath, for cleanliness. Wear disposable gloves while cleaning up as needed after each use.

10. Wash hands while humming happy birthday.

Growing up, we had just one toilet in the house, and it was forbidden to close the door. As I look back now, I was blessed by this open-door policy of the bathroom. I am laughing now as I write this noticing that I keep the bathroom door open in our home today! There was no shame associated with natural body functions, including toilet time. Grandma used to pass gas regularly without holding it and called it "laying eggs." It sure did smell like rotten eggs at times, and I suspect it was from all the sauerkraut. It was Grandma who taught me as a child to wipe myself from the front toward the back to keep my genitals clean. I still teach this today to all of our clients and marvel at how many have never been told this vital information.

I remember carrying my brother, who suffered from juvenile rheumatoid arthritis and was barely able to walk, up a steep flight of stairs to receive massage and paraffin wax dips for his aching hands and limbs. We shared a bedroom, and I can recall helping him with a urinal and bedpan as a very young girl. Then my baby brother was born, and I began changing diapers at age six (before disposables). My older brother was charged with taking the buckets of dirty diapers down to the cellar for washing. This was just part of life in our home. It is crystal clear to me now as I approach seventy years that these events were truly my early training in colon hydrotherapy, natural healing, and the value of cleansing the bowel (see fig. 10.14). Little did I know that I would become an international health educator and travel the globe helping people who have trouble moving their bowels and other accompanying metabolic issues.

---

*We prefer a brand called WaterWipes as the safest chemical-free product.

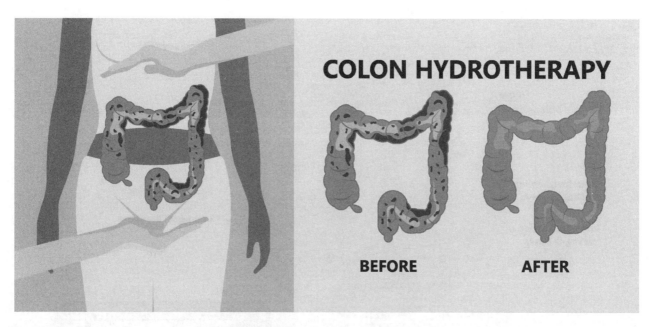

Fig. 10.14. Before and after colon cleansing

TOILET TRAINING SHAME AND NEGATIVE EFFECTS ON BOWEL HEALTH

There are many people who come to me with chronic constipation and corresponding metabolic issues. During consultations with clients, I have documented too many stories of toilet training shame. I consider this to be domestic abuse. It is far too common to hear how children are punished for soiling themselves accidentally during potty training. This cruelty has resulted in deeply rooted emotional scars and a belief that going to the bathroom is going to be painful. The vagus nerve—our connection between the gut brain and the head brain—develops a signal that the bathroom is a place of punishment (see fig. 10.15). This is a setup for a suppressed immune system due to stress and consequently metabolic syndrome. We consciously hold back what is designed to be flowing.

I believe so many of the people who seek out colon hydrotherapy need tender loving care to retrain the gut brain–head brain connection. When I hear of such abusive parenting, I sit in silent witness as these people often shed many tears. It is astounding to me that they have the courage to share such an experience. Thankfully, I know how to be with these people without any need to fix them. I simply pass them the tissues and tell them how very sorry I am that they had to endure such treatment. This kind of shame takes time to process and working with a qualified mental health counselor is necessary, so we often make that referral. It is not in my scope of practice as a licensed massage therapist and colon

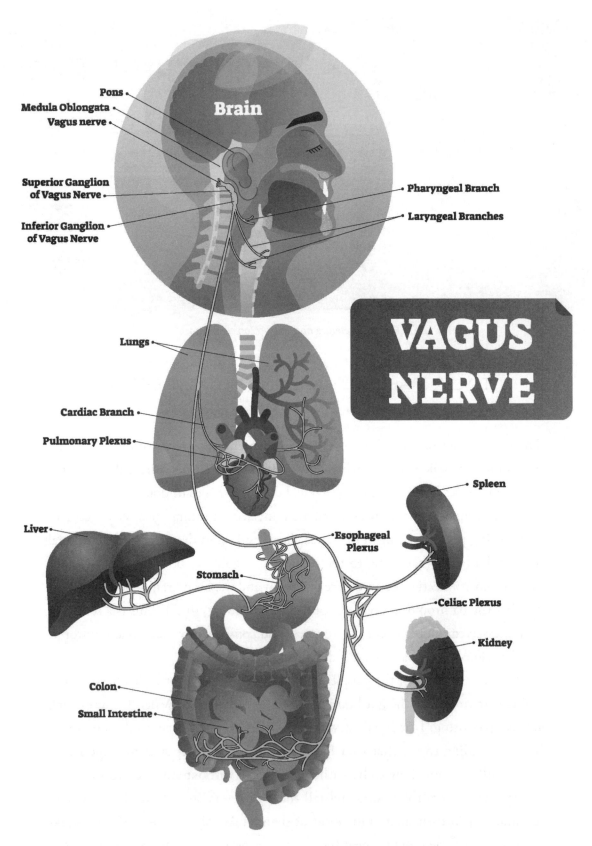

Fig. 10.15. Vagus nerve vector between the gut and brain. Colon hydrotherapy is a neurologically based therapy because it stimulates the anti-inflammatory capacity of the vagus nerve.

hydrotherapist in the state of Florida to do emotional process work with clients. I see benefit from Emotional Freedom Technique and neurofeedback.

Toilet shame is a huge contributor to the chronic metabolic and mental/ emotional issues that are rampant in our Western world. It is not my intention to cast blame on parents here. We can't know what we don't know. Everyone does their best with what they learned from their parents and the enormous generational patterns before them. If they knew better, they'd do better. Blame and shame bring no gain. As therapists, it is vitally important to remember that the issues relating to the client's health that we hear from our clients are complex and multilayered. Also, the mother's nutrition and lifestyle choices while they were gestating in utero deeply affect the person's adult health.

If the gut is not right, the body will not function well. There are many over-the-counter laxatives and other digestive remedies that line the shelves of the drug stores and health-food stores. These are short-term fixes for long-standing problems and simply mask symptoms without getting to the source. Laxatives ultimately stop working and send many people looking for a different answer or something chemically stronger to heal their constipation. Research has shown that nerve damage results from long-term laxative usage; this leads to a weak intestinal muscle system and thus a decrease in intestinal peristalsis, which interferes with a proper bowel movement. It is a vicious cycle that creates more stress. If we cannot relax and immobilize without fear, we simply cannot release appropriately on the toilet. Magnesium will often assist with relaxation since it is the mineral that supports muscles. It also draws water into the colon, and we use a particular brand* since it never causes cramping. Magnesium is better than a laxative because it strengthens the muscles of the large intestine rather than irritating the colon as most laxatives do, especially those that include the herbs senna or cascara sagrada. We always recommend beginning with just one capsule before bed to assess its efficacy. The dosage may be increased as needed for daily, complete bowel evacuation. Please remember to add soluble and insoluble fibers to your food choices with ample water. The fiber creates a coral reef effect (solidity) with the bowel movement.

As we explore the gut and its complexities, it is evident to me after so many clinical hours that there is a strong emotional component related to gut issues. The stories I've heard convince me that it's not just what people eat; very often it's what is eating at them emotionally. The stress of life is often a huge contributor

---

*We use the Oxy-Powder brand of magnesium.

to gut issues, particularly if there was toilet training abuse in the person's child-hood or different forms of trauma at any age. It may have been some simple message given by a figure of authority that going poo is taboo. It certainly isn't a topic of conversation that is allowed in social circles, unless you grew up in my household!

In the Buddhist tradition of mindfulness, the practice is to notice that we have been captured by the thought before it cascades into an emotional reaction. It is helpful to simply be a witness to the thinking process when loads of thoughts are stuck together. By witnessing, we can let go into a grounded awareness of one's body and breath. Thoughts do not really go away; they can fade to the background of our internal experience. This supports the development of accurate empathy for self and others. Every thought carries a chemical messenger of either pleasure-joy or stress-discomfort. Choose wisely and learn to move attention away from stressful thoughts. This teaching has served me well after so many years of painful constipation: your illness is wasted unless you are transformed by it.

Purification creates transformation and prevents stagnation. Elimination inspires illumination.

Constipation creates internal stagnation and happens on every level: mentally, physically, emotionally, and spiritually. People who are stuck in destructive patterns of abuse to self and others, avoidance, and/or addictions show up in my clinical practice regularly with digestive issues from early trauma. There could be an entire book devoted to these stories from my clinical case notes. Cleansing the body with the water element frees the earth element that is often static in the human body. The fire element becomes uncontrolled inflammation wreaking havoc on the body's immune and endocrine systems from the cytokine storm created at the cellular level. Inflammation is the body's way of helping the immune system to adapt, and it is necessary. Without the flow that includes elimination, we simply cannot release and give back to the Great Mother what belongs to her!

Fasting, cleansing, and purification practices are written into all ancient spiritual traditions around the globe. We have been fortunate to travel widely and witness many such healing ceremonies. A fascinating image (see fig. 10.16) shows the communal toilets in ancient Rome where people went to do their business literally and figuratively. Many cultures also had a time of cleansing typically practiced as part of seasonal change and rites of passage from one stage of life to another. We encourage a *cleansing lifestyle* that includes routine

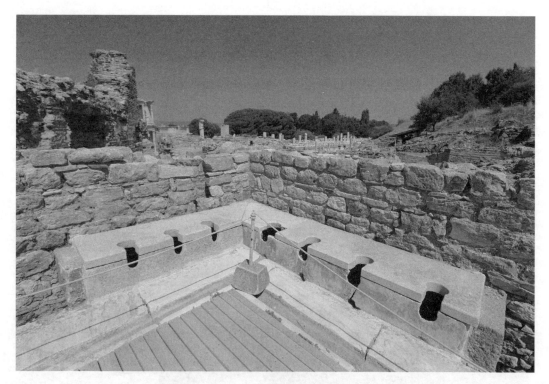

Fig. 10.16. Ancient public toilets: traditionally a place to do business literally and figuratively

days set aside for liquid nutrition, intermittent fasting, colon hydrotherapy, and days without any technology (phones, TVs, computers, cars, etc.).

The human digestive system has so many functions that are happening automatically from the intelligence of the autonomic nervous system (ANS). See figure 10.15 on page 102 for the mapping of this with the vagus nerve, which is 80 percent of the parasympathetic nervous system. The other half of the ANS is the sympathetic nervous system (SNS). Our primary goal in our practice of colon hydrotherapy is to provide *safety*. Safety is coregulated by the vagus nerve, and there is a specific pathway from the gut brain (enteric nervous system) to the head brain via the vagus nerve discussed in chapter 25. This nerve registers safety and this feeling is essential for the ability to relax and release. Providing safety includes sanitary conditions as well as emotional safety and respect for each client. Everything during the session is negotiated with the client's permission. This includes touch, timing, and permission to stop the session. The client is empowered to control their session based on their physical and emotional comfort. Our trademark SheaWay^SM/SloFil^SM methodology guarantees a gentle, comfortable colonic as we promote relaxation through safe practices (see fig. 10.17). The unique gut enteric nervous system must have relaxation for peristalsis and elimination to function well.

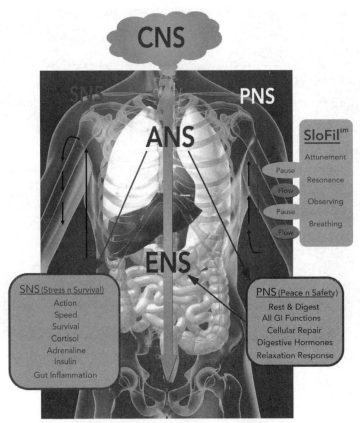

Information flows down from the head brain (CNS) to
the gut brain (ENS) and back up again. All of this communication
is regulated automatically by the ANS and depends entirely
on the relaxation response. 95% of the body's serotonin
is produced in gut cells.

Fig. 10.17. SheaWay^{SM}/SloFil^{SM} based on the science of the autonomic nervous system (ANS)
Inflamation

SHEA TRAINING

Too many clients tell me about abusive toilet training as well as abusive colonics from poorly trained therapists. I have also had negative personal experiences during my travels as I explore and have colonics from other colon hydrotherapists, many of whom were medical doctors as they are the only ones legally able to perform a colonic in many countries. My goal is to train those who are interested in this modality to be kind, gentle, and skilled at tracking the ANS of each person. I can honestly say that every session is completely different as the client expresses unique responses each time. Shea-trained therapists are individually supervised and taught how to track the ANS signals that are evident during the session. As the ANS expresses itself with the client's breathing, eye gazing, skin color changes, and other signs, the highly skilled Shea-trained therapist will adjust the session to prevent overstimulation of the ANS. Therefore we always book the first-time client for three consecutive days of colonics, one per day. On the first day a client enters with a certain level of nervousness and curiosity that is perfectly natural; the first session orients their ANS to a new experience. The second day, they are aware of the process and how gentle it will be for them. By the third day, the client's ANS has begun to repattern itself toward more relaxation. I often hear that they have never slept better!

Very often, people with gut issues have an ANS pattern of holding and ignoring the signal (interoceptive awareness) to use the toilet. We women are trained not to pass gas since it is not ladylike (unless you knew my grandmother). I remember recently hearing a client say, "I am really good at holding!" This woman has been a nurse for twenty-plus years and trained herself to ignore her body since it was often not possible to use the bathroom when needed. My coaching to her was to notice this pattern and get even better at letting go. Many people will not use a public toilet especially on an airplane. After time, this gut signal becomes weaker and begins to diminish the sensation to pass gas or defecate. Passing gas is a precursor to a bowel movement; it assists peristalsis in moving solids forward down the tube and out into the toilet. Anyone who has appropriate toilet training as a child knows that this is the sign. When we hold in the gas, we are also holding back the feces. Both of these are waste products that must keep flowing when given the appropriate internal signal. Using the toilet brings with it cultural attitudes from times when there was no indoor plumbing. On a website called The Kid Should See This, the video "Kids Meet a Poop Doctor" features gastroenterologist Dr. Marina Panopoulos revealing some funny and disturbing beliefs from children regarding toilet use and bowel movements.

Exploring how culture has evolved these negative attitudes is a fascinating study in human behavior patterns and especially how it results in ignoring the call of nature. And that is the number one cause of so many digestive upsets. We must choose to stop what we are doing to honor our body and its constant signaling.

Our posture while we sit on the toilet is vitally important to the defecation process. Modern toilets keep the hips above the plane of the knees, which makes it difficult for the rectum to relax. Simply placing a step stool, book stack, or ice bucket in front of the toilet to elevate the feet between six to nine inches (depending on the person's comfort zone) is extremely helpful (see fig. 10.18).*

---

*The travel Porta Squatty is a lifesaver for those of us who are globe-trotters. It folds down into a flat piece that fits easily into a suitcase and is very lightweight. It can be ordered at the Squatty Potty website.

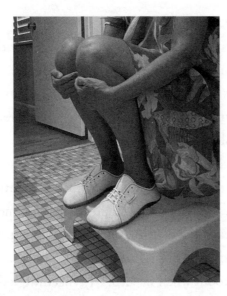

Fig. 10.18. Squatting posture that encourages complete bowel evacuation. (Photo by Evelyn Stetzer.)

This squatting position places the knees well above the plane of the hips and is the most natural state for the rectum to elongate and the pelvic floor muscles to relax and open the bowel for a more complete evacuation. Squatting is also the way women in traditional cultures give birth.

I've heard it said that having a good, complete bowel movement is often a spiritual experience. Martin Luther frequently alluded to the fact that he suffered from chronic constipation. He is known to have spent much of his time in meditation on the toilet. The sixteenth-century religious leader wrote his groundbreaking ninety-five theses while on the toilet before or after a large bowel movement. Letting go and releasing very often brings illumination. This has been true for me each time that I do any kind of cleansing protocol. It is common to notice that something from the unconscious releases, and there are insights that emerge from the unconscious nervous system. Perhaps this is why many spiritual traditions practiced fasting and cleansing as a way to encourage divine inspiration. I can honestly say that my own experience of cleansing allowed me to walk away from a long-term abusive relationship. It was so clear to me that I had to leave to feel emotionally, mentally, spiritually, and physically safe.

HOLY COMMUNION

It seems important to recognize our relationship with nature as a kind of communion. This blending of the earth body with our human body is an active spiritual aspect of life and its interdependence. Humans eat the gifts given freely by Mother Earth for sustenance, and it is necessary to return the favors with an offering of sorts. If the product we are ingesting is in a package and processed, it is not in its most natural state. It is not food for our body or soul and lacks nutrient and nourishment. This is the perpetration of separation between the human body and the earth body. It is not an illusion. This is a reality based on our food choices.

We humans sometimes deny a direct connection with our own divinity that is shared with the natural world. It is our birthright. Any intermediary (priest, guru) interferes with this direct connection and may become abusive, as is well documented in all religions. How do we learn to add fire and water to our bodies at the hearth, the center of the spiritual world in our home? How do we plant ourselves into the natural world without chemicals (glyphosate, etc.)? Can we release the earth element (feces) as an offering to the Mother Earth as a nurturing of the earth to balance what we extract from the earth? We truly compost every day when we flush the toilet. This was an insight from one of my teachers after her first experience with me during her cleansing. She spoke eloquently about the colonic being a spiritual cleanse, as the circle is complete from food grown in Mother Earth to her offering of feces given back in gratitude. Feces is a fertilizer that nurtures the origination of the generosity of the earth that feeds us in so many ways. When we take care of our body and all its components including urine, feces, sweat, and breath, we return this care to the Great Mother. It is a completion of a sacred cycle of giving and receiving and it is a gift and privilege to be born as a human being

Farmers plow under manure from animals to enrich the fertility of the land. We have seen this every season in the rural Swiss alpine villages where we have taught since 1995. There is no crop without the recycling of waste products. Then the grasses grow and become hay to feed the animals, and the cycle continues year after year. Of course, there is crop rotation to assist in this richness. The potency and poetry of the farm relies on this ancient knowledge, and it translates into variety in our kitchens, the hearth. Most people eat the same food day after day without much thought. This behavior often results in food sensitivities. Many do not cook at all and rely on prepared food every day. Fast food is not food. It is corporate junk created in a factory, not grown in the earth. The key to strengthening our immune system in the gut is feeding the variety of organisms with Real Foods in the prebiotic and probiotic families (see fig. 10.19). This variety is what gives the stool super structure and makes it easier to pass out of the body.

The earth requires biodiversity for sustenance and so do humans, especially

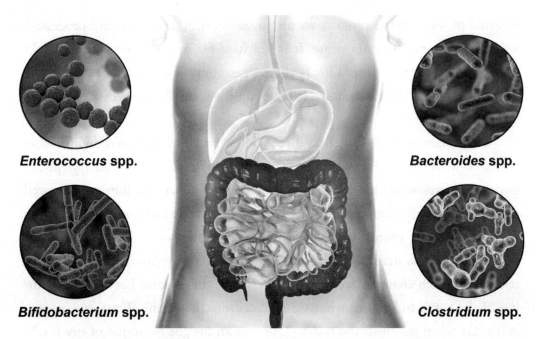

Enterococcus spp.

Bacteroides spp.

Bifidobacterium spp.

Clostridium spp.

Fig. 10.19. Feed the numerous microbes in the gut for optimum well-being.

in the gut microbiome. Current guidelines suggest that we eat a minimum of five to eight different fruits and vegetables per day to strengthen our body's immune capacity and feed our cells abundantly. Where do we start to climb what seems like a mountain of fresh produce? Begin in your garden and bring it into your kitchen. Be sure to avoid plastics, as they take hundreds of years to decompose in the landfills. Each day I burn the paper and boxes as a gesture of gratitude in prayer. Save your eggshells and teabags for the renourishment of the soil. Composting is easy and fun as you explore this on YouTube videos. Give back to the great Mother Earth—she who feeds us so generously. Enjoy the *biophotonic* relationship between the sun, the earth, and your body as we share this delicious fellowship with the natural world. Make your kitchen a sanctuary, a holy place with gratefulness, joy, and pleasure as the guiding principles.

KITCHEN AS HEART AND HEARTH

The heart of the home is the hearth, where the five elements infuse the food. The alchemical blending of space, wind, fire, water, and earth creates this blend from the unseen world of spirit to the visible world of humanity. This is our spiritual metabolism undone by corporate food. So we teach how to bless everything we touch, everything we see, every thought we think. In this way, everything becomes sacred with the intention to bless, including the act of eating then going to the bathroom, giving back to the provider. Taking in the divine as food and transforming it into cell food that keeps our body alive and releasing waste products is a miracle of our body's metabolism of Health. It is important to honor this cycle by bowing to the source. We remember the source when we find joy in the process that includes grow, shop, wash, chop, and cook. Blessed are those who do not need to eat out much and prefer to grow and prepare their own foods! Such is the kingdom of the healthy body. Current studies prove that children who are involved in gardens from sprouting to harvest eat more veggies.* Hallelujah!

My dear mother did not like to cook. Imagine feeding twelve people each day and trying to please all of their palates! Thankfully, my dear father loved to eat, and the weekends were a culinary delight at his hands. He certainly put his heart into the preparation. It was typically meat and potatoes and his coleslaw with lots of mayonnaise and sugar added. I have a vivid memory of digging up dandelion greens in our yard on Dixon Avenue in Pittsburgh as a little girl. Dad would sauté bacon pieces and add vinegar to the skillet. Then he would blend in the *weeds* with all that good fat and create his version of *sour salad*. My German heritage was active during this moment. Guaranteed we all had hefty bowel movements the next day! When I left home at seventeen and went shopping at the grocery store in Miami, I was struck by foods that I had never seen before in my life. That is when I became curious about cooking and tasting new varieties. It is understandable that my mother cooked the same thing over and over again because she was trying to keep it simple. I grew up during the 1960s when more industrial canned, frozen, and packaged food was coming forward from the corporate food industry to make it easier and more convenient. Unfortunately, the chemicals used on the farms increased at this time along with genetic engineering of seeds, so farmers had to buy new seeds each season. Traditional cultures always had seed stored from the previous season's crop to replenish the next. We now have an exorbitant number of toxins in the earth and placed into food processing. This contributes to the vast medical issues such as metabolic syndrome many people suffer with since it creates an assault on the human immune system. Buy organic and non-GMO, please!

---

*I wish to honor a dear local friend who has been successful in setting up edible gardens at many of our public parks and schools here in Palm Beach County, Florida. She is passionate about this project and teaching the next generation how to feed themselves in a healthy way. Thank you Joseph P. Cory Foundation and Nada Cory!

Thankfully, my grandparents had a beautiful garden, and I would go there in the summer and help them can foods at home. They also raised chickens, and I can remember shoveling the chicken manure out of their little coop to spread on the garden. This was long before "organic" was even a commonly used word. They had intimate knowledge of the cycles of nature and how to grow an abundant variety in their garden. Yummy veggies in the jars and cans prepped the previous summer were consumed when very few fresh vegetables were available in the winter in Pittsburgh, Pennsylvania. I believe that is the other issue that is challenging. Many people live in climates where fresh fruits and vegetables are not available several months out of the year. Flash freezing and canning are the answers to this dilemma. Most homes up north also had a cold cellar where root veggies and fruits would be stored in the winter out of the elements.

Thankfully, these methods are making a comeback along with the preservation of foods through pickling and fermenting. I truly believe that my grandmother lived to a ripe old age because of the friendly microbes in the sauerkraut despite her beer drinking. There are times when it's easier to purchase the kraut, and I prefer the Trader Joe's brand since they add pickles like my grandma did. I do enjoy my Sunday at-home time making ferments.

Dairy products in the United States come from cows who are held in close quarters and given antibiotics as well as growth hormones for fast fattening. When we ingest dairy, we are also getting the residual of these drugs and chemicals. In addition, all dairy products carry a specific protein molecule called beta-lactoglobulin, and it is one of the most common reasons why people are allergic to milk products. I first learned about this from Thomas Rau, M.D., my mentor in Switzerland. When you couple this protein with the residual waste product metabolites from the medications that the cows are given, even organic milk can become problematic simply because of the protein molecule. Commercially prepared milk products are made from a blend of milks from many, many different cows. This contributes to the problem. There are numerous studies proving that a high percentage of people with digestive issues find relief after eliminating all dairy products and all gluten-containing products.

I heard from a woman recently who has a three-year-old that is now attending day care while she works. This little boy was getting sick every single weekend after enrollment and, of course, she thought he was adjusting to the new environment as his immune system managed it. When this continued for four weekends in a row, she became alarmed as his symptoms worsened. She took this child to four different medical doctors who all pronounced him "healthy" despite his suffering with stomach aches, mood swings, sore throats, earaches, and other maladies. She finally found a doctor who asked about his diet and what they might be feeding him at day care. The mother inquired and found out that all the children were required to drink a carton of whole milk each day. Thankfully, when they stopped the milk, all of this child's issues resolved quickly. He is now a dairy-free, happy little boy who is taking a specially formulated probiotic each day as prescribed by the doctor.

OUR HOME KITCHEN

When the food is not grown locally but on farms somewhere in the distance and most likely GMO, they may contain untold poisons from chemicals. If a package has ingredients you cannot pronounce, it is very likely a chemical from a laboratory somewhere. Over many decades, there has been government-sanctioned chemical warfare (glyphosate, etc.) that has poisoned countless lives from a tainted food supply. Untold numbers of chemicals are also added to the public water supply that further diminish the human immune system. As families grew larger after World War II, the food industry capitalized on this trend by offering convenience foods that were cheap and plentiful. I remember shopping with my father and siblings on Saturdays. He would buy ten Swanson TV dinners for one dollar each, and that was an easy meal for one evening for our brood. It was the beginning of an acculturation to fast food. We found out later that identifiable nutrients in these early versions of processed foods, such as carbs and protein, were grown in soil tainted with leftover stores of nitrogen used in the making of munitions in World War II! These were neither nurturing nor wholesome, but convenient and filling for busy baby-boomer families trying to feed lots of children. This points out the collusion between the government, chemical companies, and the food industry. And so continues the deeper destruction of the earth and its people that in many ways has led us to this time of widespread illness from suppressed immunity and loss of a spiritual center in the home.

Michael and I have found simple ways to make it easy in our kitchen, so we offer these ideas to our readers:

We sit and do meal planning at least twice a week, covering all meals for ourselves and our office manager usually for three days in advance. We discuss what protein, what carbohydrate, what fat, what veggies, and so forth to serve. As we travel, we always rent an apartment with a kitchen and work this routine as we forage in the green markets that are available everywhere. Our water comes from our well since we declined the offer to hook up to the city water system full of chemicals. We filter from the tap through an ionizer that also creates alkalinity.* It is a good investment and pays for itself in less than one year. Buying water in plastic bottles is like drinking water with chemicals no matter what the label says. We each have several large stainless steel or glass bottles we use to manage our daily hydration needs.

We have a daily confirmation usually in the morning after waking up. There is usually a check-in around the timing for the different meals that day to determine when we are going to eat, what we are going to eat, and if we are going to eat together. Eating together is a priority when possible. Sharing at least one meal together per day and sometimes two or even all three, depending on our individual schedules, is a great gift to our relationship.

Shopping is done almost twice per week to maintain an abundance of fresh Real Food. We generally will sit down and go over the shopping list briefly or text it to each other. We always inform each other when we think we might be stopping at a store to gather. Almost all fresh fruits and vegetables coming into our home are organic, and we also wash them thoroughly in ozonated water after removing the containers they came in. Check out the "Dirty Dozen" and "Clean Fifteen" lists on the internet, since that will guide you about what must be organic in the larder. We transfer veggies into green bags, glass bowls, or jars, since plastic and Styrofoam leach chemicals into the food rendering it poisonous. There are over ten thousand chemicals allowed into food and its packaging. Glass and stainless-steel containers are better and keep the foods better preserved for a longer shelf life by reducing the chemical exposure and pollution of foods. Real Food is better preserved in chemical-free containers. This practice makes short order of cooking up the veggies quickly for our meals. It's the preparation that takes most of the time in the kitchen, so we do this on Sunday for the week ahead. We also drop these chopped or shredded veggies into my homemade broth for a sumptuous quick soup when adding miso to the broth. This sharing of the bounty as a family is fabulous! I remember as a child finally being a "big girl" and my mother showing me how to use a butter knife to cut soft foods. As I look back now, this was one of my initiations, and I felt so grown up helping her. She needed help for sure with our clan!

---

*The BioMat and ancillary health products can be purchased in the products section of Cathy Shea's website.

Meal preparation involves several cycles to complete. The initial preparation involves:

- washing
- cutting
- chopping
- storing extra foods for future meals

We use high-end Japanese knives and serrated-edge knives for most of the cutting and chopping. This means keeping the knives sharp, and my husband sharpens them at least twice a month. He says the cutlery in the kitchen needs to be Samurai quality since that is where the training for the warrior began.

All veggie cuttings are saved in a large bag in the freezer and simmered in the slow cooker for soup broth. It is easy to add bones to this mixture to make gut-nurturing and restorative bone broth, which I use for soups, stews, sauteing, or sipping. The slow cooker is perfect for this process or the Instapot.

Cleanup etiquette is a very important cycle. We only use ecofriendly products including essential oil products, white vinegar, and baking soda. Differentiating what goes down the disposal and what gets thrown away or composted is vital. Some dishes are hand washed and others go into the dishwasher. When the dishwasher finishes its ECO cycle, we usually put away the dishes together as a shared ritual in the morning. All counter tops get a good scrub every night, including the stove. The kitchen floor is mopped two or three times a week. We live with a lot of different critters in South Florida and do our best to keep temptation to a minimum. I found some nontoxic boric acid tablets that do the job of repelling insects and are safe around pets and children. Cleanliness and good hygiene is essential in any kitchen and must be a priority. Spreadsheets are kept of all the stores locally where we purchase our fruits and vegetables, especially organics. The spreadsheet shows price comparisons between stores and quality recommendations for brand products such as nut butters, organic whole grains, and so forth.* The gluten-free grains and quinoa (a seed, not a grain) are steamed gently in our stainless-steel rice cooker. It has an automatic shutoff so we can get it started, go to the beach for a swim, and when we return, it's on the warm cycle. A big part of meal planning involves the timing of preparation. That is why my freezer is always full of frozen mango, berries, soups, and broth. Grab and go!

---

*Good mail-order resources for dry goods include Swanson Vitamins and Vitacost; see their websites.

It is wise to purchase quality meat online.* We found out that the vegetarian industry's claim about industrial animal farming as a major contributor to greenhouse gasses is false. A 2020 documentary called *Sacred Cow* by Diana Rodgers makes this falsehood abundantly clear.

Recipes are discussed regularly to create variety in our meal planning. We like to experiment with different recipes and use the internet as well as the numerous cookbooks and images from other people's cookbooks to provide diversity and flavor at our table. I have a large herb garden that adds a tasty garnish to our meals daily. I also enjoy the sprouting process in the glass mason jar with the screen lid. In just a few days, the quart jar is full of live greens that are full of biopotency. It is also much more economical than purchasing sprouts in plastic containers that often carry mold. They are also luscious in a green smoothie.† The human gut microbiome thrives on diversification of foods to support the growth of wholesome, friendly microbes. More is better! Check the appendix in this book for yummy ideas for breakfast, smoothies, and meals.

Sometimes the ingredient list in a particular recipe is discussed for substitutions. My husband avoids added sugar like the plague but can tolerate stevia.‡ He eats much more fruit than I do, but he always has. Since we have a dozen mango trees with that many varieties, he eats up to five mangoes a day during the summer. Several summers ago he had his microbiome tested at the end of mango season and found that his microbiome was in the top 99 percentile for diversity. Sometimes people are afraid of eating too much fruit because of the sugar. Not all of the sugar in fruits and vegetables ever enters the bloodstream. It is always chelated with numerous other metabolites. Michael claims that mangoes are a superfood and recently edited a book called *Maturing with Mangoes* by Walter Zill.

As I close this chapter, I implore you to please involve all of the people in your household with these suggestions and ideas and embrace the wisdom and practices of our elders. Preparing and dining together is an ancient, deeply rooted behavior that encourages intimacy and strengthens the family unit. A commitment to this process will yield many benefits for your body, mind, spirit, and community. Create a relaxing environment so that each person is calm. Never eat when you are

---

*We use Slanker Meats or ButcherBox.
†I like the Blendtec or Vitamix brands of blenders.
‡I like the Trader Joe's brand of powder for baking or liquid for drinks, since it does not taste bitter.

upset, especially angry. Never eat with someone whom you do not feel emotionally safe with. Keep the meal conversation wholesome and light since we swallow the words we speak. At our table, the daily news is not discussed. It is bracketed for later or the next day. Give cravings for that special treat a twenty-four-hour pause. I have found that I usually forget all about the treat. If it's still on my mind, then I bless it and enjoy it—even better if I share it with someone that I care about. The guilt will do more harm than the treat so please, relish your reward! Don't keep it in the house. Sometimes if it's an inconvenience, I decide it is not worth it to go out to the store and get it. When I do make that choice, I always buy the best quality treat I can find. Mine is Italian tiramisu! Then I bring it home and sit quietly to relish every single morsel. The occasional measured indulgence is a gift I give to myself so I never feel deprived. Deprivation leads to cravings. My discipline is gentle and mindful and includes pleasure as an essential part of my self-care practice. Twenty percent of our population eat in the car, and 33 percent of Americans do not know how to cook, and we wonder why it costs Americans one trillion dollars a year in medical bills to overcome poor food choices. Some clients say that organic food is so expensive, but so are repeated medical and hospital visits. Just say no to fast food joints and processed and packaged foods and eat foods in their most natural state. Find a local fisherman or hunter who has humane attitudes for the animals. Research grass-fed meats from local sources if you are a carnivore and support the small businesses that provide them. Always look for wild-caught fish instead of farm raised, since the latter is often laced with chemicals. Decide to turn off all electronics during mealtime. We do enjoy some music during meal preparation if it is quiet and soothing.

Remember, food has energy and will absorb nutrients that are seen and unseen. What vibes do you want to ingest? Think of the love in your grandmother's voice and how she supported your family. This is the essence of the kitchen as hearth. Similar to the movie *Like Water for Chocolate,* be mindful of thoughts and ideas that are wholesome while preparing food in the kitchen. Follow the pleasure principle as you put heart into your meals at your hearth.

Feel free to visit me on my Cathy Shea Channel on YouTube for some fun, easy video recipes!

RECOMMENDED READING

Breaking the Vicious Cycle, Intestinal Health Through Diet by Elaine Gottschall (Kirkton Press, 2007).

Deep Nutrition, Why Your Genes Need Traditional Food, Featuring the Four Pillars of the Human Diet by Catherine Shanahan, M.D. (Flatiron Books, 2017).

Colon Hydrotherapy: The SheaWay by Michael Shea and Cathy Shea (CreateSpace Independent Publishing Platform, 2013).

The Second Brain by Michael Gershon, M.D. (Harper Perennial, 1999).

The Swiss Secret to Optimal Health by Thomas Rau, M.D. (Berkley, 2009).

Gut and Psychology Syndrome, Natural Treatment for Autism, Dyspraxia, A.D.D., Dyslexia, A.D.H.D., Depression, Schizophrenia by Natasha Campbell-McBride (Mediform Publishing, 2004).

The Compassionate Kitchen by Thubten Chodron (Shambhala, 2018).

Gut, The Inside Story of Our Body's Most Underrated Organ by Giulia Enders (Greystone Books, 2015).

Pocket Peace, Effective Practices for Enlightened Living by Allan Lokos (Penguin, 2010).

The Fourfold Path to Healing, Working with the Laws of Nutrition, Therapeutics, Movement and Meditation in the Art of Medicine by Thomas Cowan (NewTrends Publishing, 2004).

11

COVID-19 and the Rule of the Artery

By Mary Monro, B.Sc. (Hons) Ost., M.Sc. Paed. Ost., FSCCO

Mary Monro graduated from the British School of Osteopathy, now the University College of Osteopathy, in 1999. In 2009 she was awarded an M.Sc. in Paediatric Osteopathy at the Foundation for Paediatric Osteopathy in London. She is a Fellow of the Sutherland Cranial College of Osteopathy and has had work published in the *British Osteopathic Journal* and *International Journal of Osteopathic Medicine* as well as delivering a webinar on the pathophysiology of COVID-19 for the Osteopathic Alliance. She treats human and animal patients in Edinburgh, Scotland, and teaches internationally.

One of the founding principles of osteopathy covered in part 1 of this book is that "the rule of the artery is supreme," and since it has become clear that COVID-19 is primarily a disease of the blood vessels (Libby and Lüscher 2020), this chapter will review the pathophysiology of COVID-19, with particular emphasis on the role of obesity as a risk factor and how the vascular endothelium provides the virus with access to the body. The endothelium is the interface between the fluids inside the blood and lymphatic vessels and the fluids in the rest of the body. It could be thought of as the nervous system of the whole fluid body, since it reaches everywhere and has intelligence and executive powers.

COVID-19 BASICS

COVID-19 is caused by a novel virus called Severe Acute Respiratory Syndrome Coronavirus 2 (SARS-CoV-2). SARS-CoV-2 seems to be particularly aggressive and has been likened to a "dirty bomb" causing damage and dysregulation to a variety of systems (Ball 2020). Intensive research done since 2020 is clarifying how the virus works, building on what was learned from the previous coronavirus outbreaks of SARS (2003) and MERS (2012). SARS-CoV-2 resulted in a global pandemic and an unprecedented public health crisis. By the end of 2021 it had infected more than 300 million people and killed over five million worldwide (WHO Coronavirus [COVID-19] Dashboard, January 15, 2022). Clinical features vary from a mild, asymptomatic state to a severe state with respiratory dysfunction, thrombotic complications, and multiorgan failure. Up to 20 percent of patients require hospitalization (Chernyak et al. 2020), and the death rate is thought to be around 2 percent. It is likely to be lower, as many sufferers are asymptomatic or unrecorded. Typical initial symptoms include fever, cough, shortness of breath, fatigue, and loss of a sense of taste or smell.

Vaccines appear to be effective at reducing the risk of serious disease and death from COVID-19 (Connelly 2021). However, there remain risks from novel vaccine-evasive variants, unknown long-term side effects of the vaccines, unknown duration of immunity, and the possibility among vaccinees of acquiring infection and transmitting it. There is also the possibility of antibody dependent enhancement, whereby a high level of antibody response to the wild virus actually worsens the severity of the disease (García 2020; Lee et al. 2020).

An understanding of the pathophysiology of COVID-19 enables us to help minimize the risk of infection for our patients and explains how to care for patients who have had COVID-19 or who are still suffering "long COVID" with symptoms lasting more than twelve weeks. It is clear that COVID-19 is a syndemic—a confluence of an infectious disease that interacts with noncommunicable disease factors such as poverty, obesity, Black, Asian, and minority ethnic ethnicity, and old age (Horton 2020). As community therapists, we need to educate patients to enable them to help themselves and the wider community and encourage and support initiatives that address these societal risk factors at national, local, and individual levels.

RISK FACTORS

COVID-19 patient statistics reveal a higher risk of severe disease and mortality for older people, men, people with comorbidities (especially cardiovascular disease, type 2 diabetes, autoimmune disease, liver disease, kidney disease, and chronic lung conditions), people in lower socioeconomic groups, smokers, and people in the Black, Asian, and minority ethnic communities (CDC, "People with Certain Medical Conditions"). Obesity, defined as a BMI of 30 kg/m² or more, is a major risk factor for serious disease and death, particularly among people under sixty (Kompaniyets et al. 2021). It is difficult to specify the unique role of obesity, as many people may combine several of the risk factors identified above.

In their "Obesity and COVID-19: Policy Statement," the World Obesity Federation states

> overweight and obesity seem to be risk factors for worse outcomes in those who are infected by COVID-19. Studies overwhelmingly show that obesity is associated both with a higher risk for intensive care unit (ICU) admission and poorer outcomes for COVID-19. In the UK, a report flags that out of 10,465 patients critically ill with confirmed COVID-19, 73.7% were living with overweight or obesity. Meanwhile, a report from Italy suggests 99% of deaths have been in patients with pre-existing conditions, including those that are commonly seen in people with obesity such as hypertension, cancer, diabetes and heart diseases. Overweight and obesity also seem to be risk factors for worse outcomes in younger populations (<60 years old), with patients with a body mass index between 30 and 34 being twice as likely to be admitted to ICU compared to individuals with a BMI under 30.

Another risk factor for people with obesity is that as BMI increases it becomes more difficult to treat effectively for severe COVID-19. For example, intubation, prone positioning, and effective ventilation are all more difficult in the morbidly obese (BMI 40+) patient.

The problem may have worsened as the pandemic led to many people sitting more, exercising less, comfort eating, or changing their eating behaviors because of anxiety, all leading to weight gain. Also, the job losses and low income that came with the response to the pandemic made high quality, nutritious food more difficult for many to afford.

The table below shows various countries in terms of COVID-19 deaths per million population, prevalence of adult obesity, and the percentage of the population whose household income is below half of the median. Clearly there are other factors at play—the table doesn't show deaths as a fraction of infections, for instance, because the data on infections is poor—but they might indicate general well-being level, the effectiveness of health care, and the effectiveness of government response to the pandemic.

TABLE 11.1. COMPARISON OF COVID DEATHS, OBESITY,
AND POVERTY IN SELECTED COUNTRIES

Country	Covid-19 Deaths per Million Population (to Jan 2022)*	Prevalence of Adult Obesity BMI 30+ (2018–20)†	Population living below half median household income (2020)‡
Japan	146	3.6%	15.7%
Germany	1387	19.0%	9.8%
Spain	1925	16.0%	14.7%
UK	2257	20.1%	12.4%
USA	2567	42.7%	18.0%

*Source: Statista
†Source: World Obesity Federation
‡Source: Organisation for Economic Cooperation and Development

COMPLICATIONS

The CDC states that complications of COVID-19 include organ failure in several organs (kidney, liver, pancreas), heart problems, acute respiratory distress syndrome, venous thromboembolism, central nervous system injury, septic shock, and additional viral and bacterial infections.

Understanding the risk factors and the complications gives some clues about how SARS-CoV-2 works and explains why some people suffer longstanding medical issues after the initial infection.

IMMUNE RESPONSE

The innate immune system responds first to any infection, reacting as soon as it detects a pathogen. With SARS-CoV-2, as with many other infections, the response is better among young people than among older or unwell people. Initially there is a cytokine (including interleukins, interferons, and tumor necrosis factor) and noncytokine inflammatory mediator (especially ferritin and C-reactive protein) release, along with pro-inflammatory complement activation, to destroy the invader and summon the white blood cells. In COVID-19, this response can be excessive, leading to a generalized inflammatory state, dysbiosis, endothelial damage, a prothrombotic environment, and to the so-called "cytokine storm." In extreme cases it leads to acute respiratory distress syndrome, a common cause of death in severe COVID-19 cases.

The T cells summoned by the innate immune response include killer cells that destroy viruses and helper cells that stimulate the production of antibodies and memory B cells. In COVID-19, the virus binds with the T cells via ACE2, deactivating them and compromising the immune response. In addition, when there is an excessive cytokine response, this can destroy T cells in a paradoxical autoimmune response. Reduced T cell availability then interferes with the production of antibodies and memory B cells, reducing immunity against future attack (Bernard et al. 2020).

THE ROLE OF ACE2

It seems that SARS-CoV-2 accesses our bodies via Angiotensin-Converting Enzyme 2 (ACE2), using this enzyme as a portal to cross from the air into the respiratory tract and from the blood vessels into the tissues (Varga et al. 2020). However, further research has shown that this is an oversimplified view, given that ACE2 expression in the respiratory tract is low relative to the intestine and kidney, and yet this is the primary route of entry. It seems likely that other receptors may play a part in ways that are not yet fully understood. Certainly, SARS-CoV-2 seems to have a greater affinity for ACE2 than its predecessor, SARS-CoV (Cuervo and Grandvaux 2020).

ACE2 was discovered in 2000 and is part of the renin-angiotensin system that regulates blood pressure, fluid, and salt balance. ACE2 also has local regulatory roles in the heart, lungs, kidneys, liver, brain, and gut. It is found in high concentrations in the tongue, and this is thought to be the reason symptoms often include ageusia (the loss of the sense of taste) (Jasti et al. 2021). ACE2 is found throughout the vascular tree in the lining of the blood vessels, the endothelial cells (Hamming et al. 2004; Li et al. 2020). ACE2 seems to oppose the action of ACE1; ACE2 is anti-inflammatory, vasodilatory, antithrombotic, and supports vascular endothelial health. Essentially, SARS-CoV-2 attaches to ACE2, reducing its availability to the body and thereby creating an imbalance between ACE1 and ACE2, which leads to systemic hyperinflammation, endothelial activation, suppressed immune response, and thrombosis.

Adipose tissue is a reservoir of ACE2, provides a plentiful supply for the virus to use, and is also a source of many proinflammatory mediators and adipokines. High baseline C-reactive protein, interleukin 6, hyperleptinemia with leptin resistance, and hypoadiponectinemia (all associated with obesity) explain the preexisting inflammatory state in obese individuals. In addition to the compromised immune function that chronic systemic inflammation brings, obesity is characterized by insulin resistance and lipid deposition in lymphoid tissue, both of which profoundly affect the function of the immune system (Mohammad et al. 2021; Villapol 2020).

Inflammation is at the forefront of COVID-19 research, and major complications of COVID-19 infection are directly associated with systemic inflammation (García 2020). Recent studies have indicated that disease severity and outcome of COVID-19 patients are directly associated with dysregulation of pro-inflammatory cytokines. Therefore, it is plausible to suggest that acute inflammation arising from COVID-19 may exacerbate existing chronic inflammation secondary to obesity and, along with compromised immune function, lead to more severe disease and poorer outcomes.

THE MICROBIOME AND
THE GUT-LUNG AXIS

The microbiome is the ecosystem of bacteria, fungi, and viruses that inhabit our respiratory and digestive tracts. It widely affects host well-being and greatly correlates to a variety of illnesses, including metabolic, digestive system, and respiratory diseases, along with mood and mental health. The human intestinal flora contains over one thousand different microbial species but, on average, each host contains about 160 dominant bacterial species, depending on genetics, environmental factors, and dietary habits. The human microbiome is a highly dynamic microecosystem that interacts with and regulates the immune system. Immune cells induced by a variety of antigens can move between the gut and the lungs through the lymphatic system and/or blood, resulting in the regulation of immune response of both organs. The crosstalk between intestinal and pulmonary tissues mediated by the microbiome and immune cells is called the "gut-lung axis" (He et al. 2020).

Obese individuals and older people have a less healthy microbiome than others, with fewer microbes, a different balance of species, and a higher level of harmful bacteria, tending toward a pro-inflammatory profile. In addition, obesity is associated with a leaky gut and poorer vitamin D uptake, vital to immune health (Belančić 2020). People with digestive symptoms of SARS-CoV-2, such as diarrhea and vomiting, have been shown to have more severe disease. Gut dysbiosis can occur when infection disrupts the microbiome and inflames the intestinal epithelium (causing diarrhea), releasing cytokines into the circulation and thereby adding to the systemic inflammation provoked by the infecting virus. The ACE2 imbalance generated by SARS-CoV-2 infection exacerbates this picture, further disrupting normal microbiome function (Villapol 2020).

MEDICAL TREATMENT

There is a subtle balance that is not fully understood (Guo et al. 2020), and so it's not a simple matter of treating with ACE1 inhibitors or boosting ACE2 production to redress the balance (though patients taking ACE1 inhibitors are advised to continue with them). Drugs that show benefit in the treatment of severe COVID-19 include anti-inflammatories (corticosteroids such as dexamethasone), IL-6 inhibitors (such as tocilizumab, usually taken by sufferers of autoimmune disease), and remdesivir (the drug used to treat Ebola) (NIH, COVID-19 Treatment Guidelines). Vitamin D may be helpful in reducing risk, especially for Black, Asian, and minority ethnic and older populations, by supporting immune function (Vimaleswaran et al. 2021). Given that the inflammatory state provoked by SARS-CoV-2 triggers systemic oxidative stress, it is reasonable to suppose that antioxidants may be of benefit in reducing the severity of disease (Chernyak et al. 2020). Probiotics may be of benefit to tackle dysbiosis and its impact on the immune system and to counter the negative effect of dexamethasone on the microbiome (Din et al. 2021).

THE RULE OF THE ARTERY: VASCULAR ENDOTHELIUM

A. T. Still was prescient when he said in his autobiography: "In the year 1874 I proclaimed that a disturbed artery marked the beginning to an hour and a minute when disease began to sow its seeds of destruction in the human body. . . . He who wished to successfully solve the problem of disease or deformity of any kind in every case without exception would find one or more obstructions in some artery, or vein. The rule of the artery is absolute, universal, and it must be unobstructed, or disease will result." The lining of the blood vessels, the vascular endothelium, has been much studied in recent years and is now known to be an intelligent, organizing, feeling, planning, responsive, communicating organ—a body-wide web lining every vessel and reaching every part of the body. It is intimately connected with the health of the whole being, just as Still observed. It has a central role in regulating complex physiological processes, comparable to the role of the brain, such that we might call it "the nervous system of the fluid body." Researchers say "endothelial activity is crucial to many if not all disease processes" (Ramcharan et al. 2011) and it is "a powerful organizing principle in health and disease" (Aird, "Endothelium: II," 2007).

The nature of the endothelial cells varies from organ to organ and from arteries to capillaries to veins in terms of morphology, permeability, and secretory activity. Until quite recently this heterogeneity was ignored, but with new imaging techniques, the diverse range of endothelial structure and function is beginning to be fully appreciated. It may even be that each of the sixty trillion or so endothelial cells is a unique individual with its own structure-function character (Aird, "Endothelium: I," 2007; Aird, "Endothelium: II," 2007). In health the endothelium is still, quiescent, and only activates in response to insult or injury (Deanfield et al. 2007).

Shear stress—especially turbulence—and oxidative stress (inflammation) are the main activators of endothelial cells, provoking them into changes in permeability or secretory activity, damaging or even destroying them. Venous endothelial cells are associated with more mast cells (white blood cells that contain histamine, involved in the allergy response, wound healing, and inflammation) and histamine receptors (histamine activates the endothelium, leading to leakage and tissue swelling) and are more permeable than arterial endothelial cells, allowing for extravasation in the case of insult or injury.

The vascular endothelium has been described as the "chief governor of body homeostasis" (Simionescu and Antohe 2006). In this regard its functions include regulation of perfusion; regulation of fluid and solute exchange; equilibrium between plasma, interstitial fluid, and lymph; regulation of permeability and lumen patency (via fibronectin, heparan sulfate); regulation of leucocyte adhesion and migration (Steyers and Miller 2014); secretion/signaling with a wide variety of electrical and chemical (autocrine/paracrine/endocrine) factors; hemostasis and coagulation (thromboplastin, tissue factor)/blood liquidity (thrombomodulin) balance; antioxidant and anti-inflammatory promotion; regulation of vascular tone (vasoconstrictors include angiotensin converting enzyme ([ACE1]) and endothelin-1); vasodilators include prostacyclin and nitric oxide (prostacyclins also inhibit platelet aggregation, and their production reduces with age, raised blood pressure, diabetes, and nicotine usage) (Pries and Kuebler 2006; Epstein et al. 1990).

Most endothelial cells have a fuzzy, sticky, brush-like luminal surface, called the endothelial surface layer, which is metabolically active in its own right. The dynamic structure is made of a proteoglycan core bound to the endothelial cells, with glycosaminoglycan chains (mostly heparan sulfate) attached and floating soluble elements. Functions of the endothelial surface layer include modulating fluid shear stress effects on the endothelium; barrier and sieve functions; supporting red blood cell survival in the capillary beds; binding ligands and enzymes to support cellular signaling; reducing oxidative stress and maintaining nitric oxide availability; modulating adhesion of inflammatory cells and platelets; retaining anticoagulation factors (e.g., antithrombin, tissue factor inhibitor); modulating immune reactions via glycoproteins such as integrins, selectins, and immunoglobulins; regulating oncotic pressure and preventing leakage of fluid out of the vessels; and maintaining a net negative charge to repel platelets, red and white blood cells, and albumin (but albumin is amphoteric—both positively and negatively charged—so this relationship is complex) (Pries and Kuebler 2006; Alphonsus and Rodseth 2014). Chronic hyperglycemia, as seen in diabetes, destroys the endothelial surface layer and interferes with its important anti-inflammatory, antioxidant, and anticoagulant activities (Dogné et al. 2018).

The microvasculature represents about fifty times the surface area of all the macrovasculature combined. The heterogeneous endothelial cells of the microvasculature play an important role in innate immunity, adaptive immunity, coagulation, and inflammation. Their ability to direct and regulate leucocyte trafficking, interact with platelets, release and respond to cytokines, control vascular tone and permeability, and maintain an anti-inflammatory environment are key to their role (Danese et al. 2007). Inflammation and its impact on the vascular endothelium is at the root of all chronic diseases (Khansari et al. 2009).

THE ROLE OF VASCULAR ENDOTHELIUM IN COVID-19 AND LONG COVID

In the case of COVID-19, the vascular endothelium is activated by oxidative stress via the reduced availability of ACE2, leading to vasoconstriction, systemic inflammation, altered immune response, and a procoagulant state. It cannot produce nitric oxide (NO) or hydrogen sulfide (H_2S), so-called gasotransmitters, both powerful vasodilators and anti-inflammatories. The gut microbiome produces some of the H_2S (which keeps the vascular endothelium healthy) as a metabolite of cysteine breakdown (Sun et al. 2020). In patients with a limited microbiome (such as the elderly and people with type 2 diabetes and hypertension), its circulating immune and anti-inflammatory functions are restricted, making these patients more vulnerable.

Activated vascular endothelium, so-called "endotheliitis" in COVID-19 (Varga et al. 2020), causes havoc around the body, featuring generalized vaso-dysregulation. Evidence suggests that hyperglycemia and insufficient glycemic control could be associated with increased oxidative stress and hyperinflammation in severe infections, potentially promoting endothelial or organ damage in patients with obesity and diabetes (Osuchowski et al. 2021).

Long COVID, where symptoms continue for more than twelve weeks, has yet to be fully understood, but systemic inflammation, a compromised immune response, and endothelial dysregulation can have severe and prolonged effects on the body. Metabolic syndrome takes years of gestating before full-blown symptoms may appear. It is thought that long COVID affects about 10 percent of COVID-19 patients and is more prevalent among women and younger people, in contrast to the people more likely to be affected by severe acute disease. People who have more than five symptoms in the first week of COVID-19 seem to be at higher risk of getting long COVID (Sudre et al. 2021), but the etiology is not fully understood. Long COVID is a catch-all term for a diverse range of symptoms, which may include ongoing symptoms from the acute phase, chronic fatigue, chronic organ damage, worsened preexisting conditions, and new symptoms, such as autoimmune disease. There are several theories about the cause of long COVID: continuing presence of the virus, reinfection (the same or possibly a different strain), dysfunctional immune response leading to a chronic inflammatory condition, and/or a condition like myalgic encephalomyelitis/chronic fatigue ("Living with Covid19—Second Review," 2021). Autonomic dysregulation, gut dysbiosis, chronic inflammation, and microvascular damage are the common denominators for all symptoms of long COVID.

HEALTH CARE

Post-COVID and long COVID patients need a holistic, integrated approach to support their recovery (NIH, "Living with Covid19—Second Review," 2021). Standard medical tests often return normal results in people who are obviously unwell, making it difficult to specify pharmaceutical therapy. Restoring normal autonomic function, reducing inflammation, supplementing the microbiome, and supporting endothelial health and ACE2 balance are all key to physical recovery.

COVID-19 has been accompanied by a pandemic of fear, loss, and mental ill health. Depression, sleep loss, the stress of social isolation, and anxiety about health and financial security compound a suppressed immune response (Segerstrom and Miller 2004) and a feeling of being unwell. "Brain fog" has left people feeling diminished and has sometimes affected their ability to return to work. Some sufferers experience post-traumatic stress disorder or post-intensive care syndrome (Nalbandian et al. 2021).

Osteopaths and other natural health therapists are in a good position to help these patients. We offer a holistic approach that includes compassion, listening, connection, therapeutic touch, dietary advice, and techniques to improve the mechanical function of physiological systems and support metabolic health.

By providing a reassuring and supportive presence, we begin to normalize the autonomic nervous system, as the multivagal system can utilize social coregulation to destress (see Stephen Porges's polyvagal theory discussed on page 266) before we even start our treatments. The heart, arteries, veins, and lymphatic system are all accessible to palpation, so we can access the vascular endothelium via any of these vessels. Treatment can help to quiet the vascular endothelium and support its return to equilibrium. This "nervous system of the fluid body" also gives us access to the organs and tissues that the vessels supply and to the whole fluid body. This is a good opportunity to practice "divided attention" looking both at a local issue and how it manifests in the whole. This vascular approach integrates our existing skills in working with other systems affected by COVID-19, such as breathing mechanics, the musculoskeletal system, digestive system, psycho-neuro-immuno-endocrine system, and the autonomic nervous system.

It takes us back to our roots, making us palpate the normal and the abnormal in the whole body and seek to support the body to find health. Nobody is an expert on treating post-COVID and long COVID patients, and medical tests won't give us much guidance. Like our forebears, we must learn what is going on in the body via palpation and use our understanding of physiology to treat patients effectively. The vascular endothelium brings Still's wisdom into the twenty-first century, focusing our attention on the health of the whole person based on the quality of the blood vessels, the origin of the disease cascade.

We can help patients to influence their ACE2 expression by suggesting that they reduce intake of or avoid: smoking; a diet high in fats, salt, sugar, or meat; and alcohol (Li et al. 2020). A high-quality, mainly plant-based diet, particularly including sulfur-containing vegetables (e.g., brassicas), can support and improve health. Probiotics to support the gut microbiota may be helpful, and the nutraceutical *Ephedra foeminea* is a powerful antioxidant and antiapoptotic (Khalil et al. 2020). Vitamin D to support immune recovery, along with folate, B12, and magnesium, which underpin methylation (Pruimboom 2020) and thereby epigenetic effects, can also usefully be supplemented. This dietary advice to support the vascular endothelium sounds familiar, as it is also relevant to general health—as A. T. Still said, "the rule of the artery is supreme." All disease starts with a disturbance in the vascular system, most commonly inflammation of the vascular endothelium.

Many of us are now seeing patients with long COVID, and we are learning to appreciate the complexity and individuality of the symptom picture. People are not necessarily only suffering from long COVID; they may have other stresses affecting their lives and other health issues complicating their recovery. Their internal resources may be limited, making it a challenge to treat them enough but not too much, to help them pace their return to normality, and to provide the right support to enable them to cope with the distress that they may be experiencing. We must deploy all of our sensitivity, skill, and experience, exercise all of our compassion, and use our networks of skilled therapists in a range of disciplines to provide patients with the care that they need for "mind, matter and spirit" (Still 1899). This is the moment to show that a whole-person approach is the path to health, not just for COVID-19 but for the major public health issues of our day—metabolic syndrome, cardiovascular disease, and cancers.

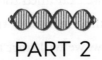

PART 2

THE FLUID BODY

Biodynamics and Embryonic Healing

12

Levels of the Fluid Body

In the first section of this book, we examined the deep metabolic disturbances in the human body that plague human beings on the planet right now. Here, with this chapter and those that follow, we will start to work with different solutions and antidotes. All the images and visualizations suggested in this part of the book, and the remainder of the book, are to create a sensation of metabolism in your own body for you to begin to know what that feels like. It is the ground from which interoceptive awareness is cultivated—consciousness of the instinctual urges in the systems of the body for hunger, elimination, connection, and nurturing. This is necessary because metabolic movements in the client's body have a broad perceptual spectrum much beyond what is taught in many manual therapy trainings and mindfulness practices. This is the pro soma movement at its heart, sovereignty and agency over one's own body. While these images can be very healing as a practitioner begins to incorporate them into their own somatic awareness and lifestyle, they also organically bring a clarity about the culture and society of corporate interests in maintaining addiction through greed. Sensing one's one metabolic health is a fundamental basic human right and includes knowing what to accept and what to reject for the well-being and self-regulation of our body and mind. It is simply about sensing our body and its health, and now we know from the state of the world body, we must be able to start by sensing individual metabolic health and all of its nuances and voices. Otherwise biodynamic work is only palliative care. We cannot really help anyone in the sense of fixing them or removing their symptoms; rather we are serving someone without any such agenda. Our agenda should instead be to confront our fear of not-knowing, bearing witness, and waiting for compassionate action to arise patiently.

But first we must find a different metaphor for relating to our body. In her book *Crystals, Fabrics, and Fields: Metaphors that Shape Embryos,* Donna

Haraway tells us that all transitions in scientific paradigms begin with the use of metaphors. We are now in that time of a transition to understanding the human body differently. I have been a student of Tibetan medicine for almost forty years, and although I am not a Tibetan physician, I understand and work with the Eastern science of the human body being constructed of elements. In the case of Tibetan medicine there are five elements: space, wind, fire, water, and earth. I will be using this metaphor not in a retroactive way but in a more contemporary integration and phenomenology for a deeper, richer, and more therapeutic effect for those who are reading this and implementing it into their clinical practice or their life in general. So we start with the fluid body.

I cannot say exactly what the fluid body is. This is because the fluid body is a biodynamic metaphor, which for me in the arc of my career is now a very personal experience of the five elements in Tibetan medicine and the embryo. It is not possible to understand the complexities of the contemporary challenges inhabiting the body without a felt sense of the elements and the spiritual and medical traditions that see the human body through the elements. The water element is just one of the five that constitute the human body. However, the term *fluid body* was originally coined by Dr. Jealous. The term, as Jealous used it, referred to the embryo as described by the embryologist Erich Blechschmidt in Germany starting in the 1940s. Blechschmidt describes the embryo as being mostly fluid containing a variety of biokinetic and biodynamic forces (purposeful movements) that are acting on and within the fluid of the human embryo as illustrated in the color insert. It is known that the embryo and human body in general is over 90 percent biological water. It must be remembered that at the same time in history, Dr. Sutherland was discovering organizing forces of healing that were "in the fluids but not of the fluids." According to Jealous, the fluid body is said to be our *original* body. I love the metaphor that our fluid body as the embryo is our original body, which lends itself to healing methodologies associated with a return to origins to reclaim our original condition of wholeness as it was in the beginning. Now for the remaining part of this chapter and those that follow in this section on the fluid body, please take time to look carefully at the images in the color insert. Friedrich Wolf purposefully drew the embryo with watercolors, and I will be referring to those images in the practices I am offering here. We are perpetual embryos as fluid bodies. This is an invitation to explore your own body and its originality for healing.

In a morphological understanding of embryology, the growth of the whole is biodynamic (see figs. 12.1–3 starting on page 135). Figure 12.1 is a glossary of terminology regarding the academic field of morphology that describes biodynamic and biokinetic growth and differentiations of the human embryo. Likewise, figure 12.2 describes in detail the four stages of morphology as they are classically defined. The first three stages are each about a week in length, and the fourth stage consumes the remaining embryonic time through weeks eight to ten. These four stages are like the four directions in a medicine wheel or sacred mandala. In this mandala the heart is at the center of that which is sacred in the body. Figure 12.3 provides additional detail for those practicing or wishing to practice biodynamically regardless of their therapeutic methodology. To practice biodynamically is to develop a felt sense of one's own fluid body and therapeutically come into relationship with the client's fluid body. I recommend the reader take time to integrate the images and their descriptions in the color insert, with these three figures providing a glossary of terms and an academic scaffolding for the imagery. This is a major component of the return to origins for healing and the retrieval of one's undifferentiated wholeness present at the moment of conception. It forms the basis for exploring the origin of the universe in the remaining sections of this book. Detailed explanations of figures 12.1–3 can be found in my books *Biodynamic Craniosacral Therapy,* volumes 1–5.

In the first two weeks postfertilization there is only a fluid body that is contained by several membranes. Consequently, in the five-element construction of the human body in Tibetan medicine, the water element is always mixed with the earth element. Only highly distilled drinking water is free of any earth elements. In the embryo there are no other body systems generated until the blood forms in the latter part of the second week postfertilization. This is how the fluid body was conceived of originally. Even after organ differentiation, the fluid body remains a constant through what Blechschmidt called the three laws of fluids consisting of three different metabolic movements: *along, through,* and *perpendicularly against* inner tissue. He called these movements *permeation, parmeation,* and *infiltration,* respectively. The first and third of these fluid body metabolic movements described by Blechschmidt are none other than longitudinal fluctuation (*along*) and lateral fluctuation of fluids (*perpendicularly against*) limiting membranes (see figs. 12.1–3). The term *perpendicularly against* inner tissue means that fluid moves perpendicular to the plane of tissue. It is very precise. Since the water molecule is the smallest molecule in the human body it can therefore move through any tissue in the human body and thus the term *permeation.* This means that our body at its deepest anatomical level is transpar-

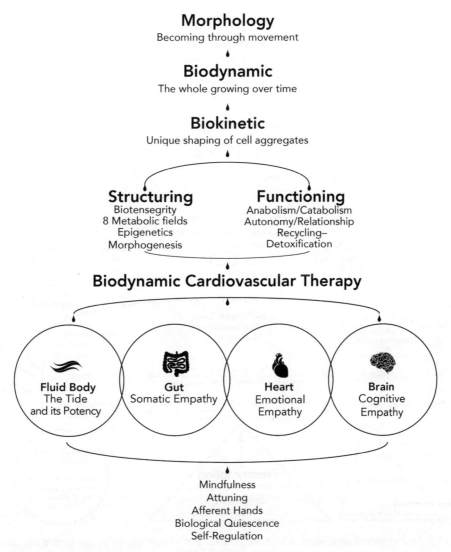

Morphology
Becoming through movement

Biodynamic
The whole growing over time

Biokinetic
Unique shaping of cell aggregates

Structuring
Biotensegrity
8 Metabolic fields
Epigenetics
Morphogenesis

Functioning
Anabolism/Catabolism
Autonomy/Relationship
Recycling–
Detoxification

Biodynamic Cardiovascular Therapy

Fluid Body
The Tide
and its Potency

Gut
Somatic Empathy

Heart
Emotional
Empathy

Brain
Cognitive
Empathy

Mindfulness
Attuning
Afferent Hands
Biological Quiescence
Self-Regulation

Fig. 12.1. Biodynamic embryonic morphology overview. This is a simple overview of the origin of the body as an embryo. Biodynamic cardiovascular therapy perceives and optimizes metabolic function based on sensing the perpetual embryo in every body.

ent, flowing, and buoyant because the human embryo develops outside the field of gravity.

The human embryo is a hierarchically structured and functioning being. This means that the fluid body is creating pathways for future metabolites to travel. The fluid body is the pre-existing original body of intelligent movement without the influence of biochemistry, cell biology, and molecules. Yet it provides the container and locomotion for all such biology. In this way, the fluid body is the core of the human organism. It is capable of mechanosensation, which allows it to explore its environment and simultaneously develop the metabolic pathways for the demand of nutrients in developing tissues and

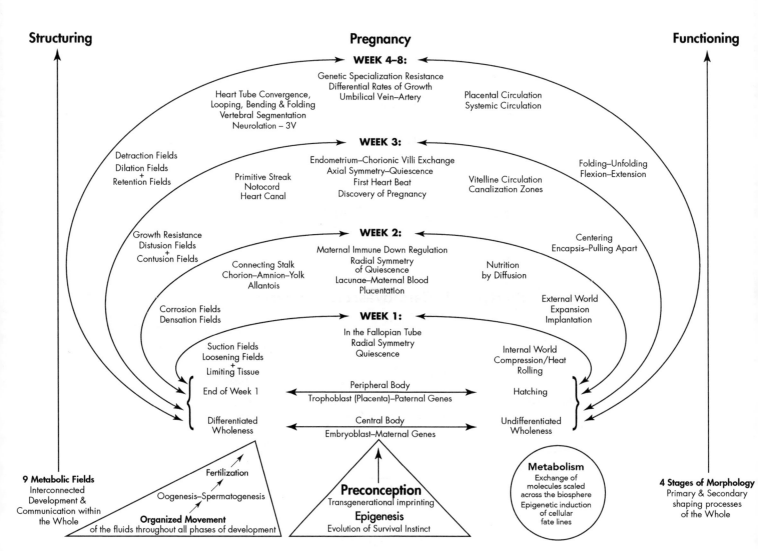

Structuring

Pregnancy

Functioning

WEEK 4–8:
Genetic Specialization Resistance
Differential Rates of Growth
Umbilical Vein–Artery

Heart Tube Convergence,
Looping, Bending & Folding
Vertebral Segmentation
Neurolation – 3V

Placental Circulation
Systemic Circulation

Detraction Fields
Dilation Fields
+
Retention Fields

Folding–Unfolding
Flexion–Extension

WEEK 3:
Endometrium–Chorionic Villi Exchange
Axial Symmetry–Quiescence
First Heart Beat
Discovery of Pregnancy

Primitive Streak
Notocord
Heart Canal

Vitelline Circulation
Canalization Zones

Growth Resistance
Distusion Fields
+
Contusion Fields

WEEK 2:
Maternal Immune Down Regulation
Radial Symmetry
of Quiescence
Lacunae–Maternal Blood
Placentation

Centering
Encapsis–Pulling Apart

Connecting Stalk
Chorion–Amnion–Yolk
Allantois

Nutrition
by Diffusion

Corrosion Fields
Densation Fields

External World
Expansion
Implantation

WEEK 1:
In the Fallopian Tube
Radial Symmetry
Quiescence

Suction Fields
Loosening Fields
+
Limiting Tissue

Internal World
Compression/Heat
Rolling

End of Week 1

Peripheral Body
Trophoblast (Placenta)–Paternal Genes

Hatching

Differentiated
Wholeness

Central Body
Embryoblast–Maternal Genes

Undifferentiated
Wholeness

9 Metabolic Fields
Interconnected
Development &
Communication within
the Whole

Fertilization

Oogenesis–Spermatogenesis

Organized Movement
of the fluids throughout all phases of development

Preconception
Transgenerational imprinting
Epigenesis
Evolution of Survival Instinct

Metabolism
Exchange of
molecules scaled
across the biosphere
Epigenetic induction
of cellular
fate lines

4 Stages of Morphology
Primary & Secondary
shaping processes
of the Whole

Fig. 12.2. Four stages of embryonic morphology. These four stages are elegantly simple and divided into the first three weeks of development and the final five to seven weeks of embryonic existence. The four stages are perceived as compression, expansion, centering, and flexion-extension. These movements are readily perceived throughout the life span.

the reciprocal opposite pathways for waste removal. Thus, the fluid body has its own therapeutics. Osteopaths say that the fluid body can lesion, meaning it can hold stress. Originally it was felt that the fluid body can lesion mainly from the overload of prescription drugs and the blockage of catabolic channels. Currently this is coupled with the stress of not being able to eliminate the metabolic waste products of complex inflammatory processes stuck in the blood, the lymph, and the interstitium of the body. A *septic fluid body,* so to speak, from metabolic syndrome is a toxic barrel of waste with no place to go but furthering the breakdown of the immune system. The body implodes on itself metabolically and leads to multiple organ failure. This is one reason why we

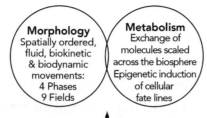

Biodynamic Differentiation
Growth movements of the whole and its differentiation over time
Every cell knows where every other cell is located in the whole embryo

Four Stages of Morphology

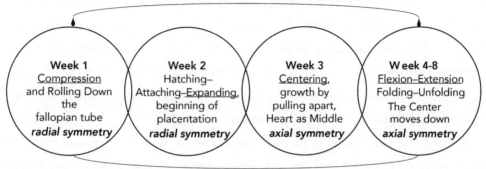

Felt Sense of Biokinetic Differentiation
1. (Topokinetics) Differential rates and direction of pressure based on position or location in the embryo.
2. (Morphokinetics) Shaping of cell groups as pressure differential determines cleavage plane of the cell and thus its differentiation into its final fate.
3. (Tectokinetics) Gelled scaffolding, a pre-structuring, occurs for all organs prior to their end function.

Spatially Ordered Metabolic Movements

Anabolism–Catabolism
Epigenetics
Morphogenesis
Growth Resistance–Metabolic Fields
Metabolism of Autonomy–Glycogenesis/Ketogenesis
Metabolism of Relationship–Vascular Placentation
Cavity Formation/Containment/Biotensegrity

Nutrition Delivery–Waste Removal
Laws of Fluids–Longitudinal, Lateral & Permeation
Water/Exclusion Zone–Canalization Zones
Nutrition: Diffusion–Umbilical Artery/Vein
Autonomy:
Apoptosis–Autophagy
Recycling–Septic Systems
Vasculogenesis/Cardiogenesis–Relationships

Fig. 12.3. Morphology and metabolism of the embryo. This image provides more detail on the four stages of morphology. This includes the developmental metabolism of building up the body and breaking it down and eliminating waste. This is key to understanding what metabolic syndrome is and how it can be repaired.

must develop a different sensibility around the fluid body and its originality.

Because the fluid body is under pressure in a growing embryo, it is said to have reciprocal tension potency, which can be palpated and influenced biodynamically. It is the potency and vitality of the fluid body that links it to the power of the Tide according to Dr. Sutherland. It is the power of the Tide that therapists synchronize with in clinical practice. It is that power that moved the embryo, me, into existence.

We are perpetual embryos because we are never quite done with our human development, no matter what age we are. We are explorers at heart with our pre-existing fluid body leading the way. Whereas all other mammals finish their development through survival specialization at the end of the embryonic period, not so with humans. Survival specialization refers to specialized structures, such as claws for digging and protecting, exaggerated noses for sense of smell, exaggerated teeth for ripping and tearing, and so forth. There is no such specialized defensive or offensive structure in the human body at the end of the embryonic period. Consequently, it is possible to say that we are perpetual embryos, especially when you consider that it takes many years of training to specialize in many things human. If you want to win a gold medal in the Olympics, it will require years of sacrifice and specialization.

To find the fluid body is to find your embryo, which is our original body still present no matter what age. Jim Jealous was my first embryology teacher in 1995. In our phone interviews for my doctoral work, he kept asking me if I had found my embryo, and I kept thinking that meant to buy more embryology books and read them. I had to shift from ordinary perception of my anatomy and physiology to a metaphorical body, which was when I finally experienced less density in my body. I learned to feel the Tide (what Jealous called Primary Respiration or PR) as described in cranial osteopathy moving through the third ventricle of my brain back and forth from the horizon. I learned to stay centered in my heart for emotional empathy. Then I experienced a sensory dimension of love and kindness as the flow of grace, the Holy Spirit, and the Breath of Life just as Dr. Sutherland experienced rather than as an intellectual concept. Altogether this is the Health that is present in the fluid movements of the body under the direction of PR. PR is thus the wind element in the Indo-Tibetan system of elements. One way to contact the fluid body as it exists in the body at this moment is through the perception of PR, also called the Tide and the Long Tide as described by Dr. Sutherland. Metaphors like this are incredibly valuable to sense the organization and repair potential of the body. In Tibetan medicine, the wind element is the most important of all the elements, and so it is in biodynamic practice. It is the most important because it causes all movement including the movement of our thoughts. It is the element that allows us to experience the world of sensation and manifestation within the element of space or the dynamic stillness in biodynamic practice.

PR is such a simple tool with which to explore our fluid body, no matter what its composition from blood to lymph and cerebrospinal fluid to urine. PR allows us to sense the fluid body as what Jealous called "one drop." This *one drop* generates a deeper sense of embodied wholeness that can be reparative to the cardiovascular and nervous systems. This is your embryo. All the elements inside the human body have complete and total continuity with the same elements outside the body. We participate in the natural world and our shared molecules communicate with each other via PR. The fluid body is a combination of the water element and the earth element. So called pure water (without the earth element) does not exist unless you steam distill it. The forces of pressure and the reciprocal tension potency of the fluid body are manifestations of the fire element. In clinical practice it is important to sense the elemental qualities of the human body. Dr. Jealous once said that the manifestation of heat and/or sweating while giving a session was the principal side effect of a biodynamic treatment. These qualities of the elements and their unique potency first manifest in the therapist and thus the adage "give a session, get a session". Thus if we come into contact with a fluid body in lesion, we have a different set of biodynamic tools to explore it.

The fluid body operates with its own unique set of movements and principles as mentioned. These movements and principles are discovered within the context of sensing the whole body and its environment with PR. This represents a paradigm shift in terms of manual therapy of any kind, but especially craniosacral therapy and the various biodynamic styles. As described in many manual therapy models, there are movements called *motion present* that are both voluntary and involuntary and associated with the various systems of the body, especially the musculoskeletal and myofascial systems. These systems of the body tend to draw the therapist into a focus on individual parts and the use of mechanical skills to enhance or increase motion present available locally. These systems are primarily of the earth element and easier to feel. The fluid body, however, constantly dissipates forces acting upon it. It is self-regulating in this way. It is of note that Dr. Jealous said that when the fluid body undergoes a stress and lesions, it can feel like soft tissue and lose its fluid quality and capacity to dissipate stress. Thus, there is more earth and less water. It is the equivalent of climate change in the body. The principle of incorporated wholeness gives biodynamic practice one of its more unique foundations as the starting point for clinical practice. The six basic dissipation movements of the fluid body are:

- **The longitudinal fluctuation:** this is a wave that typically comes from the coccyx and moves up through the entire front of the body. It cascades out from the third ventricle in the brain in a torus shape following the electromagnetic field and recoalesces at the sacrum (see fig. 12.4). At the same time it moves up and down the neural tube within the cerebrospinal fluid (see fig. 12.5).
- **Lateral fluctuations:** the therapist will feel as though his or her body is oscillating like a metronome from right to left or left to right, sliding or swinging back and forth perpendicular to the spine with micromovement or seemingly larger movement depending on where one's attention is in the body (see fig. 12.6).
- **Leaning right or left:** this is the sense of the fluid body having more weight and pulling to one side or the other. This is more like the activity of a dousing rod indicating a fulcrum of some sort in the body.
- **Micromovement:** this is a quality of vibration and minor tremoring or shaking that is subtle.
- **The spiral:** this is either a local sensation of the winding and unwinding of the pericardial sac hanging from the upper neck and resting on the respiratory diaphragm below or a global sensation of spiraling forces such as the entire vascular tree twisting and untwisting.
- **Honey:** periodically a therapist can sense PR in the fluid body and the entire fluid body (*one drop*) will have a very dense, slow movement associated with it—it is unmistakable. It is like moving in slow motion while walking on the moon.

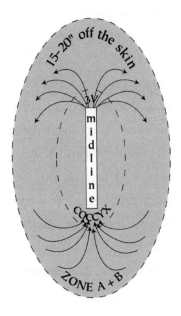

Fig. 12.4. Longitudinal fluctuation 1 cascading into Zone B. The longitudinal fluctuation is an electromagnetic torus field originating in the midline of cerebrospinal fluid (CSF) in the subarachnoid space of the central nervous system. The CSF is a ferrofluid and magnetically charged from high amounts of magnetite in the dura mater covering of the brain and spinal cord. The longitudinal fluctuation corresponds to Blechschmidt's Laws of Fluids. It is a carrier of Primary Respiration and the chi in classical Chinese medicine. Its motion and field can be explored and harmonized.

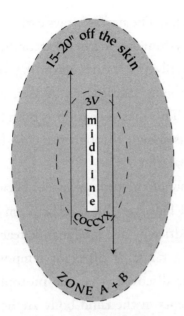

Fig. 12.5. Longitudinal fluctuation 2. Here seen moving between the coccyx and third ventricle of the brain. It also has bidirectional movement associated with the CSF. Its motion and field can be explored and harmonized. And all membranes in the human body especially the endothelium have constant longitudinal fluctuation. It is always local and global simultaneously, requiring skills of attunement.

Fig. 12.6. Lateral fluctuation. Blechschmidt's Laws of Fluids state that fluids move to limiting membranes perpendicularly, fluctuate longitudinally, and move through the limiting membrane as a permeation.

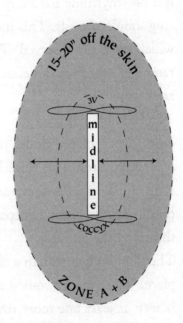

Another metaphor for the fluid body is the term *protoplasm*. Cytoplasm is a good synonym. The biodynamic community worldwide has been influenced by a 1954 black and white film from the University of Pennsylvania. The botanist narrating the film is Professor Seifritz. It is called *The Protoplasm of a Slime Mold.* The slime mold is an example of one of nature's fluid bodies in that it has few cells associated with its structure. His movie, however, demonstrates and clearly shows the activity of PR in the fluid body, both locally and globally. I have personally experienced this same phenomenon in the fluid body of my human clients. I put together a few important lessons from the movie for the reader:

- PR is seen changing phases at least ten times. The narrator says early in the film: "Note the reversal of flow with a rhythmic period of 50 seconds."

- PR is later seen breathing three dimensionally as a "heart" according to the narrator. The whole blob of protoplasm being studied can be seen to be breathing in the tempo of PR (one drop). This means that PR is both local as shown in the movie but also global as shown through the time-lapse photography of the "heart" sequence in the film.

- The various motions observed in the flow of the protoplasm in between the phase changes of PR is part of the mid-Tide (variable rates between 2–6 cycles per minute) and is called the fluid drive by one biodynamic teacher.

- The fluid body is described as having a range of different tempos all occurring simultaneously. "We made the discovery that the protoplasm is a polyrhythmic harmony." All movements in the fluid body are occurring simultaneously. This means that the therapist's perception determines which tempo is observed. The fifty-second phase of PR is considered the tempo of true Health because it is the one that never stops when all other rates stop.

- The fluid body is seen several times accessing a state of stillness (or a still-point) when placed under stress while PR continues underneath as noted by the narrator. The fluid body can repair itself while in a self-induced state of stillness. PR does not stop as the narrator mentions but keeps going on during the phase of reparative stillness as noted on a sine wave graph shown by the narrator.

- The fluid body is seen in a startle response that occurs before a shock takes place. "Note the nervous shock that occurs before. . . ." This phenomenon is seen at least one more time in the movie. In humans this is called the startle reflex mechanism.

- When two fluid bodies meet, one must be receptive to complete the joining together according to the narrator. The fluid bodies must be "synchronized . . . one or the other must give way for a fully harmonious coming together." Synchronized in this case is one fluid body being receptive to the other in terms of flow. When a therapist places their hands on a client, they immediately withdraw their attention back to their own body in order to create a receptive flow through the hands into the therapist in order to avoid overinputting to the client.

- The fluid body has different gradients of viscosity and is very elastic.

- A basic movement of PR in the fluid body is that of a spiral shown at the end of the movie. As mentioned above, the heart spiral is fundamental because of the priority of blood flow being optimized by spiral movement. Again, all of these movements attributed to PR are happening simultaneously. It is a three-dimensional matrix, so it depends on the perception of the therapist to sort out which layer he or she is observing. Thus, it is necessary to start the process of observation with the therapist's own body as he or she settles into PR and stillness.

- The narrator makes a statement that human beings "are made of protoplasm." That means cytoplasm and interstitial fluid.

More recently in the evolution of understanding the fluid body is the work of Gerald Pollack at the University of Washington. His book called *The Fourth Phase of Water: Beyond Solid, Liquid, and Vapor* is very informative and refreshing. It also created some disagreement among scientists, but the purpose here is that it provides a metaphor for understanding the body, its fluids, and their movements. This is not only because it verifies what Dr. Blechschmidt was seeing in human embryos, but because it gives us access to a way of sensing and feeling the fluid body as it exists in all of us. Pollack's work involved the discovery of what he called an *exclusion zone*. This is a zone along or on top of every membrane in the body in which water is flowing longitudinally. It's more like water molecules that are flowing. This is remarkable since his research states that 99 percent of the molecules in the human body are water molecules. This is another beautiful metaphor for a part or layer of the whole that we are not separate from.

In addition, his research showed that biological water manifests its own electricity and infrared heat. This is something that can be palpated in the client and used as a barometer for therapeutic progression. The terms *potency* and *Ignition* contain within them these qualities and meanings associated with biological water. Thus, the biodynamic teachings on integrating zones A and B (the space surrounding the body about fifteen to twenty inches and everything contained below the skin) are vitally important. I like to say that there is a warm, wet, electrically charged cloud of water vapor around the body that is in direct relationship with that below the skin. The charged cloud around us is breathing with PR. This is the fluid body.

The further evolution of understanding and sensing the fluid body as embodied experience comes from Emily Conrad. She developed a system of movement therapy called Continuum. It took her many years to evolve this paradigm shift in understanding the human body. The most basic principle is that the human body is a moving fluid body. It is constantly moving and requires a shift in perception away from traditional anatomy and physiological understandings of the body. We have been misled by a corporate, medical-industrial approach to the body as something exclusively made up of anatomy and physiology that can only be repaired by someone outside of ourselves who knows more about our body than we do. Emily's work shows that anyone can access the spontaneous rippling and undulating fluctuations of the fluid body for the purpose of healing. I sometimes like to say that we have to stand on the edge of the neural synapse or on the membrane of the cell and simply jump into the interstitial fluid or, in the case of the cell, into the cytoplasm. There is only movement as Jaap van der Wal says.

Franklyn Sills has done a lot of beautiful work describing a layer of experience in the fluid body that he calls *fluid drive* and *fluid potency*. These terms also relate to the way in which the fluid body holds and processes stress and trauma. Sometimes these collective terms are described as the mid-Tide model, which differentiates it from the Long Tide (PR) model in biodynamic practice. The Long Tide itself does not hold stress and trauma and may or may not be in relationship with the traumatic forces at all, which means that trauma issues may not be the core issue that PR is relating with. Trauma repair is a direct function of the mid-Tide model of work and is dependent on the therapist's awareness of psychophysiological issues in the client and application of trauma resolution skills. So these are different layers of experience or potential within the same fluid body. Both the mid-Tide and Long Tide models require different skills of communication, perception, and palpation. The PR model does not include a trauma resolution component as does the mid-Tide model. The Long Tide model is a spiritually based model of compassion in which the suffering of a client is held in a container of not knowing by letting go of preconceived agendas about the client's needs, bearing witness with a heart-to-heart connection via PR and compassionate engagement with right action biodynamically in order to truly serve the client and their wholeness. Rollin Becker, D.O., simply said to "Trust the Tide."

Based on the evolution of perception and understanding of a fluid body, it is simply a metaphor for a way (phenomenologically) that anyone can experience the totality of their own body that includes mind, spirit, emotions, consciousness, and perception. In this case, the totality is fluid or liquid in nature. Since we have very little knowledge of the human body from this perspective, the method of compassionate exploration of not knowing, bearing witness, and compassionate action is through the three-fold path of biodynamic wholeness:

- First, establish contact with the total surface or shape of our physical body. This includes a wide variety of body scan practices.
- Second, dedensify and soften the musculoskeletal system with a willingness to jump off the edge of the cell into the swimming pool of cytoplasm. This allows for the subtle perception of micromovement in the body, much like seaweed in the ocean undulating and moving in constant response to the ocean tides and currents. The experience of the seaweed and dedensification allows an investigation of sensation and fluid movement found in all of the teachings mentioned above. Fluids move constantly longitudinally along all membranes in the body. Fluids move perpendicular to all the membranes, and fluids can move through the membranes. These are the three basic aspects of fluid movement in the body as first described by Erich Blechschmidt mentioned at the beginning of this chapter.
- Third, the therapist contacts PR in his or her own bodily perception. PR moves through the body and intersects with three major embryological fulcrums of the third ventricle to the horizon, the heart to another heart in a connected field, and umbilicus to the earth or body of water. With these principles of movement, shape, and structure, it is possible to experience the human body in the way it is connected to nature and beyond. Fluid body perception involves a more thorough integration of the mind, body, and the natural world. Wholeness is the smallest subdivision of life as Jim Jealous said. It is the basis of the biodynamic therapeutic relationship and the biodynamic therapeutic process as I teach it.

It is important to reinforce the metaphor described above; the fluid body is simply the natural world in which everything is perceived as infinitely equal. We typically perceive the natural world as everything that is outside of us in nature, whether it's trees, the sky, the wind, the ocean, and the animal kingdom. But under the skin this natural world continues unabated. It is a world dominated by the elemental forces of air, heat, water, and tissue. It is alive and interacting not just at a metabolic level as described in cell biology, biological water, or protoplasm, but rather as an intelligence as old as the cosmos. Recent research has more than demonstrated that the human body contains the basic compounds from the periodic chart necessary for life, which astrogeophysicists have begun to find scattered throughout the cosmos. Indeed, those elements necessary for life scattered throughout the known universe live directly under our skin. That is the fluid body. It is home to the universe, all within us as the five elements described in Tibetan medicine.

The direction home is within the human body, and its fluid nature speaks a language that we can no longer hear in its continuity with the natural world. It is a forgotten language, and its voice is called Primary Respiration. The direction *in* is the direction *down* to the earth. In Taoism it is said that there is a midline going through us from the center of the earth to the north star in the constellation Ursa Major, the center of the universe. The earth is our home, where we are firmly planted with our feet on the ground and our spirit is connected to the origin of the universe. Welcome to your interconnected fluid body, your origin, you.

13

Principles of the Fluid Body

Buoyancy, Density, Dissipation, and Heat

BUOYANCY AND THE FLUID BODY

Now we have an opportunity to explore a metabolic sensibility, a lived experience of our organism, our soma as an aquarium with greater depth. Buoyancy is a basic principle of the fluid body. I frequently teach in Germany, and the translation of the word *buoyancy* creates challenges. This is because at one level of understanding buoyancy simply means to be able to float. To be able to float one needs to have what are called buoyancy organs. When I am swimming in the ocean and just rest and float, I must be very aware of my breathing, so when I fill my lungs with air, I remain buoyant on top of the surface of the water. The German translation also implies the activity of a buoy: a channel marker or a swimming area boundary marker. I remember as a merchant sailor in my twenties steering the ship through narrow channels in different river systems. The boat had to navigate inside a channel whose edges were marked by certain colored floating buoys. But the question is: How does a buoy just float?

The deeper meaning of buoyancy is related to the capacity of water to lift objects up based on their density and weight. A shark is heavy and will not float up to the surface of the ocean. Lift is a fundamental principle and activity of biological water. It acts as a counterforce to gravity. To have a felt sense of the body includes (but is not limited to) the sense of weightedness and earthiness provided by gravity and an equal and opposite effect of buoyancy that lifts the body internally, like a river flowing up the middle of the body and out the top of the head. During our prenatal development, we lived in an aquatic environment and, as an embryo, we were not subject to the forces of gravity as mentioned previously. We are conceived and develop floating in our buoyancy, our original felt sense of wholeness. My German students prefer to call it "flotility." The basic structure of the human body knows buoyancy and lift at the deepest level of the ocean. As we progress through fetal development and once we are born, the forces of gravity help further develop the musculoskeletal system and the whole body.

Sitting still and tuning into the aquarium of one's soma can be helpful in sensing buoyancy. Although the body is considered a tensegrity structure in which our upright posture is held together by a series of bones, tendons, and fascia, at the same time the water element of the body is constantly lifting us up like Old Faithful in Yellowstone National Park. Tensegrity is the earth element suspended in the water element. To experience a global sense of lift requires an intimate relationship with one's own fluid body. What is the starting point for that relationship?

I prefer to sit still and do a body scan in which I sense the totality of the surface of my skin from the bottom of my feet to the top of my head. Thus, the starting point is the shape of my body at the level of the skin. I must find the whole container, the boundaries of my aquarium. This is called Zone A—from the skin to the center of the aquarium.

DENSITY AND THE FLUID BODY

Density is another important principle. Density is related to weight. Depending on the weight and density of an object set into water, buoyancy becomes active. In other words, the water will start to lift the object depending on its size and heaviness. Of course, if the object is too heavy or too dense, such as a shark, it will sink. How can this principle apply to biodynamic practice? Once the therapist can sit and sense the surface shape of his or her body, they may then place their attention under the surface of the skin in order to sense the micromovement of the fluid body. Density is simply a matter in the human body of knowing where to place one's attention. In this case it is under the surface of the skin.

According to Erich Blechschmidt, biological water has three basic movements. The first movement is a longitudinal movement along a limiting membrane. Thus, the exclusion zone of water as named by Gerald Pollack has a movement associated with it. It is a micromovement, and the various metaphors of flow, streaming, currents, tidal movement, and waves are all accurate in terms of possible experience. These are not the only metaphors that apply to this movement. I like to suggest that students simply imagine that their skin is like seaweed, undulating in a very calm ocean. This movement is independent of the nervous system and one that Emily Conrad focused on in her work, called Continuum. Continuum work is not limited to the movement I am describing here, however.

Erich Blechschmidt also described a flow of water moving perpendicular to the limiting membrane. This type of movement is a sheering movement in which different gradients are moving laterally in the body. For example, one might feel the fluids of the pelvis shift to the right while the fluids in the abdomen shift to the left. But the most interesting movement to me is the third of Blechschmidt's so-called laws of fluids, in which water moves through and permeates every membrane in the body. This means that the water molecule, being the smallest molecule in the body, moves through every known structure, including the skin. This is a holistic movement involving a constant exchange of liquid and gaseous water through the skin in the area around the body.

To sense fluid density along different gradients as a biodynamic therapist means that a perception needs to be developed of the body being more transparent. In other words, muscles and bones need to be considered in their total fluid content that is permeating them without a boundary rather than their solidity. Likewise, all the organs of the body need to become transparent to the Tide of Primary Respiration. Yes, the element of wind also moves in the fluid body! The process of becoming transparent to the Tide leads to a greater ability to perceive the micromotion of the fluid body. It is the boundary of extrasensory perception and shamanic healing. Knowing anatomy and physiology must be discarded to have a direct experience of one's fluid body. As I enter my interiority below my skin, I gradually let go of what I know about bones and muscles and fascia and simply be with an originality of flow and movement. Buoyancy and density are polarities, sensory polarities. One is associated with gravity and the force of downwardness and earthiness. The other is a lift toward the sky or the heavens, according to Taoism. In this day and age of metabolic syndrome, especially with the prevalence of obesity for example, density is experienced as discomfort, full of emotional afflictions. With metabolic syndrome this polarity is out of balance. Lift and buoyancy as a natural organismic function of being human is lost and remedial methods such as weight loss programs, medications such as appetite suppressants, and recreational drugs are used to suppress the discomfort of being overly dense. Buoyancy becomes associated with relieving unhealthy emotions and lifting one's mental burden. In this way, the fluid body holds stress and the road to recover originality becomes an obstacle course for mystics.

DISSIPATION AND THE FLUID BODY

Dissipation is the next principle of biodynamic practice to explore. As therapists, we must consider our body to be first and foremost a fluid body, whether or not that involves the perception of the body being a majority of water or a near totality of water molecules or simply a living water balloon. Both before I contact a client and when I start a clinical session, I sit and sense my own fluid body, starting with the shape of my skin and the micromovement under the skin. I gradually wait until my attention drops down to the movement of my respiratory diaphragm and the movement of the heart that is attached to the diaphragm. I hold these two movements of the diaphragm and heartbeat to be one interconnected whole.

I ask my students to let go of the concept of respiratory diaphragm and its related function of breathing into simply being a wave that is self-generated in the middle of the body and moves in all directions from the bottom of the feet to the top of the head. This includes the movement of the heart, contributing its pulsatory and oscillating quality. After I do this, I wait for the Tide to start moving through the middle of my fluid body. I let my heart become transparent as it was in its initial development. As the Tide moves through my heart and cardiovascular system, from both the back and front of my body, the dynamic stillness in the room gradually but very clearly manifests. At some point, I will then place my hands on the client.

When I place my hands on the client, I immediately move my attention back to my own fluid body in order to sense the connection of the client's fluid body with mine. Any stress in the client's fluid body will naturally start to dissipate in and through my own fluid body. All I am required to do is sit in total attention to this process of dissipation and allow my fluid body to settle back into the exchange with Primary Respiration and the stillness. Each time I place my hands in a new location on the client, this is the initial perceptual process I follow.

Sometimes, because the nervous and vascular systems of the client and therapist are merging, I can feel tension in my respiratory diaphragm and more intensity in the movement of my heart. This is all very natural and the message here is to simply relax into that merged state of fluid body to fluid body, heart to heart, and brain to brain. It will settle as long as the therapist allows attention to be distributed throughout his or her entire fluid body. Once the process of dissipation has settled, several therapeutic processes may unfold. A deep stillness may be felt in the room, and at that point, the instruction is to connect the stillness with the literal movement of the heart in myself. This may be the holistic shift, or a Neutral, in which Primary Respiration switches to its repair function in the client's body. This can also be felt as an increase in the potency of Primary Respiration.

HEAT AND THE FLUID BODY

Now I want to mix a couple of metaphors in my explanation of heat. The fire element exists between the wind of Primary Respiration and the fluid body of water and earth. It is a type of friction, like rubbing two sticks together—one stick being space and wind, the other stick being water and earth. Heat is the most significant effect of a biodynamic session. It is an indication of a deep metabolic change occurring, not only within my body, but also the client. Thermal regulation is regulated via the heart-brain connection and the Triple Warmer meridian in acupuncture. Not only does the hypothalamus in the brain function in fight/flight, eating, and sexuality, but it also coregulates heat. Heat is also coregulated by the heart. The heart produces a lot of heat simply from its mechanical function, and it needs to be distributed and cooled by PR. At the same time, the principal fulcrums of the fire element are the superior mesenteric artery and liver in the Hara, the abdomen. This is the metabolic fire necessary for proper digestion and assimilation of food. The wind of PR moves the heat and distributes it properly unless there is a malfunction. Another way to look at heat is that it is also maintained by its friction with the fluid body. Since the biological water in a human body is saline by nature, it maintains and distributes heat through this connection to the sodium molecule. I saw a YouTube video of a physics experiment in which a tube of salt water was exposed to an electromagnetic field, and it burst into flames.

The heart as another fulcrum of the fire element has the strongest and biggest electromagnetic field in the body. It extends approximately fifteen feet around the body. According to the HeartMath Institute, the bioelectromagnetic field (ECM) shares information about the heart from inside the heart and pericardium to the outside of the soma through the fluid body. This would also increase heat in the therapeutic relationship as two heart fields become interconnected. How? Physical touch also generates heat via convection at the point of contact and a shared electrical conductivity between the therapist and the client. With this much heat in the body, then of course there would be constant evaporation occurring from the skin, which is accelerated by the two heat sources of the therapist's hands and the client's skin. In fact, three to seven liters of water can evaporate off the body per day.

This means that within the ECM we are also surrounded by a warm, wet, electrically charged cloud. Neurologically this is called the peripersonal space. The peripersonal space is a specific region surrounding the body by up to three feet. It is like a constantly moving, eccentrically shaped cloud. It is also Zone B extending from the center of the body out to the edge of the peripersonal space or the "biosphere" as Dr. Becker called it. It acts as an interface between the body and the environment for defensive and/or purposeful actions toward objects. It is a type of safety detector closer to the body, whereas the larger ECM is an emotional safety detector and field of empathy further away from the body. Neurologically it is thus an extension of the amygdala, the so-called fear detector center of the brain. But it is also an active metabolic zone filled with evaporated biological water, a microbiome sloughing off from the surface of the skin and the air being exhaled filled with different metabolites. It is charged with electricity and filled with infrared heat. It is also breathing with the Tide of PR.

Biodynamic practice is initially focused on the rehabilitation of the fluid body. This means integrating the fluid body between the soma, Zone A, and Zone B, the warm, wet cloud immediately around our body up to about twenty to thirty inches. In metabolic syndrome, the skin loses its ability to detoxify the body. It closes down like a window shutting, while the important metabolic passageways inside the body open up and become leaky. The detoxification pathway of the skin is a first order of business in biodynamic practice. One way to help integrate the fluid body that has closed its windows on the skin is to simply turn your hands palm up when in contact with a client. I like to imagine that my palms are simply holding a warm, wet cloud. Gradually, after sensing my own fluid body dissipation and settling, my attention will automatically be drawn back to both sides of my hands. Gradually, this warm, wet, charged cloud surrounding the client will come alive and breathe with PR and the window of the skin opens thus integrating Zone A with B as a single continuum. Then the deeper repair of the fluid body can take place.

Density, buoyancy, dissipation, and heat are the sensory experiences of a living body of fluid—an intelligence unto itself. Rather than initially focusing on the abstractions and concepts of anatomy and physiology, genetics, and metabolic regulation of the body, our own sensibility contacts the interior of our body in its simplest form, the elements of Eastern anatomy and physiology of a subtle body. This is our originality, our perpetual embryo that exists in and around us. It knows. And contact with such a sensibility is so close because it is never lost in its direct association with the Health. This is the starting point in biodynamic practice, the wholeness of the original fluid body before the possibility of lesioning. It builds a foundation for a bridge that can then be built to explore and influence the body's metabolism in both the therapist and contemporary client, which is suspended in the fluid body.

14
Visualizing the Fluid Body

The previous chapter gave us personal contact with the lived experience of being a fluid body and sensing the beauty of metabolism suspended in it. This is uncharted territory for many therapists and must be explored as slowly as possible to avoid creating side effects in the client, which include defensive physiology in the autonomic nervous system. The yellow warning flag is up on the lifeguard's chair indicating swim with caution. We must take the time to fully assess the basic core principles in our self gently with the grace and kindness of Primary Respiration and then explore them in our client. Maybe the lifeguard's chair has a red flag indicating stay out of the water. Once we have gained familiarity and recognized side effects bound by our own enthusiasm or boredom as the case may be, we can visit another layer of experience in the fluid body as follows in order to fully incorporate a metabolic sensibility. But we must wait for the portal to open and recognize that if we proceed, we must know, sense, and perceive when the fluid body and its wide variety of layers is reacting and contracting to our touch rather than opening and responding.

The following contemplations are based on the various practices of perceiving PR that I teach. This is a review of the more intricate practices in the approximate sequence that they are unfolded in class. They allow the therapist to deepen into the universal metabolism held by the original fluid body. The ground of perception in all of them is the ability of the therapist and client to sense and imagine her own fluid body three-dimensionally. As with all embodiment practices, the therapist is expected to move back and forth between visualizing the whole of the soma as a fluid body and then to very specific images of the parts of the soma and their fluid structure right down to the toes of the feet. All of these practices are done in the tempo and image (embryo) of PR. This blends the image with the sensation of three-dimensional shaping (or gesturing, as Jaap van der Wal calls it) and allows the therapist to reconnect with her original perfect and complete fluid body as it was in the embryo and remains today in her adult body. Consequently, when the therapist is with a client, she can then imagine holding the perfect fluid body of the client that still exists while being a fluid body herself. The perfect fluid body, the Tide breathing three-dimensionally with PR, is the preexisting condition of the body. It is the biodynamic Health and wholeness present in all people and clients.

The therapist, however, must first be able to orient to the perception of a still posture and a peaceful mind that extends to the horizon and back. Following that orientation to stillness, the therapist then senses the three-dimensional outline of the form of her soma at the surface level of the skin. An attempt is made to sense the entire surface volume of the skin or its image. Gradually, the therapist visualizes her form as a transparent three-dimensional fluid body that is made of clear living fluid from front to back, top to bottom, and side to side. It takes time to establish continuity and coherence for this three-dimensional sensibility and image, especially in terms of both the detail and the wholeness necessary to maintain an image of the total form of the fluid body.

This is followed by sensing the active shaping within the fluid body. Active shaping is three-dimensional movement from one of three basic embryological fulcrums: the third ventricle, the heart, or the umbilicus. The fluid body also demonstrates vectorial movement, vibratory movement, and midline movement (but those movements are not being discussed in this chapter). All of these processes are fundamental to the practice and experience of biodynamic practice, especially active shaping, which is three-dimensional. They are truly outside the domain of the central nervous system, yet they inform the nervous system, since these fluid body processes were present in the embryo before a nervous system was present.

THE THREE CAVITIES

The next exploration is to establish synchronization with either the inside or outside presence of PR or both together. Initially this is explored as a two-dimensional vector between the front of the body and the horizon. This is done by sensing the fulcrum of the therapist's attention automatically or purposefully shifting between the third ventricle, the heart, and umbilicus within the fluid body. The fulcrum is constantly shifting automatically, and within several moments a preferred fulcrum will manifest. It is also possible to deliberately shift one's attention as PR is sensed breathing back and forth from the horizon to each of these fulcrums in the fluid body individually and finally all together. The therapist will differentiate between automatic and purposeful shifting of perception.

These three fulcrums are then explored with various visualizations and contemplations. For example, with the heart fulcrum, a connection between the therapist's heart and the image of the heart of one's spiritual teacher or spiritual principle (such as nature) is sensed breathing back and forth at the rate of Primary Respiration, using the image of a spiritual blood transfusion. The therapist imagines that this is the felt sense of love moving back and forth from heart to heart. Then when the therapist engages in table work, the spiritual teacher is transformed into the client himself with the same heart-to-heart connection and flow of love. As is taught in Buddhism, everyone was our mother during the countless eons of life before this current one. Neurologically this practice develops empathy.

At the umbilical fulcrum a great deal of time is spent establishing the imagery of an umbilical cord connecting the therapist with her biological mother, and then to the earth or ocean, as a connection to the Great Mother. Then in the third phase of the umbilical practice, there is an umbilical connection to the Great Mother Goddess or the archetypal mother. I frequently give this practice to clients who have lost their mother. When someone's mother dies, the umbilical cord between mother and child dissolves, and some clients even report pain around their umbilicus or upper abdomen while the mother is in her dying process. This three-step umbilical meditation is especially valuable for a client who has lost their mother. When the biological mother is gone, the Great Mother of the planet earth takes over mothering as Erich Neumann says in his book *The Great Mother.* Finally, a relationship is formed with the divine feminine, such as Mary the mother of Jesus and a whole host of feminine deities found in many cultures. These are stages of establishing one's own relationship to the spiritual feminine. This is not exclusively for women but rather can also be given to male clients who have lost their mother.

Finally, with the last fulcrum, there is a connection between the third ventricle and the literal horizon of the planet related neurologically to the head-righting and orienting reflexes. The horizon is also the very edge of the visible world beyond which is a mystery. So the horizon can take on many meetings in a biodynamic session. These are important therapeutic practices for the therapist to establish synchronization with the outside to inside presence of PR based on the formation and creation of the early embryonic fulcrums in the fluid body from the first two weeks of development postfertilization. Specifically, they are the yolk sac (umbilicus), the amniotic sac (third ventricle), and the chorion (the heart and blood). They are used as client-therapist contemplations during a biodynamic session. A biodynamic session recapitulates the sequence of embryonic growth and development starting at the beginning (such as conception) in order to help the client rebuild his own creation story. This is called a return to origins. One of my doctoral program mentors, Dr. Jealous, conveyed to me clearly that contacting the perpetual embryo that lives inside every human being is vital to the biodynamic therapeutic process. This is because in accessing the embryo, we access our originality, which is our original wholeness at the moment of conception or in some cases the moment of the origin of the universe. Perception of PR and stillness, the very foundation of biodynamic practice and its essence, access this originality for healing.

Finally, I like to imagine a zipper from my forehead down to my pubic bone slowly opening all the way as it was when I was an embryo and my yolk sac was attached in that precise location. The contents of my body drift out from one or all of those fulcrums on the Tide of PR to the horizon of the natural world and return refreshed. We must sacrifice what we know about the human body because of the devastation caused by metabolic syndrome. We must be willing to expand our knowing of the body through these metaphors that I offer to the reader. Biodynamic practice is a spiritual practice. By the elements of wind, space, fire, water, and earth, we renew, revitalize, and restore the original wholeness of the human body.

VISUALIZING THE FLUID BODY

The Midline

The next two embryonic practices begin opening or deepening perception to a greater inside presence of Primary Respiration in the fluid body of the soma. The first of these practices is two-dimensional and has to do with sensing the lengthening and shortening of the notochordal midline in the spine. It is located in the very middle of the intervertebral discs of the adult spine from the coccyx up through the base of the sphenoid. It lengthens and shortens like an accordion opening and closing in the slow tempo of PR. If you have ever seen someone play an accordion, the musician appears to dance with it and move it like a snake with serpentine movement all the while lengthening and shortening the bellows of the accordion with his or her hands at either end of it. This is precisely the movement the notochord makes in the embryo. This happens in the third week of development and follows the sequence begun in the previous chapter with the three fluid fulcrums from the first two weeks postfertilization. The therapist imagines that her spine is made of seaweed, and it causes the whole spine to sway and dance like a snake.

The second practice is more three-dimensional and involves learning to sense the whole spine folding (flexion) and unfolding (extension) very subtly around the fulcrum of the embryonic heart within the tempo of PR. Folding–unfolding, expanding–contracting, and bowing–lifting the head up are some of the basic rhythms of growth and development. I ask students to bring a big beach ball or Physioball (which most everyone seems to have in their home or office these days) and put it on their lap while sitting for this practice.

The ball should reach the clavicles to be effective for this movement perception. This is proportionally the size of the embryonic heart as it extended way out in front of the body of the embryo before there was a rib cage. This folding and unfolding process represents the fourth stage of dynamic morphology in the embryo that takes place during the last several weeks (fourth through eighth) of our initial embryonic existence. Now the embryonic heart is actually suspended from the face of the embryo and its neck. This is its original position. Only gradually through the process of folding and unfolding does it grow down into the chest cavity. Consequently, the platform of the cranial base (basisphenoid, basiocciput, and petrous temporal bones) is one of the last osseous structures to form in the embryo, at which point an embryo can unfold and lift its head up, form a cervical curve, and develop clavicles. This area becomes the focus of the movement perception and is very healing for many therapists when practiced slowly.

With or without a ball on one's lap, simply bowing the head and slightly rolling forward with the forehead going toward the knee for about a minute and then reversing and slowly coming back to an erect posture with the ears over the shoulders and the eyes looking at the horizon is enough. Remember that from the third ventricle, perception can go to the horizon also in the tempo of PR. However, the therapist is mimicking the folding and unfolding on the last stage of dynamic morphology of growth and development in the human embryo. Even the simplest, slightest bow of the head signals a deep spiritual process involving humility and not knowing but rather an opportunity to bear witness to the Health and healing available through the relationship of PR with the dynamic stillness.

VISUALIZING THE FLUID BODY

The Gut Tube

Following are two important contemplations, the first of which is sensing Primary Respiration in the endoderm gut tube. These practices are usually done in side-lying (or fetal) position, which makes them easy to practice in bed. To start, the therapist imagines a straight tube from the mouth to the anus. Then the therapist senses PR moving like a tide coming up from the anus and out the mouth. Then PR reverses direction and comes in through the mouth and out the anus. PR represents the wind element in Tibetan medicine and is the cause of all movement in the human body. At the same time PR is moving through the fluid body as it exists in the gut tube. Physiologically the contents of the gut tube can move in both directions (through the processes of peristalsis and reverse peristalsis). Here the sense is that an etheric stream of fluidlike wind is coming in and going out of the gut tube unabated.

Secondly, the therapist imagines that the middle of the tube is open to a huge pouch in front of the belly called the yolk sac. PR has a dimension where it is coming in from both the anus and mouth and flowing into the yolk sac. The therapist is encouraged to imagine completely opening her belly as if there is an attached sac extended five or more feet in front of her. Prior to the heart extending out in front of the embryo's anterior body wall, the yolk sac extends even further out of the body wall for a longer period of development before receding late in the third trimester of pregnancy.

Then PR reverses direction and flows from the yolk sac into the belly and out toward the mouth and anus. This practice can be provocative for therapists holding issues in their gut such as obesity or being overweight.

The gut tube is divided into three sections embryonically: The foregut with its associated structures in the embryo, especially the pharynx down to and including the stomach, gallbladder, and liver. The midgut is the second part associated with the small and large intestines. Here, the intestines orient their growth to the superior mesenteric artery, which grows from the posterior abdominal cavity (peritoneal coelomic sac). The superior mesenteric artery will be the principal blood supply for the intestines once they get connected. Initially, the intestines then grow out of the belly, since there is not a lot of room for them inside the embryo. Consequently, they grow into the yolk sac, and while growing out of the body wall and retracting back in later, they rotate 180 degrees around the superior mesenteric artery. This is a horizontal growth orientation from posterior to anterior, from inside to out toward the yolk sac.

The umbilical cord is also present and adjacent to the growth vector of the mesenteric artery. It has a few other vascular tubes in it. Alongside the vitelline arteries and veins, which bring blood from the yolk sac outside the body wall into the embryonic heart, are the umbilical artery and vein coming from the placenta. A lot of vascular action comes in and out of the umbilicus.

Finally, the third part of the gut tube is called the hind gut, and its triple orientation is to the inferior mesenteric artery, yolk sac, and allantois. The allantois is the future bladder and protrudes into the connecting stalk and acts as a guide for the umbilical veins and arteries. Consequently, there is also a growth orientation of the pelvic floor and pelvic organs to the cardiovascular system.

PR can be sensed in multiple directions through the gut tube starting between the mouth and anus and then orienting to flowing in and out of the umbilicus. This is a practice of making friends with one's intestines and pelvic floor. A lot of history unfolds in the abdomen and pelvis regarding Health, well-being, and trauma. Sometimes it is more helpful to learn how to breathe into the abdomen to begin softening and relaxing both the abdomen and pelvis. PR is very friendly and will help you not only digest your food but also become friends with your belly and your pelvis.

VISUALIZING THE FLUID BODY
The Sea Sponge

Now a practice is taught to allow the gut tube and the entire contents of the soma to become more related to its evolutionary nature arising in the prehistoric oceans five to seven hundred million years ago. I know that many people—such as those who nearly drowned as a child—have issues with water. If this is the case, the following practice should not be attempted. If you do attempt it and become uncomfortable, please stop and move on to something different.

First the therapist imagines that her soma is attached to the very bottom of the ocean as if growing from a bed of coral. This is done by imagining that the soma itself is a tubular sea sponge submerged under the ocean. The soma is nothing but a shell of thick, porous skin like a sponge. Each of the extremities is considered in the same way as an interconnected series of ocean-filled tubular sea sponges continuous with the big, empty (of a center) sponge in the middle representing the four main cavities of the soma: cranial, thoracic, abdominal, and pelvic. Then the core or center of the soma is visualized as filled with living ocean fluid.

A flow of this living oceanic water is sensed coming in through the pelvic floor up and out the top of the head as a current or a spiral moving at the rate of Primary Respiration. The hands, feet, pelvic floor, and top of the head are wide open to the ocean ebbing and flowing in and out of those openings at the tempo of Primary Respiration. These are particularly good images to use for specific bodily symptoms. One can visualize a part of the body that is in pain and then have it be empty of any structure. With the help of PR moving the ocean in and out of a porous open sea sponge, the soma reverts to its original nature of being created anew out of the ocean.

VISUALIZING THE FLUID BODY

The Heart Spiral

The following practice—called *the heart spiral*—has several phases, which follow the sequential development of the blood and then the heart. Each phase is considered a standalone practice. I recommend looking at the images of the embryo provided in the color insert and in chapter 12 for helpful visuals and to play with each phase before moving on to the next. This is about you the reader finding your own embryo.

The first phase is visualizing the therapist surrounded by their own chorionic cavity. It is also a metaphor for Zone B as previously discussed. It is a transparent bubble extending about five feet from the body. This is where the first organ of blood is made outside the body in the second week of development. It flows and streams all around the embryo, feeding it through diffusion prior to a definitive umbilical cord. And the blood contains connective tissue cells to build the connecting stalk and future umbilical cord. Now imagine that this early, colorless blood surrounds the entire surface of the skin. It then organizes itself in a spiral current along the contoured surface of the skin. Take a few moments to sense the curvature of the body and its contours with a flow of blood curling around every inch of the body's surface and moving toward the heart and away from the heart. At the same time there is a spiral in the core of the fluid body from the floor of the pelvis to the top of the head called the longitudinal fluctuation. One spiral is on the outside surface of the skin and the other in the middle of the body. All flow reverses direction every fifty seconds in the tempo of Primary Respiration.

The heart spiral is associated with the circulation of embryonic blood in the peripheral body (inner surface of the chorionic cavity up against the placenta or outer surface). Then the establishment of a heart tube spirals into existence in the center of the embryo at the beginning of the third week of development. How does the embryo's blood get from outside of its body to the inside developing heart tube? Begin with perceiving the outside presence of PR from the horizon and back. Then the therapist imagines that her office is a chorionic cavity with colorless blood circulating at the rate of PR all over the walls, floor, and ceiling. Then the blood is flowing toward her soma from all directions and covering the outside of her soma as it does in the embryo. The fulcrum of observation in the therapist is her heart. This is where the blood is going and needs to find a way to get there. I simply sense my heartbeat simultaneously with the visualization. Here the breathing heart is filled with blood extending out to the walls of the therapist's office. Sometimes the spiral simply becomes a pulsation or a flow. The spiral has many possibilities experientially. This phase of sensing vascular function may be enough without proceeding to the following practices.

The practice may then move to sensing the blood underneath the surface of the skin in the capillary beds. Sense the pulsation and potency of the capillaries. Then imagine the whole musculoskeletal system and all the viscera as being made of a spongy material filled with blood, all spiraling and lengthening up toward the heart, neck, face, and head. The sponge is breathing and pulsing in its potency, its vitality. Again, perhaps it is enough to simply sense the pulsation of the heart and blood expanding over a larger area in one's body. Then it reverses direction and spirals down toward the pelvic floor and extremities. The soma of the therapist, like the embryo, is in the middle of the chorionic cavity. It is covered with embryonic blood on its inner surface, facing the embryo and moving at the rate of PR. Thus, the density of the blood is spiraling both around the perimeter of the chorionic fluid body and in the core of the fluid because now, in the latter part of the second week postfertilization, the connecting stalk is rooted with the placenta and has shifted from the dorsal surface of the embryo (ectoderm) to the sacral-caudal end of the embryo. Fluid pressure increases in the embryo from caudal to cranial, which initiates the axial midline discussed above. This midline is a major current of force and potency in the amnionic cavity.

Consequently, this pressure in the embryo causes the space between the ectoderm and endoderm to pull apart and form a primitive streak–notochordal canal (midline axial symmetry) and invite what Blechschmidt called a canalization zone to form laterally from this arising midline in the shape of a horseshoe. This horseshoe part of the fluid body carries cells from the banks of the primitive streak of the future heart about to be constructed in the top of the horseshoe. The felt sense of this simultaneous inside and outside spiral is like that of a very subtle tissue unwinding, because it feels like the skin is involved in the spiral as part of the larger fluid body.

Now in this phase the focus of the heart spiral is for the therapist to sense the strong spiral current of fluid coming up from the pelvic floor throughout the entire core of the fluid body. It may be enough to just place one's attention in the lower abdomen and pelvis and sense the breath moving in and out of the lower abdomen. Next comes the sense of the organization of the tubular heart in the chest cavity as the sides of the horseshoe merge together into a single tube with a loop on top for the brain to rest upon. This loop or top of the horseshoe includes the aortic sac, arch arteries, formerly the cardinal veins and arteries into the top of the neural tube. It looks and acts as a bridle. The rider on the horse is the heart and the bridle goes around the horse's head (top of the neural tube—third ventricle) to restrain it from moving too fast or to cause it to change directions. The heart grows slow, the brain grows fast. It is one spiral from the floor of the pelvis to the top of the head, from the back of the body including the spine to the anterior surface of the body. Since the form of body constantly changes, the spiral manifests as different sensations depending on which part of the body comes into sensory focus. Thus, the spiral is a broad category of possible sensory experiences. The heart and its bridle are in the middle of the spiral. The therapist may sense bulging, rotation, elongation, shortening, twisting, and side bending between the lungs, on the right side of the lungs, in the neck, and all the way to the top of the head. And the spiral just keeps lengthening and shortening at the tempo of Primary Respiration all around and through the activity of the heart tube. The best image I know of is that of a Hawaiian hula dance. Every part of the soma is moving in a circle on the outside, which causes the sensation of a spiral on the inside from bottom to top.

Originally the heart was higher up in the neck all in front of the pharynx with its original fulcrum at C3. This is where the heart tube and spiral was located in the embryo with the original fulcrum of the heart being located where the primitive node was located. It is now called the cardio-cranio-facial module in embryology. Imagine the pericardial sac hanging from the third cervical vertebra, holding the heart and resting on the respiratory diaphragm. Sensing the breath is a critical part of the spiral, and it is from the breath that the spiral gathers some of its potency. The adult heart also moves in a spiral within the pericardial sac, and focusing on this area is a shortcut I use while treating clients as I sense my heart spiraling and unspiraling in the tempo of PR. There are many images on the internet showing the spiral arrangement of the muscle fibers of the heart. When the left ventricle squeezes the blood into the aorta the muscular contraction is a spiral like wringing the water out of clothes that have just been washed. Developmentally, the heart tube comes together in the middle and is initially a loosely connected cluster of cells, then an elongated tube, then it appears as having an S-shaped curve, and finally in the fourth phase of heart development the heart turns itself downside up as the atria are at the bottom of the tube and need to get into proper position. These four phases of heart development are usually where a large amount of sensation manifests in the heart spiral when staying in the tempo of PR. In our adult body, these phases may consume the entire space of the trunk, neck, face, and head as a perception of a spiral with bending, looping, folding, and unfolding sensed in the trunk and torsioning and side bending in the neck and head.

Feelings and emotions in the therapist tend to greatly expand the heart tube. This frequently feels like a stronger heartbeat or more potency expanding across the front of the chest. The front of the heart is like a balloon whereas the back of the heart is more fixed and stationary. Its natural movement is in direct relationship with its embryonic growth, which is in direct relationship with the mother's heart. The human heart is always in relationship with the hearts around it. These are subtle movements that are associated with the fluid body containing a heart shaping itself as a growth process rather than an unwinding process in the tissues. It is through the perception of PR that these distinctions can be made therapeutically in oneself and in others. Such perception increases empathy and compassion.

The next phase of the heart spiral has to do with the therapist's contact with the client. The initial contact with the hands and arms is visualized as a connecting stalk from week two of development and then an umbilical cord from weeks three forward in the pregnancy until the cord is cut after birth. The therapeutic relationship involves the metaphor of an embryonic circulatory system (see figs. 14.1A–B). For the convenience of the reader, the therapeutic relationship is divided into four zones of awareness—A, B, C, and D as shown. The heart and cardiovascular system of the therapist will always respond when in proximity to a client or anyone else, for that matter, who is in a relationship with the therapist. This is called an interpersonal cardiovascular system. Once the preliminary practices of reorienting to stillness and synchronizing with

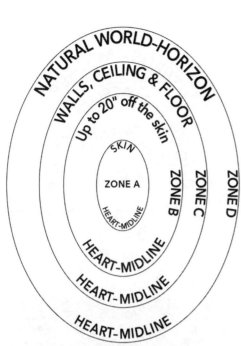

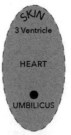

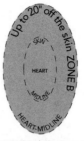

Zone A

Zone B includes Zone A

The three horizontal original fulcrums initiating perception of Primary Respiration and stillness.

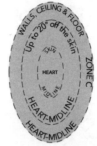

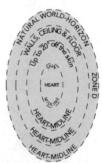

Zone C includes Zones A & B

Zone D includes Zones A, B & C

Zones are boundaries of awareness that gradually disappear leaving a single continuum of perception in the therapeutic relationship. Practioner suspends attention between the zones sensing the rhythmic balanced interchange of Primary Respiration and stillness. The heart-midline as used here represents a fulcrum of this interchange.

Dashed lines indicate permeable boundaries. The Zones are one integrated continuum that contain the biodynamic therapeutic relationship for transformation.

Conceptus

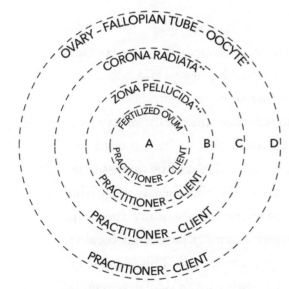

The therapeutic relationship is a two-person biology based on pre- and perinatal metabolism. The practitioner and client rhythmically exchange places among the zones during the course of a session.

*OOCYTE: Unfertilized ovum
**CORONA RADIATA: Nutrition/waste removal cells surrounding ovum
***ZONA PELLUCIDA: Shell around ovum that cracks open for implantation

The Embryo

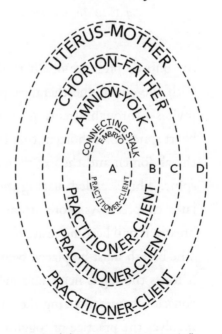

Any metabolism in one zone can automatically exchange function with another zone between the practitioner and client. The therapeutic relationship is in constant flux.

Fig. 14.1A. The therapeutic relationship: metaphors, definitions, and zones of awareness

Epigenesis

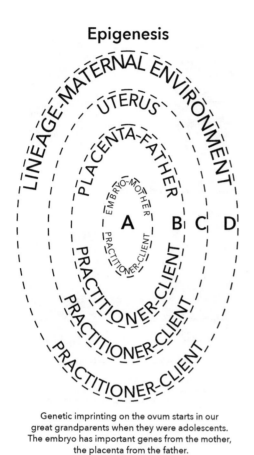

Genetic imprinting on the ovum starts in our
great grandparents when they were adolescents.
The embryo has important genes from the mother,
the placenta from the father.

The Fetus

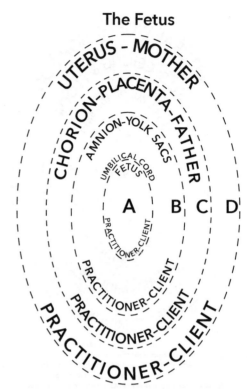

Focus on the movement of the heart in one's body, because the
therapeutic relationship is an interpersonal cardiovascular system
The therapeutic relationship depends on the practitioner's perception
and attention being evenly suspended in all the zones.

Fig. 14.1B. The therapeutic relationship: metaphors of epigenesis and the fetus

the outside presence of PR in the therapist are reestablished following contact with the client, the therapist places her attention in her own fluid body. She invites—through attention in her core and on her skin—the perception of the heart spiral. One shortcut that I like to use is to sense how the inhalation expands the abdomen and the exhalation causes the abdomen to relax back toward the spine. This is called placing the mind in the Hara, which will be discussed in later chapters. As more attention is established in the abdomen through the breath, it will become easier to sense the spiral of the fluid body in any direction. The breath must be placed below the heart, which is correct physiology because it tones the vagus nerve and moves the lymph properly as well. This is a way of consciously metabolizing the client's stress load in their cardiovascular system. It involves the practice of toggling back and forth with my attention between my fluid body and that of the client inside the perception of the Tide of PR. "Trust the Tide," as Dr. Becker would say.

This joint practice allows the client to circulate freely into the therapist's yielding and receptive heart and blood. In his book of the same name, Thich Nhat Hanh calls it the practice of "Interbeing." This is a much easier biodynamic method for relating with shock and trauma in the client without overstimulating the autonomic nervous system of the client. Through the cardiovascular resonance with the client, the therapist naturally absorbs and metabolizes stress and trauma held in the cardiovascular system layer of the fluid body. This is all done by focusing on the heart spiral in the therapist from the macroview of the whole soma and its core fluid body to the actual or literal heart spiral itself within the pericardial cavity. Consequently, in the first ten to fifteen minutes of physical contact with the client, the heart spiral in the therapist can go through all sorts of interesting shaping processes associated with the basic movements of the tube bending, rotating, elongating, shortening, twisting, and being turned downside-up. This includes the carotid arteries, Circle of Willis in the brain, and vertebral arteries all responding to the spiral. Head turning is also directly linked to heart development.

Another image I like to evoke in the heart spiral is a flame of heat moving through the blood coming from the extremities *in* and from the abdomen of the body *up* and permeating the whole soma and fluid body. The perception of heat is crucial. The therapist scans their body and senses differences in heat versus cool and any variety of temperature variations from the surface of the skin that is covered with clothing to that which is exposed, such as the arms and hands. By focusing on the sense of heat, the fire element in the body is perceived and in conjunction with the spiral may rehabilitate metabolic challenges, especially if there is too much inflammation in the body. The heat needs to be distributed properly in the core of the body and in the sleeve of the musculoskeletal system. There are two different but interrelated thermal systems in the body, which are spoken of at length in classical Chinese medicine, especially the Triple Warmer meridian. However, it is the venous system of the body that forms an interface between the two thermal regulatory systems in the body. The veins are like a car's radiator and when the body heats up the veins dissipate the heat and those on the sleeve of the body move closer to the surface to discharge excess heat from the core.

It is the responsibility of the heart to warm the blood and, of course, the blood coming from the periphery of the embryonic body has already been warmed by contact with the uterine wall. So the warmed blood is associated with a spiraling flame, a central spiral in the fluid body during the second week of development. This becomes joined on the inside of the embryo with the primitive streak at the beginning of the third week. From the primitive streak future blood cells differentiate and move in between the layers of the ectoderm and endoderm to create the mesoderm. Mesodermal cells move outward to the periphery of the embryo to connect with the blood cells already circulating on the outside of the amnion and yolk sac. The more lateral mesodermal cells encounter the canalization zone or current that when mixed together now become the cardiac fields and future heart tube. All this shaping and connecting is directed by the core spiral in the fluid body.

The primitive streak itself is made up of the future cells that will become the primordium of the various chambers of the heart. But before they do that, they must be moved into place by the central spiral in the fluid body moving at the rate of PR. It is PR in conjunction with the natural tensile strength, the reciprocal tension potency, and the aliveness of the fluid body to move in a spiral shape that creates the heart by directing future heart cells into the horseshoe-shaped canalization zone that will become tubes and join together in their dance of becoming heart.

In review, the therapist contemplates these three stages of the heart spiral:

1. The peripheral movement of the current of PR, such as the embryonic blood in the second week of development moving over the skin of the therapist and causing a spiral or undulation in the skin to subtly occur.
2. The joining of the peripheral blood spiraling on the outside surface of the skin with the central spiral current of the fluid body going from the coccyx to the third ventricle.
3. The central spiral being filled with a flame-like heat that causes the various movements of the heart to shape and form in response to the metabolic dynamics of the therapeutic relationship, such as conduction and convection of heat. This activity is sensed in the whole inside of the trunk, neck, face, and head. It is frequently experienced as beads of sweat trickling down the spine of the therapist.

This chapter is a biodynamic buffet based on the lived experience of a constantly moving and pressurized fluid body that continues to support differentiation from conception through the life span. The practices covered are listed on the next page from the simplest to the more complex.

1. Attunement
2. Form
3. Shaping
4. Three shifting fulcrums
5. Three mothers
6. Structural midline
7. Flexion–extension of the whole
8. Gut tube in three parts
9. Sea sponge
10. Heart Spiral

Some of these practices the client and therapist will find valuable, but it is not my intention to have you master all of these possibilities. It is my intention that you find your embryo and perhaps one or more of these contemplations will lead you to find the pre-existing flow of grace and love in your body. In the next chapter, I will continue the exploration of our perpetual embryo in terms of specific gradients of biodynamic and biokinetic processes still very much alive in our body. The perpetual embryo is the infinite embryo.

15

Embryology of Growth Resistance

My favorite embryology professor, Jaap van der Wal from the University of Maastricht, made a profound statement in class one day. He said there is "no growth without resistance" in the human embryo. Whether you gestate in a womb, in an egg, or as larvae on the surface of a scum pond, the growth of the whole and the development of the parts in living organisms requires resistance from inside and outside. The whole organism facing outside expands, while the parts inside differentiate at different rates and tensions depending on their position in an eccentrically shaped organism. Within moments of conception all organisms form an inner boundary layer and an outer boundary layer of tissue in contact with the environment. To take the *form* of a human we must first build our body with *two layers* of tissue: a surface layer facing out and an inner layer facing in.

The entire organism is always expressing connection and expansion as the outside layer receives nutrient first before passing it through the inner layer. The organism must meet forms of resistance based on tensions and flow dynamics from the outside environment. Likewise, the organism must meet the constantly changing and growing inner terrain. The constant changing of the inner terrain of organs, membranes, and blood vessels depends on their respective positions in the embryo. Think of this as a geography lesson. Each organ has its own unique shape, and its structure has its own unique rate of metabolism. Position, shape, and structuring of the inside terrain is called biokinetics. Biodynamics and biokinetics constantly express both purposeful and eccentric movement with multiple tempos.

ENCAPTIC GROWTH

Encaptic growth is a principle in which this basic bilaminar structure, the boundary between inner and outer, progressively builds and multiplies many bilayers of complexity over the life span. A good example are the coelomic sacs. At about four weeks postfertilization, a sac forms to hold the future inner organs of the body. This sac differentiates into three compartments: the pleura, the pericardium, and the peritoneum. Each of these three sacs also has two layers, one to manage the metabolism of the inside organs and one to manage the metabolism with the outside consisting of the musculoskeletal system and the head and neck. The fascial system of the body is another perfect example of this encaptic bilayering principle. The outer layer grows faster because it has access to more nutrition. Already there is resistance in any of the bilayered membranes because of the nutrition differential. This means that sometimes for proper growth the two layers pull apart from different tensions. Even in the pulling apart cells are ripped and torn, spilling their contents in the milieu providing more nutrition. From the microcosm to the macrocosm there is always this yin and yang, a polarity, a polarization, an organic differentiation on a broad spectrum and hierarchy of boundary formation and being fed.

THE FULCRUM

This bilaminar boundary, however, is always automatically *shifting its fulcrum,* its point of organization within the whole. This is an important principle of biodynamic and biokinetic differentiations. Thus, the tempo of growth and development is always changing just like the speed limit on a two-lane road and the switchbacks going up and down a mountain pass. And when we are driving on a superhighway, some of us are always changing lanes to go around slow traffic. The embryo is a master of changing lanes to support optimum growth and development. A good example in the embryo is how fast the brain is growing and how slow the heart is growing. What makes the shifting fulcrum interesting is that it is identified and perceived by its intrinsic stillness. There is always a point or state of balanced tension. There is a tension field between the brain and heart in the embryo that is dynamically still. This means that all movement is organized around a fulcrum of stillness and thus making stillness a vital component of growth and development. This biological principle is accurate all the way down to molecular transformations and all the way up to spiritual practice.

THE DOUBLE BIND

Professor van der Wal also said that anything that begins in the *metabolism* of the human embryo becomes *physiological* shortly before and after birth. Finally, he said that this evolution of form and function that starts metabolically becomes *psychospiritual* in the postnatal and subsequent stages of life. Thus, we see the origin of the psychological term *double bind*. The double bind is an intolerable tension between two dynamic forces emotionally and spiritually. If we look at the original principles of growth and development morphologically, we see that one of those emotional forces (originally membrane) will be relatively fixed, and the other emotional force (originally membrane) will have a degree of flexibility. But this fulcrum of the metabolic/psychological organization is also shifting its fulcrum moment to moment with different thoughts, sensations, perceptions, and conceptualizations. Concepts are stories rooted in strong beliefs mentally and emotionally. It is the *conceptual level* of the double bind that makes it feel like it is set in stone; a rigid, life-threatening, catastrophic pulling apart—a dismemberment. Each layer of the double bind needs to be examined mentally and physically. The brain processes quickly and the rest of the body processes more slowly, just like the growth differential of the heart and brain mentioned earlier.

Encaptic growth will also cause the psychospiritual double bind to intensify because, as we age, we are given more complex situations to integrate psychospiritually. We are all facing our death. In the embryo, local movement activity along the borders is described as a metabolic field. It is a field or an area of purposeful directional biokinetic movement. It is quite active with two basic types of growth movement. One is a pulling apart, and the other is compression. In the embryo, such compression causes the boundaries to dissolve and the compressed cells to die, which leads to a perforation such as the constant remodeling that the vascular system must do to keep up with all the growth. Blood supply is built one day and disintegrated the next day as the embryo evolves its structure through numerous phases in each part of our growing body. For example, the heart goes through four phases of development, each requiring a different blood supply. The gut does not get a full blood supply until after birth.

GROWTH BY PULLING APART

Growth by pulling apart the two layers can happen in different directions such as shearing, torsioning, and side-bending—cells are frequently ripped and torn apart. The embryo is constantly being pulled in different directions as we also find ourselves throughout life after birth. The contents of the cells are recycled or used as nutrient locally like the way the embryo implants on the uterine wall and secretes an enzyme that kills the cells of the uterus (see the color insert).

THE FLUID BODY OF THE EMBRYO

Art by Friedrich Wolf

The newness of the spiritual life, its autonomy, could find no better expression than the images of an "absolute beginning," images whose structure is anthropocosmic, deriving at once from embryology and from cosmogony.

MIRCEA ELIADE, *RITES AND SYMBOLS OF INITIATION: THE MYSTERIES OF BIRTH AND REBIRTH*

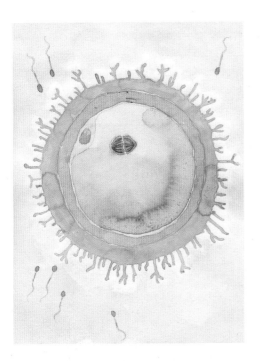

Plate 1. *The embryo is a fluid being. She is a fluid body. The sperm is attracted by the egg. The inner mantel in light blue is the zona pellucida, a hard shell protecting the egg in her perfect roundness. The green outer mantel is the corona radiata, which provides nutrition to the egg and removes waste products through microvilli extending from inside the egg to the corona radiata. Anabolism and catabolism is present from fertilization.*

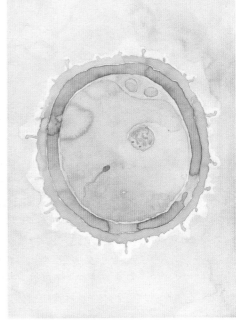

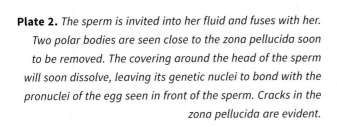

Plate 2. *The sperm is invited into her fluid and fuses with her. Two polar bodies are seen close to the zona pellucida soon to be removed. The covering around the head of the sperm will soon dissolve, leaving its genetic nuclei to bond with the pronuclei of the egg seen in front of the sperm. Cracks in the zona pellucida are evident.*

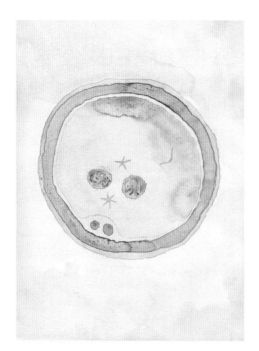

Plate 3. *The pronuclei (genes) of the sperm approach the genes of the egg.*

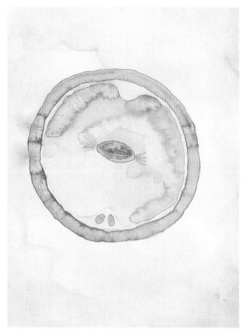

Plate 4. *A human being is conceived. The human body is now a whole single-cell fluid body. The morphology and shape of the human being at this stage is different than all other mammals. Vigorous metabolic activity is taking place directed by the blueprint of wholeness in the fluid body.*

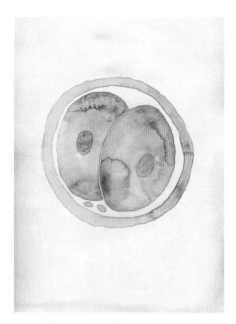

Plate 5. *The first cell division into two. Each cell (blastomere) is capable of becoming a full human being when raised separately. The further development of each cell depends entirely on its future position in the embryo. Each blastomere carries its own unique genetic signature for health and disease.*

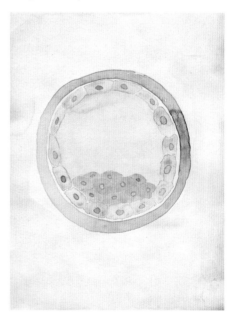

Plate 6. *The end of the first week of morphology. After a week of compression, the first division into two different types of cells. A cluster of cells called the embryoblast that will become the body and encircling the embryoblast is the trophoblast, the beginning of the placenta. The zona pellucida still covers the embryo prior to implantation in the endometrium of the maternal uterus.*

Plate 7. *A human being is liberated out of its shell at the beginning of the second week. The embryo "hatches" and is ready to implant in the uterus.*

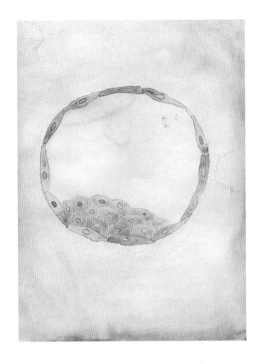

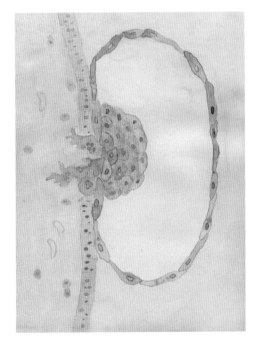

Plate 8. *The embryo negotiates contact with the uterine wall. The embryo secretes enzymes that break down the endometrial cells in order to take in the nutrition from their cytoplasm.*

Plate 9. *The embryo grows rapidly into the uterine wall. The embryoblast differentiates into a layer of cells here, colored green. It is the future gastrointestinal system (endoderm) surrounded by a yolk sac of fluid. Adhering to the endoderm is the newly formed ectoderm, the future nervous system. The amniotic sac can be seen. The dorsal surface of the ectoderm is attached to the rapidly expanding trophoblast. This is the next phase of placentation. The embryo now has grown from a single fluid pocket to a double fluid being (yolk sac and amniotic sac).*

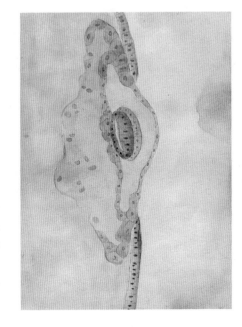

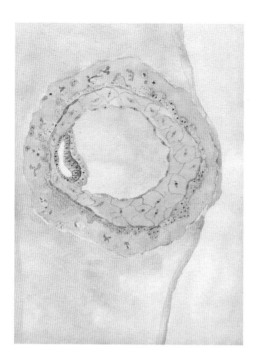

Plate 10. Two fluid cavities are well defined in and around the future visceral system and brain. Still lagoons (lacunae) of fluid form in the placenta, which, because of their stillness, invite maternal blood vessels to connect with the placenta for nourishing the embryo. The green colored network is the extraembryonic mesoderm, the beginning of blood formation containing connective tissue to help build a connecting stalk and umbilical cord for the embryo to secure its connection to the placenta in between the ectoderm and placenta as shown.

Plate 11. A third cavity forms so the inner embryo can be connected to its peripheral body. It is the large chorionic cavity as the green yolk sac becomes well defined. The three cavities of amnion, yolk (umbilical vesicle), and chorion are now present in their anabolic and catabolic metabolic function, especially as acting as a septic system for waste products. Nutrition delivery is still by diffusion into the ectoderm and endoderm.

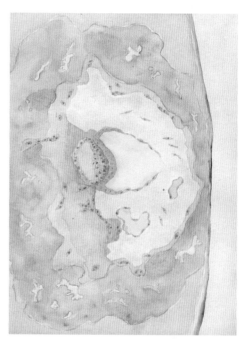

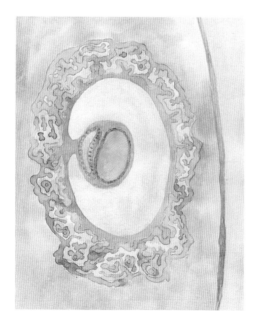

Plate 12. The three cavities become a differentiated fluid body. The back side of the embryo is rooted into the periphery. The embryo has a greater chance of survivability now. The connecting stalk then becomes a template for the umbilical cord. Notice the initial placenta surrounds the embryo. Nutrients flow along the yellow borders.

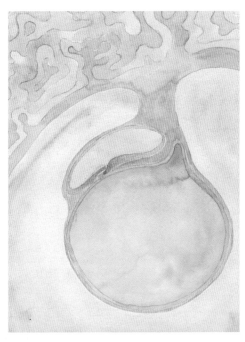

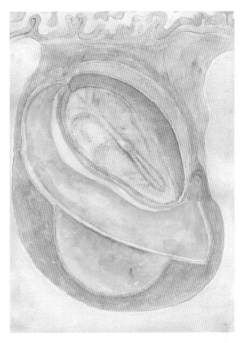

Plate 13. *The embryo rotates and becomes grounded at its caudal/sacral end. A bulge in the yolk sac extending into the connecting stalk called the allantois is shown. It will become the bladder much later in development.*

Plate 14. *The amniotic sac is opened to show the arising of a fluid midline called the primitive streak. The beginning of axial symmetry is shown. The primitive streak forms from pressure in the fluid body of the amnion. From the edge of the primitive streak, heart cells will differentiate to become the heart.*

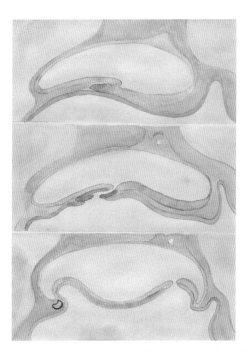

Plate 15. *The median plane of the embryo shows the development of the notochord as a folding under at the end of the primitive streak, then a canal, and, in the bottom image, the primitive heart is seen.*

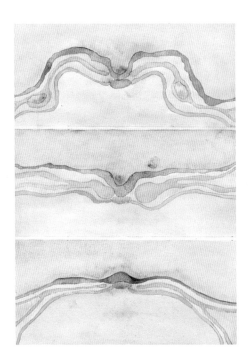

Plate 16. *A transverse plane through the future shoulders. Now three layers can be seen. A middle layer (mesoderm) arises from the perforation caused by the primitive streak pulling apart the endoderm and ectoderm. Heart cells can flow toward the apex or cranial end of the embryo. In blue can be seen the gradual closing of the neural tube from the floor of the ectoderm. Pockets of cardiac cells can be seen in the yellow mesoderm.*

Plate 17. *A transverse plane through the base of the head showing the neural tube cresting and finally closing. The top image shows the tip of the notochord as a circle of cells. All three images show clusters of cardiac cells in the early plexiform phase of heart development.*

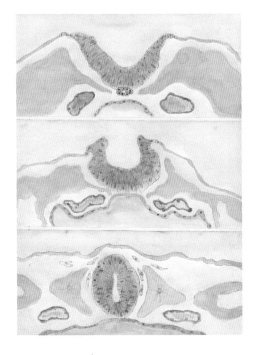

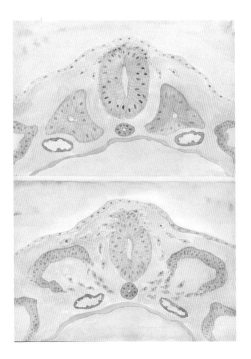

Plate 18. *The neural crest sprouts the future cranial nerves, especially the vagus nerve. Shown here are neural crest cells moving toward the heart tubes lateral of the tip of the notochord. This differentiation is occurring down the whole length of the neural tube. Neural crest cells move through the mesoderm toward the endoderm to facilitate the growth of the enteric nervous system and dorsal vagus in the gut. Growth is now oriented to the stillness of the notochord.*

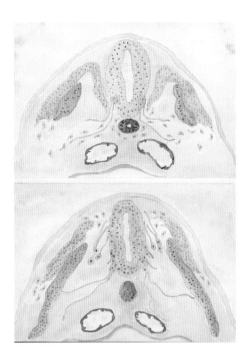

Plate 19. *Spinal nerves grow out from the neural tube like the tentacles of a jellyfish. The lateral heart tube can be seen in cross-section along with the central location of the notochord in these images.*

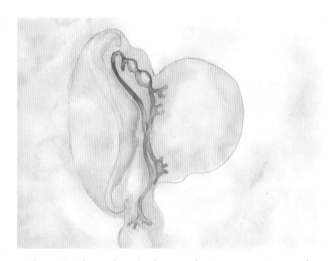

Plate 20. *The embryo is shown to be transparent to see the temporarily complete and functioning cardiovascular system. The embryo is the size of a navy bean and yet has a functioning cardiovascular system. The heart tube becomes a two-chambered heart.*

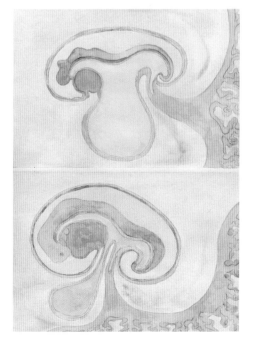

Plate 21. *The median plane of the gut tube forming with its yolk sac and allantois. The heart grows down and into the center of the embryo. The embryo continues to rotate and in the bottom image can be seen the final location of the umbilical cord in the middle of the ventral surface of the embryo. Blood cells are generated in the yolk sac and move into the embryonic heart at this stage. The allantois is shown.*

Plate 22. *The heart becomes the center of the human being. The head bows down and touches the heart with its face as the top of the neural tube, the future third ventricle appears to touch the bottom of the neural tube. The early arm and hand buds can be seen. The liver in brown is shown. It forms from the epicardium of the heart.*

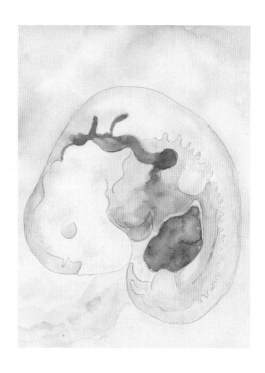

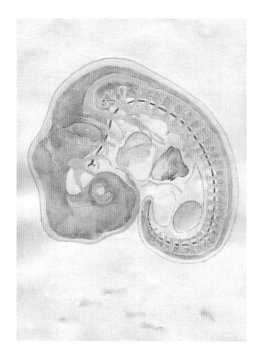

Plate 23. *The neural tube circles around the heart and liver. The cranial nerves, especially the trigeminal and vagus, and somatic nerves grow. The notochord, appearing here as a line anterior to the neural tube, will become the center (nucleus pulposus) of the intervertebral discs of the spine.*

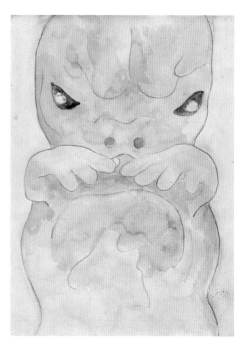

Plate 24. *The face of the embryo embraces its heart. The hands form by this embrace. Since the ribs are not formed yet, the heart balloons out at this stage.*

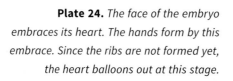

This provides both nutrition and a perforation from the compression of burrowing into and implanting in the uterus. By pulling apart or compressing, local cells die or are torn open and release nutrients to feed surrounding tissues in the growing embryo.

Thus, we see that the biology of *growth by pulling apart* is natural and cells are dying. It is encaptic growth because it increases in complexity over time in our aging bodies. We live on the precipice of death and dying every moment of our life. Each layer of the boundary can be pulled in different directions depending on its location and timing of differentiations, and thus the intense biological metabolism and felt sense of resistance and tension in two directions occurs. Each layer can have powerful compression/tension and then switch to freedom/opening.

DEATH AND DYING

It feels like certain death if one tries to change a complex emotional double bind. Yet we are already dismembered, pulled apart, with cells torn open and the nutrient distributed to serve local tissue. It is organized around senescence. Senescence is a condition in human biology in which successive cell division is accompanied by a progressive decrease in the growth and reproduction of each new generation of cells. The genes necessary to reproduce the cell decrease, and gradually the cell cannot reproduce. It is a gradual dissociation and dying process leading to death. The emotional double bind is, in essence, a constantly shifting biological dissociation and reassociation organized by the interchange of Primary Respiration and the dynamic stillness as the metaphor for the spiritual conditions that normalize the tension field. The growth resistance constantly shifts its organizational fulcrum, its point of orientation from the body to the mind, to the emotions, and to the sacred. The sacred contains the interconnection between all fulcrums. This constant shifting of orientation has seemingly no firm ground to settle upon. The resistance itself is centered by the constant interchange of PR and the dynamic stillness, the psychospiritual sacred ground of the double bind. It is the ground even though it feels like there is no stability with the constant shifting. The states of resistance and shifting growth seem intolerable, suspended between life and death—the scent of life fading and the abyss of death widening. This is our natural embryonic metabolism that transforms into physiology and ultimately psychospirituality. And thus, we are perpetual embryos. We are constantly living and dying simultaneously. Dr. Sutherland and Dr. Becker were fond of saying, "Be still and know," from

Psalm 46. They meant being still in order to know there is a direct channel to the Holy Spirit guiding their sessions and their lives. Every cranial practitioner learns this quote in school. The perception arising from being still is the first and last practice biodynamically. From such stillness, a connection to the sacred and the spiritual can be made regardless of one's religion, which brings us now to the next part of my book.

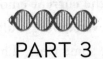

PART 3

BIODYNAMIC SPIRITUAL HEALING

Death, Distance, the Soul, and the

Influence of COVID-19

16

The Cycle of Moral Distress

Moral distress is the result of the current emotional plague in our inner and outer environment. There are overlapping multiple distress signals in our culture that have been present for some time. There is a pandemic of metabolic syndrome in which the majority of the world's population in developed countries is metabolically dysregulated. People are primarily suffering from diseases related to eating processed food, which cause metabolic syndromes such as diabetes, cardiovascular disease, cancer, dementia, obesity, and many other disorders. In addition, a worldwide viral contagion resulted in COVID-19. Then, in the United States, seven out of ten Americans experienced election anxiety and generalized fear of violence following the November 3, 2020, general election.

Moral distress is a cycling through helplessness, irritation, anger, rage, hopelessness, and despair, and it is deeply polarizing regarding the discernment of right, wrong, and integrity. In her book *Standing at the Edge: Finding Freedom where Fear and Courage Meet,* Joan Halifax defines integrity as "having a conscious commitment to honor one's own strong moral and ethical principles. Morality refers to our personal values related to dignity, honor, respect, and care. Ethics refers to the codified sets of beneficial and constructive principles that guide society and institutions and to which we are held accountable. When we cause suffering to others or ourselves, our integrity is violated. When we alleviate the suffering of others, our integrity is affirmed." The word *moral* ultimately refers to the nature of human rights as defined by the United Nations in 1948 and subsequent changes in the definition of human rights.

Moral violation is a new term describing certain forms of trauma such as combat trauma, sexual abuse, and obstetrical violence. The United States has a very poor record for maternal health outcomes, especially among Black and Latina women, who suffer a 60 percent higher risk of adverse health outcomes for themselves and their babies. Self-regulation, autonomy, and agency is gradually lost.

Moral injury is the result of a moral violation. It is a lack of differentiation between behaviors on a broad spectrum of right and wrong. Consequently, all therapeutic responses are unique and focused on the present moment. Moral injury frequently requires a spiritual solution to rebuild integrity, morality, and ethics. I have a very personal experience of a moral injury as detailed in chapter 6 because of a terrorist bombing attack.

Moral engagement means that one is naturally morally engaged in the community in which one lives. Given the amount of moral distress and moral violation in our culture now, it is vital to wake up the need to engage appropriately and as compassionately as possible. It starts with our autonomy and agency as we experience our own moral distress and have deep and profound self-compassion. New ways of helping people are needed by simply listening and bearing witness with nonattachment.

Moral independence is a call to action for a sane and just society. It is a call for appropriate autonomy away from the center of a materialistic culture and hedonistic society. To be ethical and morally independent is produced by one's inner spiritual development. Each situation in our life needs to be held in the present moment by relying on body sensation using a method of conscious breathing into the belly called *bringing the mind into the Hara* and clear thinking. Then attention is brought to the outside world with somatic, emotional, and cognitive empathy. We can no longer completely rely upon moral formulas and rules that try to fit all occasions. At this time, we must become independent of what the crowd on social media, the internet, the TV, and news media are promoting. We must also become independent of religious authorities, political authorities, and others professing infallible knowledge. Through one's own spiritual practice and healing with the natural world, one's own body, heart, and mind becomes the arbiter of morality through self-regulation and somatic knowing of what to accept and what to reject. It simply means that we meet each moment as it is and sort out what needs to happen in that moment. As shown in the first figure of the introduction, the current dilemma is a spiritual disease that demands spiritual healing as a partnership and grounded attitude permeating the mind and body of our planet and all its inhabitants. This exploration is spoken of eloquently by Dianne Connelly in her beautiful book *All Sickness Is Homesickness*. Contemplate that.

Zazen (and meditation in general), exercise, and Real Food are critical for recognizing the portal (the "Way") to the present moment: the supreme spiritual teacher is the present moment. This moment expresses a Middle Way (or the

"Way" according to Taoism and Zen) between extremes of good and bad, eternalism and nihilism, right and wrong, and so forth. The "Way" is moral independence, which requires effort to maintain.

In *Zen Mind, Beginner's Mind,* Suzuki Roshi said, "form is form, emptiness is emptiness." The spiritual life is already present as a united body and mind. The totality of originality, cosmology, enlightenment, and the ground of being are already totally present. Build ethical autonomy and then a sane society around shared goals of happiness and full, appropriate self-expression: spiritual self-regulation first; moral engagement (coregulation) follows. This section of this book explores these possibilities as preparation for the subsequent chapters that deepen the understanding and practice of spiritual healing.

RECOMMENDED READING

Medical Nemesis, The Expropriation of Health by Ivan Illich (Pantheon Books, 1976).

Standing at the Edge, Finding Freedom Where Fear and Courage Meet by Joan Halifax (Flatiron Books, 2018).

17

Aspects of Biodynamic Practice
To Palliate, the Second Pair of Hands,
and Not Knowing

TO PALLIATE

To palliate: 1. to reduce in violence; to lessen or abate; to mitigate; to ease without curing; as, to palliate a disease.
  2. to moderate; to cloak; to shelter; to hide.
To mitigate: 1. To render to become mild or milder; to moderate, become less severe or painful; to soften, diminish or lessen.
  WEBSTER'S NEW INTERNATIONAL DICTIONARY (2ND ED.)

If I say biodynamics is about incorporation, then that is only half of biodynamics. The other half is disincorporation. This means death. Inside each of us is a death instinct, a death metabolism, and a mind of death. We all periodically have thoughts and contemplate our death or suicide or even think about others ("I just wish *so and so* were dead!"). To have a mind of death is natural. It is the instinct of ending and dissolution. As sure as one thought or emotion ends, another begins. Birth and death are right here 24/7. These three are linked: the death instinct, our thoughts, and their cessation.

We are constantly being primed for death in the simplicity of the Buddhist teaching of impermanence. Sitting meditation is a death meditation. We can sing the praises of mindfulness and compassion, but what guides us is the fear of death, and we avoid it at all costs even if we support hospice and shop in their resale stores. We are afraid of death because we accumulate so many things to make our life and our body seem solid, but they are not. Life is very fluid. It is a flow that goes on and merges with the ocean of death. Thus, the infallibility of impermanence. Nobody gets out alive.

Contemporary biodynamic practice must integrate a type of palliative care to reduce a person's deeply instinctual fear of death. We simply help patients relax their minds and bodies as one thing. We serve rather than fix. This is the gift of Primary Respiration and the dynamic stillness. It allows nature to take its course. They are self-directing elements in Eastern medical traditions (such as Tibetan medicine). We need to include the elements as described in Eastern traditions and the spiritual practice of sitting meditation to make biodynamics a complete practice of embodiment and disembodiment. The yin and the yang: this is the way of the natural world and a source of healing—to acknowledge these realities inwardly and outwardly. Thus, embodiment includes disembodiment. It is one thing. I declare that correct biodynamic practice is a death practice.

It is fishy that biodynamic practice has focused so much on conception, pregnancy, and birth. But that is not all of life. To hold our client as if they are a newborn baby, as Dr. Jealous suggests, begs to be balanced with equally holding each client as if they are dying or dead already. This is not some morbid zombie fantasy or a flowery, romantic view. It is having a clear sense of gentleness, kindness, and delicateness necessary to hold someone, who is both a baby and a corpse at the same time, with our hands, our body, and our mind. This is the image of the *Pietà* that Michelangelo carved when he was twenty-one years old. This is biodynamic wholeness. This is correct biodynamic practice. Your mind of wholeness is located in your heart, which beats seventy times a minute. This is the simplest practice to create empathy and balance in biodynamic practice. Feel your heartbeat and center your attention there while you are dying or do it now all the time. One of my favorite practices is to say a prayer nonverbally in the cadence of my heartbeat. Sometimes I simply talk to my heart in the middle of the night or during the day when I feel its incessant potency pounding and vibrating in the middle of my chest. I say, "Hello my old friend, my heart. How are you today?" Then I listen for the answer.

It is incomplete biodynamic practice if we only consider the client's originality from a cosmological perspective or as an embryo or fetus or a newborn baby. Yes, we are told by our biodynamic teachers that PR touches one's origins, and it is the origin. Origin also implies death, the void that is the absolute ending of the previous universe. What starts as life will die. We birth in with our mother and birth out at death.

Now, however, the balance scales have tipped in this new era of metabolic well-being and metabolic syndrome. Not only are 88 percent of Americans metabolically dysregulated, but 60 percent have at least one chronic disease. The emergence of a complete biodynamic practice integrates an attitude of serving the end-of-life care, palliative care, and compassionate care for the contemporary client. We are not limited to exploring this with only those who have terminal diagnosis, but rather we synchronize with the priorities of PR and dynamic stillness in the client's totality—spiritually. When we hold both the beginning and end of life for ourselves and our clients, this is complete biodynamic practice. This is spiritual practice.

In Buddhism it is understood that there is no-self. This is called emptiness. It is not nothing, and it is a mistake to think of it this way. We meditate to achieve nonthought, however briefly, in order to be fearless and watch the solid self and ego dissolve, element by element, thought by thought and emotion by emotion while sitting in a still posture. Meditation posture is the posture of stopping to watch the dissolution of our thoughts and concepts about life. Why not start now rather than waiting for death? We have all heard the stories of yogis and yoginis sitting and meditating in the charnel grounds! Our mind is a charnel ground of compulsive thinking that blocks our deepest knowledge. Our health care system is a charnel ground treating symptoms rather than causes. No-self simply means wholeness in its fullest sense. It means we are all interconnected. We all intellectually know that we are interconnected to all things, or as Thich Nhat Hanh says: "We inter-are." But do we feel this viscerally, elementally? Is it heartfelt?

In biodynamic practice we are merged with the client automatically in our hearts and brains. We know this from the research in interpersonal neurobiology that we are coregulating each other metabolically and physiologically. We know this because this is the way it was during pregnancy, and that capacity remains with all beings throughout life. But at the same time, we maintain a balanced contact with our metabolism of autonomy. We periodically move our attention to our own body-mind, our breath, our heartbeat. Therapeutic attunement involves a constantly repeating cycle of moving attention between self and other until we get tired of it and rest in the dynamic stillness of space beyond self and other.

Ultimately, we die alone, and death becomes our autonomy. Autonomy is a form of spaciousness like a good night's sleep. Meditation is a celebration of autonomy. We must withdraw from the world to rest and repair, to practice self-care, and to explore our perception of reality to reduce our collection of fears to zero. Thus, we self-regulate socially and autonomously. It is a pendulum swinging 24/7. It is a continuous practice moved by PR and dynamic stillness.

This is correct attunement in biodynamic practice because each of us constructs a solid self differently, and thus the deconstruction of a compulsive connection must be gentle and palliative for our own joyful discovery of aloneness rather than depressive loneliness. We facilitate the discovery of such for the client simply by being present to our own suffering and compulsive habits. Compassion means to be totally present for someone and at the same time nonattached to any outcome of the social/therapeutic connection. We cannot know the inner reality of anyone but ourselves, and do we really know ourselves?

In biodynamic practice we can focus on our own no-self, which is a much deeper autonomy. We do this through sensing the transparency of our fluid body, calming our mind and letting PR and dynamic stillness establish the priorities for the client and supporting as gently as possible their own dissolution of a solid and false self with nonfright. This is considered transcendental patience or simply patiently waiting. Self-regulation and respecting the client's agency, as well as having the ability to perceive the environment accurately and the power to change one's environment, are the primary ways to serve a client. Our autonomy becomes a simultaneous offering with connection to our client for them to self-regulate in whatever way is possible relationally or autonomously without imposing anything at all but kindness, tenderness, and warmth. Biodynamic practice is palliative care. It is learning to serve and sit at the side of someone who is suffering.

When we finally understand that we cannot help other people, we can ask ourselves; What is my motivation? What is the nature of my spiritual intention? When we examine ourselves this way, we may recognize the need for help from a spiritual source. The very nature of the manual therapeutic arts is that it constellates a connection to the sacred if we know how to open ourselves to that possibility and recognize it in the moment. Above all it is important to have no fear when in the state of not knowing how to proceed or even what our motivation is. From these experiences and perceptions we can clearly embody a set of biodynamic values that include empathy and compassion based on not knowing.

THE SECOND PAIR OF HANDS

There was a long pause, which represented my unknowing. This pause, this kind of emptiness, remained for a considerable period of time. . . . I found myself just waiting and breathing; there was only the movement of air and time passing. Slowly, the emptiness became complete. There was absolutely no afferent activity in the perceptual fields of the patient's nervous system. It was still, very still. There was the presence of integrity; my eyes closed. Slowly, it seemed that something was happening. I perceived a vague movement in the patient's body. I was aware only of this motion, and then, as if from nowhere, like a ship appearing out of the fog, another pair of hands appeared in contact with the patient's body. . . . If this had been a singular event, I would say so, but it has happened on a regular basis and is becoming more common place.

JIM JEALOUS, D.O.

The above quote from Dr. Jealous was from an article called "The Other Pair of Hands" published in *Alternative Therapies Magazine* in 1998. I mention this because everything mentioned in that article occurs in my clinical practice. We must increase our spiritual capacities; our contemporary world and the contemporary client demand it. These instructions I offer to you. This is the way *the second pair of hands* manifests in my practice and my everyday life.

The Second Pair of Hands

The context of the practice is "Be still and know" according to Jealous. It is the felt sense of stillness permeating the treatment room.

1. There is no afferent activity in my hands coming from the client while in contact. My body also enters a neutral, deep stillpoint.
2. I usually wait until the last ten minutes of the session, usually while treating at my favorite endpoint such as the feet.
3. Upon feeling the stillness in the room, I nonverbally invite a "benevolent second pair of hands" into the room. Sometimes they are there already, and sometimes an invitation is necessary.
4. I allow my mind to enter an *active imagination* around the appearance of the benevolent figure. A spiritual figure, alive or dead, or a family member that we

do not recognize but is nonetheless benevolent, may arrive. Or a stranger may show up. If the figure does not appear to be benevolent, send them away until your heart feels benevolence toward the second pair of hands.

5. I wait for this *benevolent other* to place their hands where he or she deems appropriate. There is no need to suggest, invite, or direct the second pair of hands. They will go where necessary. Just observe their process of choosing their fulcrum.

6. Be still and know.

Your hands will immediately sense this *benevolent fulcrum* and its activity at any number of sensory levels, including the visual. You might witness the benevolent other's hands dispensing a form of grace that is visually apparent in some form or another. I once observed a baptism of water being poured over the forehead of my client by Jesus. There is no need to engage or assist this process as it is rather quick—maybe a minute or two. The two sets of hands become connected through the client's body.

I make nonverbal mental contact with the benevolent other as an acknowledgment of being in an equal partnership rather than submitting to a higher authority. This is still your session over which you have sovereignty. The second pair of hands arises from your own enlightened heart activity and the spiritual healing power of Primary Respiration.

Maintain awareness and then the second pair of hands of the benevolent figure will fade away. This whole interaction does not take long, and the therapeutic fulcrum will shift. Grace does flow in the body and can be felt. I then wait several minutes before ending the session.

The few clients I have verbalized this to (family members only) have all recognized and felt the potency of the Health from this benevolent interaction. If unable to see clients in person, this can be done over the phone or Zoom by setting an appointment in which you and your client are in a designated space of relaxation for the distance healing to manifest. I am so grateful for these experiences that I will be filled with tears of joy or struck speechless by the power of the sacred image. This is not a process that can be duplicated exactly each time. It is a living, moving, and sacred aspect of biodynamic practice. As Jim Jealous once said, the therapist should learn something new in every session. Every session is different. It starts and ends with feeling one's own heart. We must overcome the fear of not knowing. Not knowing is a portal to the deeper heart essence of empathy and compassion.

NOT KNOWING

If You Want To Understand
You Don't Understand
If You Attain Don't Know
That Is Your True Nature

ZEN MASTER KO BONG, 1890–1962

Biodynamic practice is the study of perception and the incorporation of wholeness. It is plain and simple from our teachers. In a world that has been reordered by pandemics such as metabolic disease and COVID, it is important to name a third aspect of biodynamic practice. We should make it the first and most important part of our practice. Biodynamics is now the study and practice of compassion and compassionate action. Compassion includes acknowledging our own pain and suffering from social distancing to the deeper states of mind that keep us locked down in compulsive behaviors. We have an innate longing to transcend our suffering and to help others with their style of suffering. Everyone desires to be free of the natural fear of change process that is so deep. We cannot control the way the world changes, and we don't know the future because the present is so painful. If we can recognize this awkward movement within ourselves, we can then feel what everyone else on the planet is feeling inside their body and mind. We can wake up the heart of compassion and engage in compassionate action.

So the priority became to open to our heart of compassion in a time of social distancing and daily death counts, surges, waves, and lockdowns. We must take refuge in our heart at seventy beats per minute and lower the beats per minute if it is higher! We must drop our breath down deep into our belly of not knowing. Compassion involves the willingness to feel sad and humble from not knowing. It is vitally important to feel sad and feel the warmth and tenderness that this sadness brings to our cardiovascular system and body-mind in general. It softens the mind and creates humility from the not knowing rather than chaos.

Two years ago, I spoke at a biodynamic craniosacral therapy conference in Spain. I was asked what I thought was the most important part of biodynamic practice. I answered that the therapist could periodically bow their head when they have their hands on the client. It is the gesture of humility, a gesture of sacrificing one's ego and entering the not knowing. The Health is underneath the suffering and intact as the preexisting condition. In this gesture of bowing there is a recognition of mutual sanity. We bow to the Health in each other. The term

Health has been capitalized since the time of Dr. Still, as it represents the spiritual foundations of osteopathic biodynamic practice since its foundation. What better way to make a client feel safe than to bow in recognition of their own Health and well-being, which is inside of them already operating under the guise of Primary Respiration (wind) and dynamic stillness (space)? This bow is also a short prayer in which we offer our own helplessness and state of not knowing as a compassionate action. Such a truth will set us free from the compulsive mind of needing to fix the client rather than serve the client in their wholeness and Health.

When we bear witness to our own pain and suffering, we more fully recognize our own not knowing. It can greatly decrease the amount of wasted time, energy, and technique to try to fix ourselves and others. It invites and gives the more potent spiritual aspects of Primary Respiration and dynamic stillness complete freedom to transform what needs to be transformed in one's body and mind. This is the gesture of transformation. It is simply a bow of the head. As the Dalai Lama said during a teaching of his I attended some years ago, "Humility is the greatest way to change the mind."

Since many of us did not treat clients during the period of social distancing, when we reflect on all that has happened to the planet, we can simply bow our head in the space of a fearless not knowing. This act deeply engages the potency of the Health intrinsic to PR and dynamic stillness. We must understand that the dance and interchange of PR and dynamic stillness is a metaphor for not knowing. Trust the Tide. Now we must trust the dance of PR and the dynamic stillness in their deeper transformational state, the simplicity of not knowing free from fear and hesitation. It is a state of resting the mind and emotions.

To trust the not knowing means to give up trying to control the world. It gives us freedom from the compulsive thinking of trying to accomplish something more. It activates the very core of compassion and compassionate action to accomplish less: less thinking, less conceptualizing. It can prevent emotions that are unwholesome. It is an essential time for discovering one's deeper values with which to navigate life. When in the experience of not knowing, find out what is important in your own body and mind. There is stress in not knowing if we allow it.

At the same time, we can recognize its spiritual value when we feel our heartbeat and feel our breath slowly fill our belly. In Japan, this type of belly breathing is called "placing the mind in the Hara." The Hara is the abdomen. Keep it simple. Stay with your literal heart and mind in your Hara. That is the center. Do not move until the Health of the client requests your attention. Do not move until your Health requests your attention. This is a foundation of a compassionate response.

18
Biodynamic Compassion

It is a different world out there since coronavirus arrived. And it will be a very different world when the coronavirus passes. We biodynamic therapists and all healers have our work cut out for us. Andrew Taylor Still recognized the spiritual component of manual therapy. He said: "I love my fellow man, because I see God in his face and in his form." Is this how we see our clients? Is this how we see the cashier in the grocery store while checking out? Is this the way we feel when reading about all the people who died alone and were buried without family members present? Every week during the height of COVID we saw pictures of body bags filled with patients who died. We then meditated on the global charnel grounds of COVID from a distance in our own home. We practiced distance healing by default. We must therefore increase our spiritual healing capacities to meet the new demands of our clients. We must realize that biodynamic cardiovascular therapy (BCVT) is a compassion-based practice.

∞

A Compassion Meditation

I practice and teach a compassion meditation called Tonglen from Tibetan Buddhism.

- It starts with twenty minutes of calm abiding or zazen meditation, with strong back and soft front, belly breathing, and using mindfulness to return to the breath when our attention has been captured by compulsive thinking.
- Then there is a moment of open awareness where thoughts, breathing, and posture are all suspended equally within the wholeness of the natural world.
- Then there is a phase of recalling an event in my life that allows me to feel sad. I always think about going to the mortuary and seeing the body of my dead father and then some years later the body of my dead mother before

they were cremated. I visualize those scenes until I feel a tear in my eye or a sadness in my heart.

- I then work with a sense of breathing in a dark color and exhaling a light color.
- With a sad heart I can begin to contemplate my own fears and challenges and allow my heart to transform my dark fear into light courage. I simply create a space for my own hope and fear to coexist.
- I then extend this practice to family members, clients, and loved ones. I imagine them one at a time sitting in front of me. I bring in their challenges as a dark color when I inhale, and I exhale a sense of lightness and well-being to them. I simply create a space for their hope and fear to coexist.
- Finally, I take in the whole planet, everyone suffering, especially emotionally and physically. I imagine I am an astronaut in orbit above the earth. I breathe that in and allow my heart to transform it into a sense of well-being to the entire planet. I simply imagine a space for planetary hope and fear to coexist and transform in the sense of "Thy will be done."

Tonglen is an ancient form of distance healing. It is also a form of shamanic practice that I will speak to shortly. I am always aware of this reality whenever I treat a client or walk through my daily life. Wholeness is the smallest subdivision of life. Compassion is also free from desire. It is based upon bearing witness, being totally present for someone yet completely nonattached to an outcome. It is humbling to feel helpless and be nonattached during the contemporary situation. This is the birth of great compassion.

INTERCESSORY PRAYER

Distance healing is also called intercessory prayer. It is well researched, and people with medical conditions whom we do not even know can get better when their names are given to prayer groups thousands of miles away. We can help people feel better and not even know them! Imagine such easy and effortless compassion. This is distance healing in the metaphor of intercessory prayer. Such prayer is based on devotion and humility, the hallmarks of compassion. It is also enough to pray for the highest or deepest good to emerge during a pandemic. Or perhaps a pandemic is the manifestation of a higher or deeper goodness? How does each of us pray for the planet and its well-being? In what form does that prayer take place (such as with words or visualizations)?

BIODYNAMIC SHAMANISM

A central premise of this book is the evolution of biodynamic practice into a contemporary form of shamanism. This is based on the evolving needs of the contemporary client experiencing or needing spiritual healing because of the colossal failures and iatrogenesis of the medical system in general. Distance healing is also seen in shamanism, which is a category of perception outside normal sensory experience. It involves a type of extrasensory perception. Shamanism is the original healing methodology on the planet developed in traditional cultures. It is what I call the Way of the Natural World. It is an innate or latent set of instincts for healing oneself and others found in all sentient beings. It is the most natural medicine on the planet and the oldest. Shamanic skills evolved from cultures that were completely integrated with the natural world. Isn't this component of integrating the natural world into biodynamic practice what Dr. Jealous, the godfather of biodynamic osteopathy, insisted upon for a long time while he was alive? One of his favorite books that he always recommended was *Heart of the Hunter* by Laurens van der Post. It is a story of the !Kung people who live in Africa's Kalahari Desert. They could see Primary Respiration moving back and forth from the horizon into their awareness.

To practice shamanism requires a phase of separation from the ordinary world. Isn't this social distancing? Everyone could feel the deeper energies stirring due to being separated from each other during the early days of the COVID pandemic. The deeper energies are death and dying at many levels. This is the second step in biodynamic shamanism: to acknowledge the depth of our current experience. The charnel grounds are multidimensional and ever present.

Biodynamic shamanism means to be familiar with death by having had a near-death experience and been initiated by it. Many modern births are near-death experiences, as are car accidents and a host of other traumas. We can also work with death through palliative care training as a spiritual aptitude. We relax around death. All clients are dying as we are, too. Our contemporary situation demands we look at death in the eye without fear. We turn our face into the wind. In this way Ignition, which is integral to biodynamic practice, becomes an initiation via the wind of Primary Respiration that emerges from the heart and the space of dynamic stillness that centers our heart. This is the final stage in our biodynamic shamanism.

THE GIFT

Each biodynamic therapist has their own gift, their expression of the potency of the Primary Respiration and dynamic stillness. We must integrate the skills that are given to us from outside via our teachers and those that emerge from inside from a devoted spiritual practice. Just because you have a license to practice manual therapy or any other healing art does not mean you are working on your personal spiritual formation. Continuing education is required both for our licenses and our spiritual formation. Each of us is charged with forming our own method to heal ourselves and each other under the biodynamic guidance of Primary Respiration and the dynamic stillness. Our unique individual therapeutic gifts are linked to our spiritual capacities. This is the dominant invitation of our time. The clear intention of biodynamic practice, as I teach it, is to evolve one's practice spiritually from decade to decade as we all grow and evolve toward our death. Primary Respiration is the Breath of Life. The Breath of Life means we are being spiritually guided by it while we work and live on this planet. We are always *receiving* a treatment from the Breath of Life and the dynamic stillness.

Dr. Sutherland said in 1943 that the cranial concept could be "religious in nature," which would now include valid forms of distance healing, compassion meditation, and intercessory prayer. These forms are not learned overnight but through long processes that ensure the ethics and morality of not harming others or causing fear. We must have a clear heart. The spiritual dimension of BCVT and its roots in craniosacral therapy is something that is rarely discussed. It is now unavoidable except for the atheists, the control group in the experiment. The portal to increase our spiritual capacities is now wide open. We must enter it in a way that does not scare people unnecessarily but rather increases our own gift of compassion and enhances our healing gifts. Can we make a vow to ourselves to increase our spiritual capacities in whatever way possible? The real question is: If not now, when?

19

The Breath of Life, Reverence, and Devotion

Intercessory prayer is the meditation on what is ultimately true, good, and lovely. It aligns the current reality we exist in with that higher reality through our thoughts, feelings, and words. Intercessory prayer is powerful from a distance as you can speak life into a situation and exude hope for someone or something that lacks it. However, we must not discount the power of laying on hands and interceding without thoughts, feelings, or words. The hands hold the power of compassion as we connect with another human being, assigning dignity and worth to them. This act, as well as intercessory prayer from a distance, interrupts pain and suffering with light and allows healing to take place.

EVELYN STETZER

My niece Evelyn wrote this for me during the height of the COVID pandemic. She is a mystic just like my mentor, Dr. Jealous, and she amazes me every time I am in her presence. Thank you, Evelyn and Jim, for singing the praises of the Divine during plague time and forever after.

I opened this chapter with my niece's quote because I feel it illustrates concepts at the basis of biodynamic practice: compassion, reverence, devotion, and the Breath of Life. This chapter will cover these as well as offer tools, practices, and information that the biodynamic practitioner can utilize in later parts of this book.

This chapter is also a natural extension of Dr. Sutherland's life work. In 1948, Dr. Sutherland observed the release of a lesion by the Breath of Life, and it surprised him. He declared that *reverence* must become an aspect of treatment. He felt the Tide at the death of a client. He writes, "Get as far away from your physical touch as possible. Deep touch will lead you to the primary site." He sensed an "otherness" appearing. He then said that the whole idea, even his initial thought of the cranial concept in 1898, came from God.

It is now time to allow these germinal thoughts and initiatory experiences from him and his teacher, Dr. Still, to arrive at another level of fruition. With all due respect to Dr. Sutherland and his lineage holders, I offer the following thoughts in the hopes of assisting contemporary therapists, clients, and all beings on the planet. I also offer this in honor of the life of Jim Jealous, D.O., who died in February 2021. He also focused on the spiritual dimension of biodynamic practice.

Let us look at what biodynamic practice could be at this time on the planet as a biodynamic spiritual glossary. As Dr. Sutherland said in his final lecture in 1948, "What I am about to say is not a religious talk, but it may appear to be" ("Seminar in Cranial Osteopathy," Des Moines, Iowa, April 25, 1948).

SPIRITUAL

Spirituality is most readily recognized by its branches—connection with creation and Creator through practices like prayer, serving, and loving—but the root of spirituality is knowing.

And not just the kind of knowing a mind does, but the knowing that comes from your gut, your soul, the very essence of who you are, connecting to its Source.

Once the knowing begins, then comes the ever-expanding nature of spirituality—the more you think you know, the more you realize there is to learn.

Knowing quickly turns into a perpetual longing to experience more of Who, What, Where we come from, until we return.

EVELYN STETZER

Spirituality is the aptitude for being relaxed in the present moment, for gratitude for each breath we take, for humility in not knowing, for kindness when we smile, and for searching for our heart when it is lost.

INTERCESSORY (INTERVENTION)

Act of interceding; mediation; interposition between the divine and human realms with a view to reconciliation; prayer, petition, entreaty in favor of compassion and healing for self and all others.

PRAYER

A prayer is an earnest entreaty or supplication addressed to a higher or deeper power that is invested with authority and respect, such as the living reality of the Breath of Life (or PR) and dynamic stillness. It is made by someone in a state of humility. In this way prayer is an offering of devotion, reverence, respect, and gratitude to a higher or deeper power inside the body and continuous with the natural world and beyond.

BIODYNAMIC INTENTION

The conscious thought for the spiritual motivation for biodynamic practice is that *laying on of hands* is a form of intercessory prayer. This simply means reverence. Furthermore, this interaction between myself and my client is dedicated to consciously being of benefit for each of us on the whole planet. This is the generation of the spirit of altruism and the awakening of the highest form of moral development in human beings. It is a practice of nonfright according to the Dalai Lama. It is a basic human right to generate safety for oneself and others to prevent moral injury and moral violation. The physiological pandemic is in the human autonomic nervous system. It is the full spectrum of posttraumatic stress disorder displayed in the variety of ways described in the work of Stephen Porges and his polyvagal model of safety. The polyvagal model suggests a hierarchy of responses to stressful situations and trauma, from the oldest and most primitive to the newest and most sophisticated in the ANS hierarchy of structure and function. We can see the primitive in our society and must enhance the new through compassion and empathy as a foundation for biodynamic practice. *Safety first* is the most practical exploration of this altruistic intention. Safety cannot be accomplished without kindness in our body and mind, especially our hands as extensions of our heart.

BIODYNAMIC PRACTICE

Biodynamics is a study, an experience, and a perception of the uninterrupted rhythmic, balanced exchange of the Breath of Life with the dynamic stillness. Primary Respiration is equated with the Breath of Life. The Breath of Life starts in the heart and body then extends out to the natural world and beyond. It is more tidal than the breath of air according to Sutherland. It originates in the literal heartbeat in a revolving protocol of breath awareness, heartbeat awareness, mental awareness (mindfulness), and the Breath of Life moving between our hearts. Through this practice we can perceive the effects of the Breath of Life and the dynamic stillness on the ANS and clinically pass through the eye of a needle otherwise known as the *Neutral*. It is the Neutral that deepens the prayer of biodynamic practice. The Neutral is the stillpoint. As Dr. Becker said in a lecture, "The therapeutic process does not begin until the will of the patient (ANS) yields to the will of the Breath of Life." This is the sacred Neutral and the first step in a biodynamic rite of passage for spiritual healing.

COMPASSION

Bearing witness is being utterly present for the moment-to-moment experience in the therapeutic container. At the same time, being utterly present to ourselves and to our client, we are completely nonattached to the outcome of the prayer that we offer to the client with our body, hands, and mind. These two aspects of compassion, bearing witness and nonattachment, require training and practice through meditation, contemplation, and joyful effort. To be totally present for someone begins with not-knowing mind. It includes mindful listening, the capacity to bear witness. We need to notice the thoughts we are thinking while we are engaged with a client (or anytime, for that matter).

The *first* stage in such a connection is to notice a preoccupation with all of our personal feelings, emotions, and storylines that fill our mind and distract us from being with the other person. We sometimes are completely disengaged mentally from the client.

The *second* stage is to try to be present and hear the other person even if mentally we are feeling an urgent impatience to move on and get away from that person. It is a kind of attentional whiplash that happens in our minds: I'm here; I'm not.

Third, we arrive at a sense of somatic, emotional, and cognitive empathy. Our mind calms down. We are able to feel our way into what the other person is communicating, which includes eye contact, facial expressions, and body movement. This is how we register neuroception, the feeling of safety, and the giving of safety. It decreases the unconscious need for the client to feel the need to protect himself. It is the most basic foundation for achieving a Neutral in biodynamic practice. It is facilitated by turning off all electronics a half hour before a client arrives. With luck, the client arrives, and you are already in an empathetic state of heart.

Finally, we rest our attention in the back of our heart, breathing into our belly and waiting for the Breath of Life to move between our two hearts. We become more comfortable in sensing the stillpoints that occur in the relationship, without having to react to their emptiness, and just let the stillness be the stillness. We must also be nonattached to the dynamic stillness. We let go of our senses, moving out to the horizon and back, allowing the stillness to permeate the atmosphere.

IGNITION (INITIATION)

Our practice includes the retrieval and remembrance of the *lost midline* of peace, serenity, grace, and love. Jim Jealous simply referred to these qualities as a hollow midline extending to the horizon and filled with dynamic stillness. These are the inhabitants of the precious biodynamic midline. They are missing in the context of PTSD and contemporary society in general. The embodiment of empathy and compassion is a growing and deepening process rather than a single immutable state. Compassion is the instinct of altruism and as strong as the survival instinct at the other end of the spectrum. It is optimized when the mind and body decrease their polarization and finally synchronize following the Neutral. This requires the noble virtue of patience, as we do not know the client's inner spiritual process. Thus, with nonattachment, this not knowing is critical.

Ignition in this context means *initiation.* It is the experience of passing through a portal whose roots are in the ANS of the body. The portal mimics the experience of death, but we remain alive. The vagus nerve transforms its sensory and motor messaging to one of spirituality on the other side of this portal. This is sometimes called the kundalini, but it is the movement of spiritual energy in the biodynamic midline. The Breath of Life and the stillness rehabilitate and reinhabit the midline. Where is the middle, the center of your body from this viewpoint? At the same time, Ignition refers to the complex inflammatory conditions involved in metabolic syndrome as detailed in the first part of this book.

INCORPORATION

Incorporation in the context of this book derives from Arnold van Gennep's book *The Rites of Passage.* He describes incorporation as a return to or an inhabitation of the body following an ordeal or initiation in the biodynamic sense of Ignition. The end point of a correct and appropriate Ignition is to be more fully incorporated in the body and have a direct relationship with the Health at a spiritual level. We know that biodynamic practice has physiological benefits. The work in general is very relaxing, and a case is being made within our biodynamic community that it increases vagal tone, optimizes immune system function, and increases self-regulatory capacity. Incorporation, a cross between embodiment and incarnation, is the main side effect of biodynamic practice. It is the ability to consciously recognize the client's initiatory experience of life and silently bear witness to it. This includes the felt sense and *intrinsic value of the Neutral* when ANS hierarchical activity recalibrates and becomes more resilient. The background of serenity and equanimity (effects of compassion) comes to the foreground of our mind and body. But we cannot rely solely upon the vagus nerve, new or old, to complete the healing. It is the decision of the Breath of Life, as Sutherland's metaphor for divine intervention came to be known and perceived. It is a lifelong process. As clinicians how often do we actually let the Breath of Life decide on the therapeutic process?

OUR HANDS

Our hands are a prayer unto themselves. They are afferent. They are a *bridge to wholeness*. They are a mudra of nonfright. They can kill (think flies and mosquitos, please). They can heal. They interconnect us intimately. How do we do all of this? With an equal amount of attention on our hands, heart, and perception. The message of the Breath of Life and the dynamic stillness is very simple and very clear. It is the message of slowing down (Breath of Life) and stopping (dynamic stillness). How could anything this simple be effective? We center our attention on our heartbeat. It is because it is imbued with a sense of the spiritual, a light, and an interconnection with all the natural world and beyond. This flows through our hands as an extension of the mind in the heart.

When we are compassionate in the treatment room and outside of the treatment room at the grocery store, we must recognize not knowing. This is an important aspect of the initiatory portal. As Dr. Jealous said in his 1998 article "The Other Pair of Hands" (see chapter 17), helplessness is a fundamental part of the practice that generates empathy and mindfulness throughout our mind and body. When we are not attached to the outcome, the not-knowing mind is a fountain of creativity. We are not letting go of our knowledge; we are simply putting it on pause momentarily. Our hands are an invitation for a spiritual dimension to open from the shamanic (extrasensory perception) to the ordinary. What do *hands as prayer* feel like?

A VOW OF SAFETY

Vow to yourself to *deeply care for yourself and your safety*. We all know this, and we have all learned many practices to fulfill this vow already. Spiritual practice is about maintaining and keeping a vow, a candle lit for our own safety first to be of service and benefit to oneself and the world. *Be devoted to safety.* Safety has many meanings. At this time, we must learn to take refuge in our very heartbeat (literally) and placing the depth of our breath in our belly. We must make the inside of our body a safe refuge first.

We can see all thoughts as equal and notice that thoughts dissolve by themselves. To become mindful of the simple, natural cycle of thoughts arising and dissolving brings relief, albeit temporarily! So the vow, to *take refuge in your heart,* requires a little bit of effort to nurture and allow thoughts to dissolve before behaviors arise that make the thoughts seem solid and permanent. It is the essence of self-compassion. We must practice mindfulness, including the frequent observation of our own distracted, recreational mind. Compulsive thinking is the actual enemy of tranquility and the main driver of karma for those that traffic in that term. Then we generate a sense of conscious gratitude that opens the brain in the heart. Gratitude is a portal to the deeper dimensions of the heart, spiritually.

SPIRITUAL TOOLS

The Breath of Life and the dynamic stillness are spiritual tools for the biodynamic therapist. They always have been, according to the teachings of Dr. Sutherland, Jim Jealous, and the original lineage holders. If we only sense anatomy and physiology changing while we work, we might miss another, deeper dimension of our clinical practice that can integrate anatomy and the physiological change process across the entire spectrum of human spiritual experience in ourselves and others. When we touch the sacrum, we know it as the *sacred* bone. Isn't every other contact we make with a client's body during a session equally sacred as well?

This is the antidote to our plague times. Our ministry is one of *laying on of hands.* It is an intercessory prayer guided by the Breath of Life and the dynamic stillness. Our hands are an extension of our heart, as we know from embryology. And our mind can rest in our heart to nurture the compassion reflex, and our breath can rest in our abdomen, the source of Ignition at birth and the origin of the cosmos according to the Taoist tradition. The biodynamic therapist becomes the ultimate spiritual tool. Thank you, Drs. Sutherland and Jealous, for your inspiration! Thank you, Evelyn Stetzer, for your inspiration! May the whole world be free of pain and suffering. May we truly learn to serve biodynamically those who are in need.

REVERENCE AND DEVOTION: THE STILLPOINT

Biodynamic practice is the study of perception and our fluid interconnection with the natural world. It is plain and simple from our teachers and their teachers in this splendid lineage of natural bodily Health. Now, as our world is reordered both inside and out, it is important to name another aspect of biodynamic practice. It needs to be the first and most important part of our practice: *reverence*. Biodynamics is the study and practice of complete reverence for stillness, the intelligence of Primary Respiration, safety, and compassionate action.

As we navigate an emotional plague (I am using this term metaphorically and not politically), we are constantly faced with impermanence. Whether it is the death of someone we know or our own reactions to social isolation, the effect has polarized our family, friends, and community. Everyone seems to have an opinion, whether it is well informed or not. The middle way is absent. If we can recognize this awkward and painful backward step within ourselves, we can then feel what everyone else on the planet earth is feeling inside their body and mind. This is the heart of compassion, and it is deeply humbling. Then we can learn to navigate between the extremes of views being expressed.

The priority is to have reverence for the plague, the pandemic of illness in all its myriad forms, the fear, the impermanence. The plague is the teacher. We are the clients. We are receiving a deep biodynamic treatment. Reverence further implies devotion to a spiritual practice. Dr. Sutherland was fond of saying that his cranial concept could be considered religious in nature, and certainly the founder of osteopathy, Dr. Still, was a deeply spiritual human being and perhaps even mystical, as was Jim Jealous. Reverence is the spiritual practice of discovering the stillpoint in our heart or, if that is unavailable, the stillpoint in nature. We must form a personal relationship, a type of devotion, with the natural environment around us until our thoughts about the past and future are suspended into space. *Devotion* is a determination to relate with sanity to the roadblocks in our mind and body in order to reach the heart of stillness in its vastness and its potency.

Our times present us now with a perfect teacher to step back and settle just as we do in a biodynamic session for another person. Why not give ourselves a biodynamic session by sitting outside and looking at the sky? We can treat ourselves as we treat our clients. We open to our heart and contemplate "to socially distance or not socially distance" (that is the question), "to wear a mask or not wear a mask" (that is another question not unlike the first). We contemplate daily death counts ("to be or not to be"). Reverence and devotion mean taking refuge in our heart at seventy beats per minute and lowering the beats per minute when encountering a roadblock in our mind. Likewise, with nature we can take refuge in the oak tree in our backyard, the rain, or the clouds that make us pause and not think, if only momentarily. In my case, my yard is full of mango trees, and my mind truly stops when I am with them and they are with me.

In Zen, the instruction is to bring the mind into the Hara. We drop our breath down deep into our belly of not knowing. Not knowing involves not thinking, the improvisational dance between our thoughts and their periodic cessation. Not knowing is simply a state of stillness, a stillpoint after we remove the fear. Then we can experience empathetic sadness that links all human beings. It is vitally important to feel sad and feel the warmth and tenderness that this sadness brings to our cardiovascular system and body-mind in general. It softens the mind and creates humility from the not knowing rather than chaos of anger, polarization, and tribalism. This sadness is free from depression and fear.

When the state of dynamic stillness is perceived, it is because there is a gap in between our thoughts. This gap is the space of not thinking. It is both a space from an elemental point of view in Eastern cosmology and a loss of cognition and knowing at an intellectual level. That is why the dynamic stillness is so important and so valuable in the healing process, because we actually experience a suspension of ordinary thinking and knowing. It may last several seconds or several minutes depending on one's aptitude and comfort with such states. Imagine how joyful it could be without so much thinking and pondering so many emotions.

THE NEUTRAL

To complement Dr. Becker's idea that "the therapeutic process does not begin until the will of the patient yields to the will of Primary Respiration," I say the therapeutic process does not ignite until the therapist becomes nonattached to the dynamic stillness and Primary Respiration.

Through this quality of bearing witness without mentally fantasizing a fixed end point or even the next moment of the treatment, the dynamic stillness and PR are liberated from our mental focus and helping intentions. We become present to the suffering of our client. This freedom ignites the self-existing and self-directing Health composed of the potency of PR. We synchronize our attention with nonattachment to any outcome in the therapeutic relationship because the treatment is being given by PR and the dynamic stillness.

The therapist is totally and completely present. She is aware of being in stillness and bearing witness. The combination of one's presence, mental discipline, and synchronization with the present moment is the ground of the practice. When combined with the attitude of nonattachment, the heart ignites. Then the skillful engagement of participating in the wave of Health moving through the therapist and the client becomes unimpeded by structure and function.

The therapist naturally becomes aware of their Self-Neutral. It is perceived through nonattachment to PR in oneself and others. The recognition of the state of dynamic stillness and its implications in the therapeutic process co-emerges with the perception of PR and its therapeutic potency. The implication of the dynamic stillness is that its potency builds the state of not knowing. This is a recognition of something benevolent (what Sutherland called the Breath of Life) that moves through everything unobstructed, including the therapeutic dyad. Thus, the Neutral is a state of bearing witness to the self-directing potency of PR and dynamic stillness in both the client and therapist.

Bearing witness is characterized by a choiceless awareness. Even if thoughts arise there is a distance between the perceiver and the thought that does not solidify the thoughts and ramp them up into a storyline. Thoughts are allowed to simply dissipate as they naturally do anyway. So there is no need to choose between one thought or another, a good thought or a bad thought, a therapeutic thought or a selfish thought. Choiceless awareness is panoramic in that there is a felt sense of all phenomena being interconnected and suspended evenly out to the horizon without one object being more important than another. In such self-knowing awareness the subject, the *perceiver,* is already merged or melted together with the *perceived* object. This type of a Neutral, associated with bearing witness (*perceiving*) can be cultivated by simply waiting and relaxing rather than reacting and responding to thoughts, impulses, and motions. Our thinking, seeing, perceiving hands and mind when in contact with the client are also bearing witness. In many of his lectures, Dr. Jealous exhorted us to "wait, watch, and wonder."

As I mentioned in a previous chapter, I spoke at a biodynamic craniosacral therapy conference in Spain several years ago. I was asked what I thought was the most important part of biodynamic practice. I said that I periodically simply bow my head when I have my hands in contact with the client. It is the gesture of reverence and humility. It is a gesture of recognizing our mutual sanity, wisdom, and generosity intrinsic to each human being. In this gesture of bowing there is a recognition of a sameness with the client. What better way to make a client feel safe than to bow in reverence to their own Health imbued with well-being? It is the preexisting condition inside of each of us. It is already operating under the metaphors that we use of PR and dynamic stillness. This *bow of reverence* is a prayer in which we sacrifice our own helplessness and state of not knowing as a gift of generosity. Such a generosity will set us free emotionally and perceptually. This is *bearing witness*. It is the biodynamic Neutral where the forces of disorder come to a balance point and are free to be moved by the Health of PR and the dynamic stillness. It is a state of openness without attachment for any particular outcome.

When we bear witness to our own pain and suffering with reverence and devotion, a powerful Neutral emerges. The whole world is held in the palms of our hands. The perceiver, the perceiving, and the perceived become a single state of choiceless awareness. It can greatly decrease the amount of wasted time, energy, and technique in trying to fix ourselves and others. When we try to fix, we see each other as broken. Choiceless awareness is an invitation to wholeness. It gives more potency to the spiritual aspects such as the grace, kindness, and compassion of PR and dynamic stillness. Love can be ignited. There is complete freedom to transform what needs to be transformed in one's body and mind without a fixed diagnosis and prognosis but rather synchronizing with the ever-present force of becoming something new rather than retrieving something old. This is the gesture of reverence and humility that radiates an aura of a compassionate Neutral. The Neutral is about nonattachment to the forces of Health and their unique self-direction that we as biodynamic therapists are blessed to observe. Bearing witness is a profound act of self-compassion without which there can be no compassion for others. It is simply a humble bow of the head held until the Health lifts us up.

When we read the latest piece of bad plague news, whichever plague is in front of us, we can simply bow our head in the space of not knowing (stillness) and bearing witness (Neutral). This act ignites the potency of the Health intrinsic within PR and dynamic stillness. We get out of its way. We must understand the dynamic stillness is a metaphor for not knowing, and bearing witness is a metaphor for a Neutral. Again, trust the Tide. Now we must cultivate reverence for the dynamic stillness in its deeper transformational state, the simplicity of not knowing while being totally present for ourselves and others with nonattachment as we bear witness.

HEART IGNITION

Wendy Egyoku Nakao Roshi said, "the underlying intention is that the action that arises be a caring action, which serves everyone and everything, including yourself, in the whole situation" (Nakao 2017). Devotion to the stillpoint and the Neutral kindles the heart of compassion. These give us freedom from the compulsive thinking of trying to accomplish something more or better and ignite the heart from which we can engage the therapeutic process in ourselves and others with self-compassion first. We have reverence for our struggles to accomplish less, to have less compulsive thinking, to have less conceptualizing and fewer polarizing emotions that are unwholesome. To revere this state while not rejecting its opposite is to feel our heartbeat and feel our breath deep down into our belly. This is heart Ignition.

Keep it simple by periodically bowing your head in reverence for the totality of life as it exists inside and outside our body. Gaze at the sky in wonder. Bear witness with your literal heart. That is the center. The movement we sense in the heart is the front of the heart, the stillness is the back of the heart. The mind in the Hara is the pillow upon which the heart normally rests. This is the right placement of our attention. Do not move until the Health of the client requests your attention. This is knowing the potency of heart Ignition. It is the activity of compassionate action in which our hands and mind are moved by a force more powerful than we are—the "other pair of hands."

What a gift we have been given by the masters whose shoulders we all stand upon! I have profound reverence for all my teachers: the osteopaths, the healers, my mother and father, the shamans who initiated me, and all those trying to help me, including the cashier in the grocery store. Everyone I meet on the road is now my teacher. It cannot be otherwise in these holy times. Andrew Taylor Still said: "I love my fellow man, because I see God in his face and in his form." The Buddha said, "Be a light unto yourself." Sutherland called that light the

Breath of Life. That light is in your heart, and it will attract and draw forth your kindness in treating yourself with self-compassion and then extending that skillfully toward your clients. It is a simple radiance. Bow in reverence to turn on that light. Then radiate in all directions. Reverence is the switch of heart Ignition. It releases the bright light of the Breath of Life, the very breath of compassionate action for self and others.

Wendy Egyoku Nakao Roshi said in her article "Hold to the Center, Zen Advice for When Things Blow Up Around You," "Training with the tenets [of not knowing, bearing witness, and compassionate action] is a matter of taking a backward step again and again and continually discerning your internal processes in the midst of acknowledging what is happening around you." Taking a "backward step" is akin to *wait, watch, and wonder*. The idea is to be able to observe how our thoughts and concepts get in the way of empathy and genuine compassion. At the same time we apply mindfulness when we recognize too much thinking and take a backward step to not knowing.

The next chapter, written by Samantha Lotti, will build upon what was learned in this chapter and covers a topic important to the community of biodynamic practitioners regarding how to see our clients. As you read ahead, think about your client at home and how you are performing a session on them and altruistically initiating your compassion to see them.

20
Esoteric Healing

By Samantha Lotti

Samantha Lotti is a University of Chicago graduate and a practicing Taoist with more than a decade of experience working as a healthcare provider. She is a certified and registered biodynamic craniosacral therapist (BCST, RCST®), a National Association of Esoteric Healing trained esoteric healer, a licensed acupuncturist (L.Ac.), and a board-certified herbalist in Oak Park, Illinois. For more information, visit her website, **www.biodynamichealth.com**.

THE BASIC PRINCIPLES OF ESOTERIC HEALING

In order to understand how esoteric healing works as a healing modality, there are some basic principles that need to be understood first.

It is important to begin with defining the word *esoteric*. If you look up the word in the dictionary, you'll find a definition similar to "difficult to be understood" or "designed for . . . the specially initiated alone" (Merriam-Webster's Dictionary online, "Esoteric"). These definitions capture some of the inherent obscurity of the word but leave out the most important facet: that there is something there to be understood. Therefore, "esoteric" means that which is hidden within and is meant to be found.

When putting the above definition in the context of the physical body and healing, "that which is hidden within and is meant to be found" is the Soul. Esoteric healing is the process of bringing forward the inner spiritual meaning of the Soul. That inner spiritual meaning, when brought forward, can then permeate all aspects of the life of the person or animal that is receiving the session.

THE SOUL AS THE HEALER

In esoteric healing the Soul is the healer, the provider is the facilitator, and divine Source is the energy eternally available for healing. The best metaphor for this is the garden hose. The hose is the provider, the water is the divine Source, and the flower is the Soul. If a hose is left on in the middle of a lawn that has flowers on its perimeter, the water may never reach the flowers. If, on the other hand, the hose is picked up by someone and pointed at the flowers, the flowers have the option to absorb as little or as much of the water as they need to thrive.

Put back into the context of esoteric healing, the provider is the facilitator for the work wanting to be done by the Soul. The provider, like the hose, directs the energy of divine Source toward the body of the client, and the Soul of the client decides how much of that divine Source to use for healing. Therefore, healing can only come about if it is in accordance with the will of the Soul of the client. Disease is often part of the client's learning process. Therefore, it is not up to the provider to decide how or when healing occurs; rather to facilitate an opportunity for healing.

CONSENT, ALIGNMENT, AND ATTUNEMENT

To begin a session with a client, the provider must first have consent. This is usually done verbally over the phone, email, or text, but can also be done energetically by more experienced providers. Once consent has been obtained, the provider can proceed with alignment and attunement.

To be in congruence with the will of the Soul of the client, the provider must align to the divine Source and then attune to the client. Aligning allows the provider to move beyond judgment and preferences. Attuning allows the provider to see the client as a spiritual being, greater than the temporary physical form with ephemeral emotional and mental states.

STEPS TO ALIGN AND ATTUNE

To align, the provider becomes aware of the area around their heart, near the center of the sternum, and imagines a stream of light flowing upward to a space just above their head called the Soul Light. This is akin to the concept of the higher self. From there, the light continues to rise toward the divine Source. Once connected, the provider allows that divine spiritual energy to descend back down into the middle of their chest and into their Heart Center. Once settled, the provider allows for that energy to expand and rise again to the space between their eyebrows on their forehead called the Ajna. From there the energy is focused and descends into their hands, which then become the tools for healing. The Ajna is in the location of the third eye, but it is not the third eye. It is an energy center that aligns with brain energy centers and chakra centers to balance them. In this case it is being used as a place to funnel divine Source energy to allow the provider to do healing work.

To attune, the provider imagines a stream of light flowing from their Soul Light to the Soul Light of the client. Once divine Source and the Souls of both provider and client are connected, the provider asks that healing be in accordance with the will of the client's Soul. By asking that healing be in accordance with the will of the client's Soul, the provider relinquishes any credit they might want to take in the healing process. The provider becomes the garden hose through which the energy of divine Source can flow, and the provider accepts that what will unfold during the session is greater than them and beyond human understanding.

SESSION

A session begins with a check-in over the phone, in person, or over video chat with the client. Once the check-in is complete, verbal permission to do esoteric healing is obtained, and the provider aligns and attunes to the client. The client is instructed to sit or lay down quietly for about thirty minutes while the provider does esoteric healing.

During the session the provider is assessing the client as if they were in front of them. The provider evaluates all the energy centers and their minors to see which need work, and then the provider balances—in accordance with the will of the Soul of the client—the centers that are weak or excessive. The provider is able to evaluate the effectiveness of the balancing of energy centers by assessing centers before balancing them and then reevaluating after they are balanced.

Once the provider has concluded their balancing, they close the session and offer a blessing. The provider then either calls the client again to discuss findings or emails the client with findings. The entire session from beginning to end generally takes between thirty to sixty minutes.

THE PROVIDER

Esoteric healing can be done by anyone with the proper training. The key to being an effective provider is a personal meditation practice from which, through discipline, the emotions and body are calmed, the mind is quieted, made receptive and alert, and the personality is integrated so that listening stillness can be found and the intuitive senses awakened. The National Association of Esoteric Healing has qualified instructors teaching regular classes throughout the year for those interested in learning esoteric healing and becoming a provider. The certification process takes a year to complete and is pursued by those interested after four introductory classes have been successfully completed.

ESOTERIC HEALING IS AN ALLOWING PROCESS
THAT CANNOT BE FORCED

Through aligning and attuning, which is akin to prayer, the provider makes the energy of divine Source available to the client's Soul. As the flow in the client's energy centers is harmonized through balancing, the energy of the client's Soul is freed and change can occur not only in the body but in all aspects of the client's life. Esoteric healing is an allowing process. With true loving discernment and pure intentions, miracles can occur.

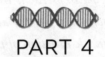

PART 4

THE STILLNESS

Inner Healing Arts and Cosmology

21

The Four Foundations of Stillness

On this nondual [spiritual] path, virtue is the effect, not the cause; the ultimate compassionate response is whatever action optimizes presence—loving-kindness is the automatic function of primal awareness.

KEITH DOWMAN, *THE FLIGHT OF THE GARUDA: THE DZOGCHEN TRADITION OF TIBETAN BUDDHISM*

THERAPEUTIC INTENTION

Dr. Becker said that the patient's body and mind contain an *inherent treatment plan*. For the inherent treatment plan to manifest, the following discernments are necessary in the biodynamic toolkit:

- Perception of a constant interchange of a background with different degrees of stillness and a foreground of Primary Respiration and then reversing
- Acknowledgment of uncertainty and not knowing as a portal to the mystery of healing
- Mindfulness to prevent attention capture and establish nonreferential awareness
- Heart-centered interoception and empathetic nonattachment while remaining totally present for the client
- Sensing the transparency of PR extending to the horizon

The longing for these qualities begins with integrating contemplative practice into biodynamic practice. It is a contemplation of body-mind unification. The therapist slows down her body and mind before a client arrives, turns off the cell phone, and stops looking at the internet for at least fifteen minutes prior to seeing a client. I will sometimes only allow five minutes between technology and client, but not often. The client then comes in and expresses himself in terms of what his symptoms and his pain are asking in the moment. A biodynamic cardiovascular therapist remembers that the parts and functions that lack vitality in a client's body also carry or have the capacity of expressing intrinsic Health.

Health is the potency of PR. It is none other than *chi* as discussed in classical Chinese and Japanese medicine. PR (on its level of chi) is doing its job. It is not in pain, nor is it suffering in any way. As therapists we contact the part in ourselves and in our clients that does not change its movement, that is slow and capable of stopping and interchanging with preexisting stillness. It is the commonality of this Health that we all share. This is the union of stillness and PR. It is the prescription for Health, the potency of its inherent treatment plan.

The inherent treatment plan in biodynamic practice is simply my perception of stillness and PR. PR is constantly writing the script of therapeutic experience, and I listen for it in stillness. It is the sound of space. I sit still and calm my mind. I open my perception to a deep place of silence and quiescence in myself that is equally suspended out to the horizon. Thoughts come and go all the time like leaves floating on the wind. I spend the majority of time during a session listening with unfocused attention to the dance of PR and stillness in my body. I must also relate to stillness or its lack in my mind. A calm mind in the therapeutic process starts with reducing mental thoughts, perception of the office space, the environment of four walls, a ceiling, roof, windows, and its principal tenant, dynamic stillness.

The stillness function involves setting an intention. Can I approach the client without needing or wanting anything from him? Can I let go of expectations and judgment and enter a still place of uncertainty and not knowing without labeling my inner experience good or bad, right or wrong? There is no conceptual goal or purpose in this activity, especially *fixing* the client. In other words, there are progressive stages to entering the felt sense of uncertainty and not knowing of my body-mind. It is a practice of nonattachment to thoughts and outcomes like getting better and helping the client improve, which interfere with the inherent treatment plan.

Stillness is often a suspect activity in any culture that places more significance on fixing the client and removing symptoms rather than discovering the altruistic intention of our hearts and integrating loving kindness and compassion into clinical practice. Stillness is the ground of compassion. PR is the movement of compassion. Even at a molecular level, cells in the body cannot function properly without a brief stillpoint. Conscious awareness of stillness can provide a rich, intimate contact with the reality in the present moment of the atomic chart living underneath our skin and the atomic chart we derive from externally. Thoughts of the past or future are distractions from being present in the now. The following statement is used in Zen: *immediate yourself or wreck yourself.* The present moment is the basis for total body safety and involves what I call the *four foundations of stillness.*

FIRST FOUNDATION

Body Sensation and Interoceptive Awareness

The first foundation of perceiving stillness is *body sensation and interoceptive awareness.* I open to and take notice of personal body sensations in the extrinsic musculoskeletal system, including its proprioception (noticing the space between the natural world and my inner organs). This quality of contact allows for the intrinsic authority of my muscles, bones, and fascia to speak to me directly. By paying attention to body sensations rather than ignoring them, I develop friendliness toward my own physical nature, the predicament of gravity, and being rooted in the earth. In this way, I share the same orthopedic sensorium of the client. Stillness of body is a settling into both body sensations and at the same time remaining curiously nonattached to the ocean of sensation in my body. We truly inhabit a fluid body, and the fascia that holds us together is intrinsically like seaweed. The body and its sensations are waves in the fluid body.

In this way of experience, I begin to gain *moral independence* from the mainstream by trusting the felt sense of my muscles and bones. My body knows the difference between right and wrong if I listen deeply. Sensations need to be unlinked from strong emotions. Emotions need to be unlinked from compulsive thoughts. It involves noticing and appreciating all the senses as they try to average all the input coherently. Everything settles in the body, including gravity pulling the mind down into the body and abdomen. It is said in Zen to "bring the mind into the Hara (abdomen)." This is a breath that continues down to where the abdominal aorta bifurcates into the common iliac arteries. Our mind needs to connect to the origin of our life close to our umbilicus.

Interoceptive awareness is a deeper sensory connection to my inner life in the viscera and organs of the body. This expands *the mind in the Hara* practice. Each organ expresses an urge that becomes conscious from breathing to eating, from urinating to defecating, to a heartbeat that is falling in love to a heartbeat that feels rage. I pay attention to the inside of my body, especially the *potency* of my heartbeat. PR is merged with the stillness in the back of the heart and, together with interoceptive awareness of the heartbeat, empathy for self and others is generated. It all rests upon the breath in the Hara.

Stillness does not cause PR or vice versa. Biodynamics does not incorporate a hierarchical model of causation. *It is only a model of how, not why.* How does body experience happen moment to moment? Causation leads to compulsive cognitions, a mental wasteland. They dance together in harmony in and around the body—a synchronized union of equality. PR is not interested in the why, only the how. Body sensations are constantly shifting and may start to settle when I maintain a balance of internal awareness and breathing into the Hara. I calm down physically, mentally, and emotionally with conscious breathing into the Hara and conscious awareness of my heartbeat as a unified whole. A body and mind at rest learn that rest and arousal are cyclical and a manifestation of the whole. This is contemplative practice. As I sit in stillness with the client, I become receptive to my body first and then receptive to impressions from my client's body. A calm mind can then begin to rest in the Hara, allowing the heart to rest on top of the abdomen. This is called embryonic breathing, a return to origins.

SECOND FOUNDATION

Nonattachment

The second foundation of stillness is *nonattachment*. It is a sense of the arising and falling away of thoughts and ideas like leaves floating down from a tree in the fall. I touch the basic state of my mind and feeling tone in my body and let go of it gracefully with a slow exhalation. This is known as the *act of stillness*. I repeat this act over and over because it requires effort to create an open space for thoughts, feelings, and emotions to simply be without interfering with them. I consciously observe my inner and outer experience without bias. This is recognizing *nonattached awareness*. I harmonize with the stillness by observing my experience without mental or cognitive expectation. Imagine sitting in a chair looking outside a window at traffic going by on the street. The traffic is the mind filled with thoughts. But I sit and observe them without contact emotionally. I just observe the traffic pattern come and go, especially the gaps where no cars come by.

- I distance from my thoughts, turning my sensory attention gently without judging them as good or bad.
- I stop cognitively naming everything that comes into my senses and my mind.
- I return my breath to the Hara.
- I sense my heartbeat.
- I attune to the space in the environment around me (four walls, a floor, and a ceiling).
- I attune to the world of nature outside the office (the window).

Repeat forever: No thought, idea, concept, belief, perception, spiritual insight, or fearful image is too big or too small to get an exemption. All such phenomena are thoughts and are consciously treated as *equal*. Thoughts rise and fall constantly and leave no trace, "like the imprint of a bird in the sky." Thoughts are not the enemy, and like a river they just need to flow unrestricted into open space before they become concepts or compulsive.

Touch and go is a stillness skill. I silently and briefly acknowledge being distracted or entertained by a thought stream. I touch it and then I drop it—I let go simply by recognizing the thought without grasping it or, if necessary, I shift attention to breathing into the Hara. I return to the midline of stillness by resting my mind on one or the other of my senses. Each sense has an object of cognition, but there is too much data from all the senses, so I do not cognitively label what any senses are reporting. I return to the home ground of my breathing in and out of the Hara. My breathing integrates all the senses in my body. It gives time for the senses to average the input into safety and open awareness.

My body contacts the chair on which I am seated with my feet on the ground. I feel gravity compel my body to the earth as I sit like a mountain. I regularly and repeatedly touch and go because *I am the host of this inner and outer perceptual simulation rather than an unaware guest*. To be the host of my inner perception requires effort at noticing my disconnection from the present moment of the therapeutic relationship. It is a practice of harmonizing with the stillness that stretches from the horizon all the way to the back of my heart and through it. This is known as *resting the mind in nonattachment*. This follows after resting the mind in the Hara. The heart must stay nonattached but responsive.

Mindfulness is a metaphor for this variety of stillness. Our attention as human beings and therapists is now being subjected to continuous partial attention by the constant use of electronic devices and the time-killing dimension of social media and all forms of media in general. Our attention is constantly being captured and held hostage by frivolous things, especially the rampant falsehoods that permeate the cultural landscape with its deep polarization. *Mindfulness is that which prevents attention capture.* It is the act of noticing being distracted and the experience of returning to nonreferential objectless awareness such as the dynamic stillness. Thus, mindfulness is both an act and an experience free from thinking about it. But it must be cultivated through the type of contemplation I am suggesting here, which would also include a variety of forms of *wisdom meditation,* as it is called in Buddhism.

Mindfulness is paying careful attention to the moment-by-moment experience of all my body's senses, the client's body, and the perception of both of us together in the office space as an interconnected yet differentiated whole. I pay attention to sensations, inner tensions and pressures, mental and emotional desires for myself, and what my hands perceive on the client. I learn gradually to recognize them, sense them, and relax my perception into open awareness. I connect to my different senses one by one. I might let all my thoughts go out into space as I exhale. Or if there is a mental struggle with a particular family story line that moment, I switch attention to other senses. I listen more intently to sound. I look more intently at what my eyes are seeing. Mindfulness is sometimes described as being a bus driver, and all the people in the seats behind you are just thoughts. Keep your eyes (metaphorically) on the road in front of you.

As mentioned, thoughts are not the enemy. The *thought police* are not necessary to manage my mind, whether alone or with the client, especially telling me where my hands need to go next on the client. I always wait until I hear the same thought about hand placement whispering to me three times before shifting there. And sometimes my hands are taken by PR to a different location absent of cognition. The thought police are especially fond of telling me, "What a waste of time this biodynamic stillness is; it's time to get doing something that will really fix the client."

Patience requires effort at this level of stillness. Effort is not totally indulging in mental fantasies, projections, or the thought police. Effort requires the potency of shifting one's attention back to one's Hara and then being nonattached in the heart. It is about the potency of transparency in the heart. No thought is so important that I cannot let go of it. You choose to stop holding on to the thought stream. You choose to do it and let go. This is becoming the host of your experience rather than being a subservient guest following a protocol.

This is the essence of relaxation. This is how I move my sensory attention within my body to stabilize a jumpy mind that acts like a frog.

Frog mind is a mind that jumps around—speedy or fixated on something needing to happen or something that just happened or something that needs to happen later at home. The past and future are eliminated. Even the present moment is eliminated by resting in open awareness. Lazy mind is a daydreamer and requires effort to descend from the clouds of dissociation and return to the earth and feel its gravity. I also call this *hangover mind* as the mind seems to be in a stupor unable to ground in the body. When I have this aspect of mind, I tend to stare at a sacred object in my office in order to move attention to another sensory organ.

I must sacrifice my erratic thoughts for the sake of a safe therapeutic container. I sacrifice my frog mind or my lazy mind by paying attention to my breathing and heartbeat. However, I need to know which quality of mind I am inhabiting when I start a session with a client. The mind, defined here as the sum of our thoughts and conceptualizations, is a sensory organ just as the other five senses. The point is that to have greater tactile acuity and perception of the Tide, I need to *gather my mind* at the beginning of a session and recognize which type of mind I have in that moment: frog or lazy. Then I move to the other senses, the breath, and the heart to allow the brain and body to average the senses together in favor of the client and my perception of the Tide in myself and the client. The mind is not reliable when it receives most of my attention in a session or in life. Be nonattached to the mind of thoughts.

I attend gently, resisting being compulsively diverted to the mundane world of desire or spacing out into the clouds of confusion in my mind. I shift my attention into open elemental space inside and outside. I can touch, however briefly, nonattachment to my mental-emotional story lines. I can see through them periodically as all the objects of senses are suspended equally in a vast field of stillness. The presence and potency of PR is then able to reveal itself as the inner garden that is swept clean, however briefly. The Health is revealed.

THIRD FOUNDATION

The Neutral of the Present Moment

The third foundation of stillness is the Neutral of the present moment. This level of stillness is the ability to recognize how states of mind and body can enter a therapeutic harmony, a balance point for Health to manifest. The biodynamic session is a three-step *rite of passage* in which the Neutral represents the first stage of establishing safety for PR to establish its priority in that moment. The ability to consciously recognize whether I am in frog mind or lazy mind is necessary to ignite a Neutral. The Neutral is a properly plowed sense field ready to be planted with PR. The stress levels in me and the client slowly harmonize with the priorities of PR. One moment I am mentally wandering, and suddenly I snap back without effort to the present moment into this field of mental relaxation, potential, and possibility. I call it the gentle whiplash of mindfulness. This quality, this state of perception and physiology after calming the mind, is called the Neutral and contains the essence, the vast potency of the present moment. The Neutral happens naturally. It is the instinctual progression of a biodynamic session. It is the natural habitat of mind underneath the frog mind and lazy mind. It is nonconceptual, nontemporal, and nonmoving, just an empty field of rich soil and great potential. The Neutral of the present moment is the stillness that expresses the potency of the Health.

My body and mind are instinctually oriented to the potency of stillness, silence, and open awareness free from the constant mental labeling of sensory objects. The Neutral is a stillness in the heart without an observer. It is the observer. It is a union, a melting together, a merging with the direct experience of being centered in the back of the heart. It is a field of intelligence and a portal to the therapeutic priorities of PR. The Neutral of the present moment is smart. This is part of the hardwiring of a settled mind to naturally recognize the Neutral—being totally present for myself and the client with nonattachment. From this place of the therapeutic Neutral of the present moment, PR is free to choose where to place its "unerring potency." I forget this innate ability frequently in sessions, however, so it requires repetitive attunement practice to recover it. Being patient and aware of thoughts thinning out invokes the Neutral. The present moment is about relaxation without any expectation. And it will shift just as the Tide does. I evenly suspend my attention between a place deep inside my abdomen and heart and as far out into space as possible, the metaphorical horizon. My umbilical cord stretches into this void. I abide in the space of this joyful moment. The Neutral of the present moment brings therapeutic clarity.

The Neutral begins the biodynamic rite of passage such that PR is now free to Ignite and direct its potency free of clinician interference or attempts to guide it. Ignition follows the entire cardiovascular system, the midline of the subtle body, and leads on to the void for renewal. The renewal brings about the third phase of incorporating as a spiritual altruistic being. This is the Health.

FOURTH FOUNDATION

Clarity and Renewal

The fourth foundation of stillness is clarity. The Neutral permeated with stillness brings clarity of the activity of PR. There is a deepening of the qualities of attention, mindfulness, and open awareness. It means slowing down the whole life process and noticing each part of PR and its exquisite precision and unique sequence of movements in and around myself and the client as a unified two-person biology. This means creating what Jim Jealous calls a metapause. I notice each effect of the interchange of stillness and PR into the foreground and background of my perception of the Neutral and the client's experience. PR eventually fades to the background when it is finished, and stillness revisits the foreground. Background and foreground shift places in their own tempo. The world is breathing through us and the therapeutic process. This is the Tide according to Dr. Sutherland.

The stillness inherent in the Neutral involves being patient for nonconceptual clarity to arise in longer pauses between thoughts. Clarity is knowing what to accept and what to reject in managing the therapeutic container with the client. It is instinctual without interpretation. There can be one or more Neutrals expressed in a single session. Many sensory impressions come to us through our hands, hearts, and minds. Some are therapeutically relevant, and others are not. Our flight simulator for helping others always seems to throw in a few side distractions to test us. Biodynamic perception of the Tide clarifies the direction of the inherent treatment plan of PR. Is the therapeutic process being advanced with PR following the Neutral? Is the Tide expanding into your being or away from your being? Clarity is spacious, open, and sharp, almost to the point of being irritating or even boring at times because of the desire to fix the client, which is a distraction.

There is no doubt, however, about where to go next with my hands and my perceptual process if I am patient. They are always guided by the constant interchange of stillness and PR from the back of the heart to the horizon. But I must be patient while in the Neutral of the present moment for as long as possible for such clarity to arrive. I practice sitting in stillness with my client as a specific biodynamic skill so I can begin to clearly recognize the interchange of stillness and PR naturally. There are moments when giving a session to a client that the fog of mind lifts and I am able to freely observe how my mind and body, the client, the office, and the natural world are suspended in a vast web of interconnectedness that extends to eternity. This is clarity. It is nonduality happening all the time. It is simple, direct perception frequently arising during a session and everyday life if the therapist can calm her mind and rest evenly in the Neutral, into the heart and/or out to the horizon. And sometimes I move my hands to an inert body location, which I recognize quickly and move on without self-reflection on being wrong. The Tide does not make mistakes when it moves my hands.

The hormone oxytocin promotes processes of multisensory integration, the so-called "glue of the senses"—the way the world typically presents itself to us as a coherent picture rather than as multiple distinct streams of sense data. It has been well known for years that safe manual therapy releases oxytocin in clients. Multisensory integration, in turn, is at the root of our sense of body ownership, the feeling that most take for granted—that our body is ours. Being still and practicing mindfully promotes our senses being glued together. The brain is like a flight simulator that pilots must practice in to maintain their license to fly. The brain is making a simulation of perceived reality from all the sensory input. It is an enormous amount of data constantly being sorted out by the brain, heart, and Hara. The brain is attempting to average all the senses together, which requires good sleep, stillness practice, and mental calm. It also requires well-bounded physical touch from loved ones and professional manual therapists. The flight simulator works best with the fuel of mindfulness!

I breathe in and then I breathe out and naturally rest momentarily in the pause between exhalation and inhalation. There is a gap right at the end of exhalation, and it is connected to the gap in between thoughts. This is the gap where I place my attention for a second before the force and potency of inhalation moves under the control of PR. From that place of letting go of mind and body, if even for a second with each breath, I drop into a void of nonthought and nonself. The void is the center (fulcrum) of stillness in the back of the heart extending out to the edge of the universe. The void is the place of renewal in biodynamic practice. The client may appear to be asleep but may actually be accessing their original state of embryonic wholeness. For the therapist, the result is clarity of perception if only momentarily. For the client, accessing their original state of wholeness is at the very least refreshing and at most transformative. It is called Ignition. Undoubtedly, this is why Dr. Sutherland said that reverence must be a part of every session. Renewal is not about feeling refreshed at the end of a session. Rather, renewal is the sense of having been suspended in a nonfearful black void and completely rebuilt from stem to stern in the body. It is a breeze of delight freely given by the Tide. It is what makes biodynamic practice so precious to me.

Finally, renewal is the present moment of eternity. Eternity is in the present moment of stillness, and the present moment is the supreme spiritual teacher. The Neutral slows down the mental process of jumping all over the place in my body and out of my body until inside and outside melt together. Wholeness is the smallest subdivision of life according to Dr. Jealous. I invite the possibility of renewal into my life and that of the client without any expectation or attachment to outcome.

ALTRUISM

I wait for stillness to move into the foreground of my inner bodily and mental life once PR fades to the background. This is a constant, rhythmic, balanced interchange of the Tide moving back and forth. There is a settling as I deepen into a clear experience. This is very personal, unique to the moment, and direct. Stillness begets stillness, the effort of being patient with open awareness and mindfulness. Mindfulness is both the act and the experience of returning and resting in the present moment from wandering thoughtlessly and recreationally (see figs. 21.1–21.2). Mindfulness requires effort (being the host as opposed to the guest of my mental and emotional experience). It is precise, and awareness is panoramic and choiceless. I do this practice with the intention to be of service to myself and all others; this is Buddhist practice.

Unfortunately, mindfulness is now part of the corporate capitalism structure to have workers become compliant and disengaged from speaking out against repressive corporate work strategies. We not only have a corporate food takeover of the body, we now have a corporate mindfulness takeover of the mind. For an excellent examination of this takeover, please look at *McMindfulness: How Mindfulness Became the New Capitalist Spirituality* by Ronald Purser. The original intention of mindfulness in terms of what the Buddha taught is altruism and moral engagement in these times of moral distress. By doing so I develop compassion, the basis of which is nonattachment to an outcome for self and other. Yet compassion at the same time involves my total being. I am totally present, lucidly still in body, mind, and heart for myself and the client. I recognize thoughts but am not swept away by them.

The union of stillness with PR is the core perception in BCVT. This is nothing other than the Tide that our teachers have pointed to. I am on the scent of the sacred with these four foundations of stillness. They are the harmonies of Health and its potency. The focus is on watching the arising process of body

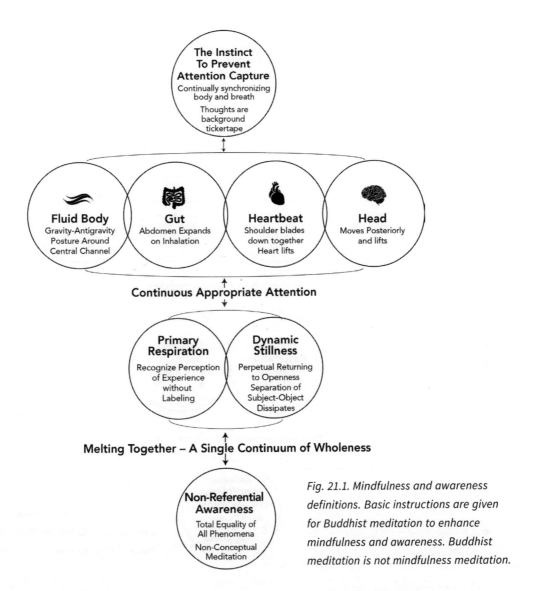

Fig. 21.1. Mindfulness and awareness definitions. Basic instructions are given for Buddhist meditation to enhance mindfulness and awareness. Buddhist meditation is not mindfulness meditation.

sensations and mental thoughts, seeing through them clearly and letting them go as a kind of sacrifice or purification of our intention to help others and be of service to humanity. It is a practice of renunciation. The Neutral of the present moment is entered like the mystery it is. You cannot solve a mystery, but you can enter it. This is what ignites the biodynamic therapeutic process. The heart naturally becomes centered in its inherent kindness and awakens the subtle emotions of compassion and love. The Tide of PR and stillness is not given in a session of biodynamic work like turning on a light switch. PR and its healing priorities are gradually uncovered by the quality of the therapist's stillness.

I am carefully observing my own internal experience like a Swiss watchmaker. I experience my senses, including my mind sense, as a constantly changing process (automatic shifting) and impermanent process. This creates a heart-centered

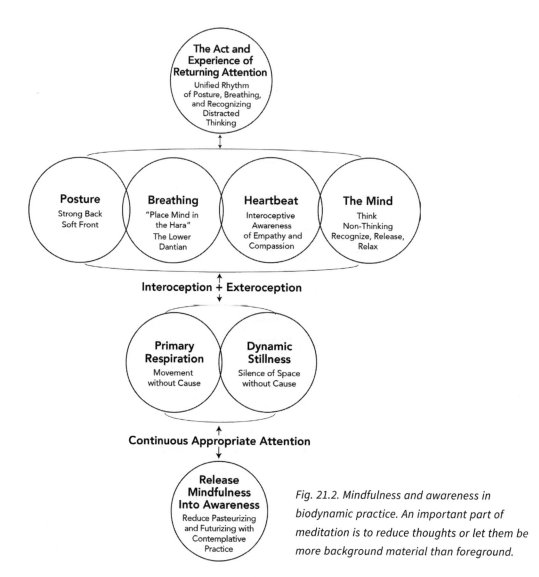

Fig. 21.2. Mindfulness and awareness in biodynamic practice. An important part of meditation is to reduce thoughts or let them be more background material than foreground.

harmony between the client and me. The right hemispheres of our brains become synchronized with one another. We share a common umbilical cord. The client's inherent treatment plan is invoked by the skills in the four foundations of stillness, by respect and reverence, by prayer and a contemplative attitude. This sets the stage for the delicious Tide to manifest its unerring potency and for change to take place outside of my control. It is the movement of Health that has no beginning and no end. It is the movement of wholeness that is in direct proportion to stillness. Thus, stillness and PR are merged and in harmony all the time because the "Health is never lost."

22

Breathing, Meditation, and Practicing the Foundations of Stillness

May all beings be parted from clinging and aversion—feeling
close to some and distant from others.
May they win the bliss that is especially sublime.
May they find release from the sea of unbearable sorrow.
May they never be parted from freedom's true joy.

THE BUDDHA

Meditation is a quintessential self-regulation practice. It is also what we do in biodynamic practice. The senses decompress and begin to harmonize with each other. The reality simulator in the brain clarifies like letting a sediment-filled glass of water settle when left alone. All the senses have an opportunity to average each other out as some work harder than others in our daily life, especially the brain. Like the gut needing time for intermittent fasting from eating food, the brain also needs intermittent fasting from sensory stimulation during our waking hours. Our brain and body cannot process the amount of sensory data coming into it every millisecond, especially while we are awake. Consequently the brain and body must make a simulation, an approximation of reality on a moment-to-moment basis. The flight simulator in our brain and body needs to access the programming for calm weather. Meditation is training for being more fully in the present moment with calmness and ease. It supports the notion of being in the biodynamic Neutral. This chapter covers aspects of meditation, including breathing and stillness, so that the brain (as simulator of reality) has time to sort out sensory input. After all, so much of a hands-on ministry is the perception of the therapist.

BREATHING

When I sit and begin to attend to my client, I bring my attention to my breath. Physiological change process in the body depends on natural organismic breathing, which is thwarted in the contemporary client for numerous reasons. The internet is awash in breathing techniques from Navy Seals to spiritual gurus. Yoga classes have their pranayama with every asana; Zen extols the virtues of sitting like a mountain and breathing like a river. Neurophysiologists tell us the importance of respiratory sinus arrhythmia, inhalation and exhalation influencing the autonomic nervous system. Vagal maneuvers to stimulate the vagus nerve with breathing are also popular these days. But how is this taught? For the most part, the missing ingredient is the direct awareness of the interior of the body. But what is breathing (see fig. 22.1), and especially what moves during inhalation?

The motion of breathing starts at conception in our physical body. Breathing starts at the beginning of our universe. There is expansion, there is contraction. This motion is associated with the element of wind or air in Eastern medical systems. To know the *breath* deeply is to sense its subtlety both inside and out.

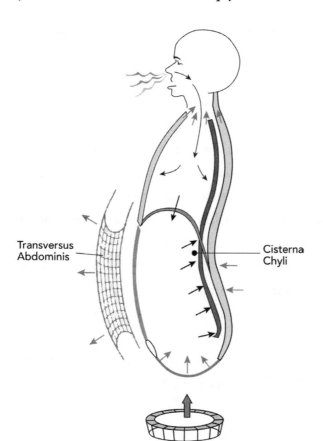

Transversus
Abdominis

Cisterna
Chyli

Fig. 22.1. The inhalation cycle of breathing into the lower dantian, also called belly breathing. The abdomen expands, the pelvic floor lifts, and the lower back is toned in its lordotic curve, which moves the lymph appropriately. Exhalation allows the process to reverse effortlessly and improve vagal tone.

Eastern medical systems have three levels of embodied meaning associated with the wind element: the ordinary physical body, the subtle body, and the very subtle body. All three levels are a unified whole interconnected with the natural world all the way to the beginning of the cosmos. Each breath is the original breath, and this book provides access to such originality consciously.

The breath of air in-forms and out-forms the shape of our body from the top of the head to the bottom of the feet with the action of the respiratory diaphragm and associated muscles of respiration, such as the transversus abdominus in the abdomen, the intercostals, and the scalenes in the neck. When we inhale, the ordinary body receives this supply of oxygen distributed via pulmonary circulation and the blood and, of course, the removal of carbon dioxide when we exhale. Oxygen delivery and carbon dioxide uptake happens in every capillary of the body. Even a single capillary is breathing. This ordinary breath is the favorite target of stress-reduction strategies and breathing techniques from different schools and teachers, such as holotropic breath work, Reichian therapy, bioenergetics, and rebirthing. However, these and other breathing techniques are principally designed for release-based catharsis or emotional release. This was a phase that body-centered therapies went through in the decades of the seventies and eighties. With the enormous popularity of hatha yoga, pranayama techniques gradually introduced a more subtle approach as emotional release with breathing became out of phase with the evolving needs of the contemporary mind and body.

Inner, Belly, and Slow Breathing

These three strategies or breathing techniques evolve slowly by gaining an inner subtle felt sense. I call this the transition from the outer ordinary breath to the inner subtle breath. The popularity of mindfulness meditation helped usher in this needed degree of subtlety by consciously paying attention to the body breathing. I ask myself "What moves?" as I inhale and exhale. The inner subtle breath is a directed breath that moves in relation to specific anatomy, such as up and down the front of the spine or the aorta. Sensing the temperature and movement of the air coming in and out of the nostrils is a mindfulness of the inner breath skill.

The inner breath becomes what I call the belly breath or, in Taoism, embryonic breathing. This is the directed placement of the breath in the lower abdomen to engage the transversus abdominus muscle. This muscle originates from its interdigitation with the respiratory diaphragm, the costal arch, the anterior superior iliac spine and inguinal ligament, as well as associated fascia in the lower back, specifically the lumbar fascia. Gradually the diaphragm–transversus abdominus muscle relationship is sensed followed by relaxation of the peritoneal cavity, which holds all the intestines via the fascia of the mesentery. Finally the pelvic floor can soften while breathing. I recommend Bill Harvey's book *Breathing, Mudras and Meridians: Direct Experience of Embodiment* for the most comprehensive treatment of breathing and the subtle body.

This muscle and related fascia expand during inhalation and relax during exhalation; this is the ordinary breath. It is the normal and natural breath—the belly breath. At a subtle level, however, the breath into the lower abdomen is directed at the lower dantian located anterior to the bifurcation of the abdominal aorta into the common iliac arteries. This is the area of the hypogastric plexi of the autonomic nervous system. This place can be visualized as an embryo or a large pearl of translucent light the size of a golf ball. It is the bottom end of the central channel of the subtle body. The subtle breath accumulates around the lower dantian and with training gradually enters the central channel to purify spiritual blockages in the subtle body, principally the ignorance of reality in general according to the Buddhist tradition. The central channel is the location of one's karmic ignorance requiring rituals of purification to be free of ignorance. In Zen, belly breathing is called "placing the mind in the Hara." The Hara is the abdomen, and the mind is the interoceptive awareness of the lower dantian, a side effect of the breath.

The inner breath and the belly breath lead organically to the slow breath or, more purposefully, by techniques such as coherent breathing and techniques associated with changing heart rate variability, respiratory sinus arrhythmia, and vagal tone. The inner, belly, and slow breath transition one's bodily attention through interoceptive awareness to the so-called subtle body in Eastern medicine. Here, the wind element takes on different aspects not only for the physical wellness of a person but also for their spiritual self-regulation and sacred well-being. The original winds existed at the beginning of the universe and at the moment of conception. They are still present. This is the birth of a whole phenomenology of breathing necessary for the contemporary client to experience self-knowing awareness of reality. The starting point is the therapist's own attention to their breathing. Every time I change hand positions while treating, I return my attention to my Hara. The essence of biodynamic practice is always returning to the Hara and then the heart. The therapist is constantly self-regulating for safety and empathy to manifest. The client naturally attunes to the safety and empathy of the therapist.

The subtle body is the world of:

1. Channels (meridians, central and lateral channels, water and life channels)
2. Energy-winds (different levels of chi)
3. Vital essences (different levels of Primary Respiration, or Lüng as it is called in Tibetan medicine or Vayu in Sanskrit, moving in the central channel)

The central channel—detailed in texts on the kundalini phenomenon, the chakra system, the three dantians, and the great ocean of chi circulating through the physical and spiritual channels of the body—is the most basic and important structure and function of the subtle body. Both the ordinary and subtle bodies operate with the common principles of nourishment and cleansing both metabolically and spiritually. However, the very subtle body is the already purified body that needs no fixing. Metaphors such as Buddha-nature, clear light, satori, enlightenment, and so forth indicate the true preexisting condition of a body, mind, and spirit already being unified. To uncover the very subtle body there is also a need for cleansing through skills and techniques found throughout this book relating to the ordinary and subtle bodies.

We are in need as a culture of a contemporary type of pranayama practice, a bridging from the old techniques to the new contemporary demands on the body and mind—a practice that opens rather than tightens the body and a practice that allows each person to discover their own ordinary body breathing mindfully. Each person will have their own unique style of transitioning to the subtle and expressing their individual aptitude for purification. Purification or cleansing is necessary to see reality clearly. That is the goal, so to speak, when a subtle breathing practice becomes a meditation on wisdom once the stress levels in the client's autonomic nervous system have stabilized.

It must be a breathing skill that is also trauma informed, as upward of 25 percent of students learning different breathing techniques can have side effects associated with overactivation or underactivation of the autonomic nervous system. So great care must be taken when we find the inner breath, then when we drop our breath into the abdomen and finally begin to experience the slow breath. It is its own intelligence, capable of knowing and directing the embodied spiritual process as it unfolds in its own time and inner body place for everyone. Chapter 34 provides a larger context for breathing. We are being breathed. We are not the ones breathing. Inner, belly, and slow are the breathing stages to practice in a biodynamic session. They are the rudder on the thera-peutic ship sailing the fluid body. At the same time we attend periodically to the client's breath. Synchronizing the pelvic and respiratory diaphragms can be done in every session to integrate any change process taking place as a result of the session.

CHOOSING A MEDITATION CUSHION

Most everyone in the East, where meditation developed over the millennia, sat on the floor or the ground outside with minimal cushioning. The ratio of hip-knee angle and lordosis of the lumbar and cervical spine is essential in the meditation posture. Contemporary practitioners or those who are aging like myself need to sit higher above the floor, such as sitting on a chair or the edge of a bed. If the hips are located higher above the floor, then the knees must remain several degrees below the plane of the hips. A seiza bench cre-ates a greater angle and sometimes increases that angle dramatically. The gauge for that angle, regardless of the sitting height above the floor, is going to be the ease of the diaphragms and the ease of belly breathing, which generates the antigravity effect of the water element. This includes the other two types of cushions typically used for meditation. The rectangular cushion is usually six to seven inches high and can be supplemented with additional cushioning with different heights. Wooden rectangular meditation benches with cushions can be up to thirteen or fourteen inches tall. The rectangular types of seating cushions and benches prevent the knees from contacting the mat. If the feet and ankles are on the mat, it will suffice if the lumbar and cervical spine is stable toward lordosis. The other popular type of cushion, the round cushion, makes it very easy for the knees to contact the ground, and they also come in different heights up to nine inches.

Since I have had both of my knees surgically repaired and have a spinal stenosis in my low back, the lower my pelvis is to the ground with one or both knees on the mat, the quicker one or both of my legs will fall asleep. That requires stretching one or both legs periodically during meditation. Finding the sweet spot for longer periods of meditation without moving them is an ongoing exploration. On the one hand, it is valuable to maintain a posture with minimal body movement; at the same time being able to make micro-adjustments in one's posture during meditation practice is necessary. It becomes a balance, especially not moving the hands to rub every itch or to swat at a fly that drives you crazy. This plays out in clinical practice with great attention placed on the therapist's posture and comfort. In this way, biodynamic practice becomes meditation practice. How can it be anything else?

THE FIVE ELEMENTS

The practice of meditation was developed through the millennia in Eastern cultures and as a function of Eastern medical systems such as ayurveda, Tibetan medicine, and Taoism, whose understanding of the human body was based on the five elements. To experience and deepen into zazen (Chinese-Japanese) or shamatha-vipashyana (Indian-Tibetan) styles of meditation, it is helpful to incorporate meditation instruction based on the five elements.

The understandings of the elements and meditation form the basis of an emerging need for the contemporary client to be viewed through these lenses. These lenses, similar to the diopters that an eye doctor uses to sharpen and clarify one's glasses, are necessary in order for the client to enter a different and ancient healing system. These are core practices and body construction data that will be continually refined throughout the remainder of the book. And the point is not to regress a client back to an era in Eastern history but rather bring this information forward into the present moment for metabolic healing.

Earth

We start with the earth element because this is the element deeply related to posture. Deshimaru Roshi said, "Sit like a mountain, breathe like a river." This begins by having both knees on the mat if possible. The pelvis is elevated on a round or rectangular cushion and/or a seiza bench with the plane of the hips above the knees. This stacks the diaphragms of the body on a tripod (knees plus pelvis) like a mountain interconnecting all the diaphragms in the body. The diaphragms are like jellyfish, and there is a potency, a current that runs through them called the kundalini in tantric Hinduism or absolute bodhicitta in Buddhism. This potency is initiated in the pelvic floor and travels up through the body via the vagus nerve with the help of the wind element in the central channel. It is typically associated with sexual pleasure and spiritual awakening. Thus meditation is associated with pleasure and is called "a self-enjoyment practice of a Buddha." It is a practice of making friends with oneself. On the one hand meditation is about calming the mind, and on the other hand we calm the mind to look at it and hear our inner voices and thus witness the fullness of ourselves, our ups and our downs, and cut through the inclination to self-protect. We ride the wave of a solid self that we have created with compulsive behaviors of body, speech, and mind. As I practice over the years, I make sure my seat belt is fastened metaphorically while practicing. There is pleasure and pain in getting to know oneself, being honest with oneself, and becoming who we dream to be. This is how a Buddha practices meditation.

The diaphragms are essential in organizing the voltage coming up through the vagus nerve especially in and through the respiratory diaphragm. At the other end of the spectrum (as detailed in chapter 25), the vagus nerve is also the coregulator of inflammation and safety. Consequently it is an intermediary between the immune and endocrine systems, which also benefit from meditation in the literature. Both pleasure and pain have strong voltage. The correct meditation posture allows the diaphragms and the vagus nerve to be unobstructed by maintaining a correct axis on and around the central channel of the subtle body. The diaphragms between the base of the neck, the atlanto-occipital joint (the two bilateral condyles of the occiput rest on and in the articular facets of the atlas or first cervical vertebra, C1) and the diaphragma sellae in the cranial base, which supports the pituitary gland, also need to be aligned. That is achieved when the chin is tucked slightly, allowing the atlanto-occipital joint to open via the suboccipital muscles and lift or float. This opens the bilateral channels of the vagus nerve that are adjacent to the carotid artery and jugular vein entering and exiting through the jugular foramen lateral of the atlanto-occipital joint.

The issue of placing the head in a position where the ears are over the shoulders in alignment is vital. Such an alignment gradually allows "breath like a river" to manifest. The river during inhalation is the breath going down to the abdomen, and at the same time there is a reverse direction of antigravity, with the river of the wind element combined with the water and earth element moving up and crossing the stillpoint of the heart and moving the head posteriorly. This then reverses upon exhalation. The river can be experienced as a wave as the breath enters the abdomen, and the wave starts there and goes out through the top of the head and then back on exhale. The position of the head depends on the orienting reflex embedded within the atlanto-occipital joint space, the vestibular nerve in the inner ear, as well as visual acuity to the horizon. The orienting reflex is also part of the head-righting reflex. This is the ability to maintain proper flexion and extension of the head, which is lost in some forms of brain disorders. Frequently when I teach, I see students with their head bowed in conjunction with a lower-eye gaze, so I always assist the student to lift their head and lower the eyes. I periodically practice by a mirror to my side to observe my alignment. Nonetheless, the instructions for correct placement of the head allow the third ventricle of the brain to be the focal point of the gyroscope of the head, the top of the mountain. The brain and cranium are still of the earth element. It turns out that the third ventricle of the brain is the axis around which the top diaphragms of the body move in their gyroscopic orientation. It is the third ventricle of the brain that perceives the connection of the wind element moving reciprocally from the horizon to the third ventricle and back.

The tip of the tongue is placed on the roof of the mouth behind the front teeth, and the temporomandibular joint (TMJ) is soft and flexible without tension or the teeth clenching. One instruction is to imagine a piece of paper can slip between the upper and lower teeth. This allows the central channel of the subtle body to exit through the top of the head at the acupuncture point called Du 20. It takes several minutes to go through this checklist like a pilot before takeoff.

Water

In the somatic stages of meditation as I am outlining here, the felt sense of the earth element is associated with a water element. All biological water is in a solution with particles of the earth element. When sitting like a mountain on the tripod, we attend to the felt sense of gravity as it comes through the body and brings us into a much more intimate connection with the earth itself. We are already interconnected with the earth via the elements. Gravity potentizes the earth element in the body with the felt sense of weightedness and density without thought, interpretation, or judgment. The water element manifests antigravity, the felt sense of buoyancy and lift through the diaphragms of the body. This groundswell of lift coming from the floor of the pelvis and lower dantian give the felt sense of floating, cooling, and clarity sometimes described as the "breeze of delight." The felt sense of antigravity of the water element usually manifests after several minutes while establishing a correct earth posture around the central channel of the subtle body. There is a moment when a spontaneous deep inhalation occurs, and lift is experienced. The water element is also associated with the perception of vitality and well-being and our inherent Buddha-nature. Nothing is really experienced in the human body without the activity of the wind element. All the other elements in the body are dependent upon the wind as the motivating factor that moves everything from thoughts to molecules and everything in between.

Dogen of the Soto Zen lineage gives minimal zazen instructions, and they include gently pendulating right to left on the sitz bones and front to back between the pubic bone and coccyx to settle the body in the field of gravity around the central channel of the subtle body. These are subtle micromotions at the beginning or at any time during a practice period. This gives the felt sense of weightedness and density in the body and activates the relationship of the earth and water elements. The posture is balancing gravity with antigravity, the earth and water elements as they exist simultaneously in the body. Earth brings us down to earth, and water lifts us up to the sky above. Thus all flow in the body is bidirectional especially in the central channel and major fluid vessels of the body, including the cardiovascular system. Even arteries have bidirectional flow, and the blood is 70 percent water. Though the fluid body can lesion—which means it is imperfect, too much earth, so little water metabolically—there is, however, a perfect fluid body in which the therapist can sense the Tide of Primary Respiration. It is called the Wisdom Wind of water. The practices I am offering here and later in the book will help a biodynamic therapist synchronize with the perfect fluid body.

Wind

"Placing the mind in the Hara" is the breathing practice of zazen. Also called belly breathing, the wind element becomes balanced between the lower and middle dantian (heart) of the central channel. The breath is not placed between the middle and upper dantian of the third ventricle or even around the heart, the middle dantian. The lower dantian is the most important because it represents the source of creation in the body. The middle dantian is the spiritual center in the heart. The upper dantian is our connection to the heavens, to the universe, and to its center point in the constellation Ursa Major. In Taoism this is also called embryonic breathing. This is because you can visualize your ever-present original embryo or a pearl the size of a golf ball radiating moonlight that is suspended in the lower dantian. This becomes the focal point for the placement of the mind as the breath in the lower dantian. The breath is initially directed into the lower lobes of the lungs, which have the most oxygen receptors. Over a period during meditation, there is a particular sequence of abdominal tensions that gradually unwind and rewind with Hara breathing. The first is the obvious tension in the respiratory diaphragm from stress, being overly vigorous in a yoga class, or too much biomechanical tension from being overweight. Remember that the respiratory diaphragm is innervated by the vagus nerve and phrenic nerve.

Then there is the tension between the peritoneal cavity, the mesentery, transversalis fascia, and umbilical fascia. This is the embryonic structural scaffolding of the intestines and digestive organs for the fire element to function properly in relation to the wind element for digestion. Gradual softening of tension could happen by exploring the breath and allowing it to touch the point of the lower dantian.

The respiratory diaphragm interdigitates with the transversus abdominis muscle, which is like a net covering the entire anterior surface of the peritoneum from the costal arch to the pubic bone and lateral to the aponeurosis of the lumbar fascia. During inhalation this muscle expands pulling the lumbar spine anteriorly, begins to stretch the related abdominal fascia, and moves the lymphatic fluid from the cisterna chyli, which collects all the lymphatic fluid from the lower extremities, pelvis, and abdomen. It is located close to the crura of the diaphragm in the posterior abdomen. It transfers all the related lymph to the left thoracic duct by the junction of the jugular and subclavian vein. Every conscious breath we take enhances the movement of lymph and the function of the immune system.

Therefore in meditation practice attention regularly returns via mindfulness to the breath in the abdomen as an object of concentration with the posture. We place our mind in the Hara over and over and over again as these various layers and levels of tension in the abdomen begin to soften. It is clear when we notice our attention has been captured by our thoughts and we have forgotten this correct placement of the breath, that upon return to the Hara, it seems as if the abdomen and trunk have been squeezed like a water balloon while thinking too much, and with the natural instinct of mindfulness, the diaphragms and the breath remove the grip in the abdomen, allowing the water back down to its natural fulcrum of the kidneys and bladder.

Breathing is the wind element. Breathing is one of numerous functions and types of wind in the human body. In a typical stressful body type, the lower lobes of the lungs are restricted by too much tension in the respiratory diaphragm, and the vagus nerve is compressed. Consequently the upper lobes of the lungs must work harder and take more air in. This causes what is called "wind heart" in Tibetan medicine, which is too much wind in and above the middle dantian.

The expansion of the abdomen occurs on the inhalation. The axis of the central channel shifts like a pendulum with a heart as the stillpoint, the middle dantian. At the top of the pendulum, the head also moves posteriorly during the inhalation. I tend to focus on the inhalation a lot because it tones the sympathetic nervous system, which can assist vasodilation of the endothelium of the vascular system. Most people have a damaged endothelium because of metabolic ill health, and the very first response of the vascular system is to lose vasodilation, which is regulated by the sympathetic nervous system via its neuro-transmitter of nitric oxide.

However, one of the ways that shamatha-vipashyana meditation is taught is to have a slight allegiance to the exhalation. This is to synchronize discursive thinking with the exhalation so a felt sense is developed of thoughts exiting back out into space with the wind element. As I said at the beginning, Deshimaru Roshi said to "sit like a mountain and breathe like a river." This is the essence of the elements coming together through the process of earth, water, and wind, the initial sense of breathing, which is simply bare attention on how the air comes in the nose and expands the body and then exits. Right posture and right breathing are an enormous playground of somatic empathy.

Fire

When the breathing becomes comfortable in the lower dantian, the Triple Warmer meridian can begin to balance, and the five fulcrums of the fire element in the body can harmonize. The wind element is synchronized with the fire element in the fulcrum of the superior mesenteric artery. It is the same structures mentioned above in the abdomen, especially the mesentery, that hold the superior mesenteric artery in place and provide the digestive fire necessary for the entire intestinal tract excluding the descending colon, sigmoid, and rectum. Placing the mind in the Hara is like using a bellows to stoke a fire. The other four fulcrums of the fire element consist of the liver, the heart, the eyes, and the skin, which radiate vitality coming from and evenly burning fire in the Hara of the body via the capillaries. This allows the heart to shine through every pore in the skin. It may seem counterintuitive to breathe into the abdomen if it is the source of inflammation in the body, yet it is precisely what is necessary at an elemental level, along with Real Food.

The spiritual voltage mentioned is part of the fire element. It is not unusual at all during practice to feel beads of sweat trickling down the spine or for the body to heat up in different areas of the body, especially the skin. This is usually a very positive sign of the elements balancing themselves unless of course it is the onset of a fever. There are usually two mudras used in meditation practice. Shamatha-vipashyana uses the *earth witnessing mudra* with hands palm down on the thighs. Zen uses the *cosmic mudra* with the right-hand palm up in the lap and the knuckles of the left-hand fingers on top of the knuckles of the right hand. The tips of the thumbs are touching. Prior to using either mudra, the Tibetan system recommends stretching the arms out palm up like vulture wings to squeeze the shoulder blades back and down toward the spine. The elbows then come down like a vulture wing to the sides of the body and the hands simply fall into place either palm down on the thigh or palms up in cosmic mudra in contact with the groin and abdomen. This creates what Roshi Joan Halifax calls "strong back, soft front." The cosmic mudra helps to balance the heart through the Heart, Pericardium, Lung, and Large Intestine meridians and thus can balance the fire element. The heart is a major fulcrum for the element of fire. The strong back represents equanimity and the soft front represents compassion with these somatic meditation instructions.

Space

There is the issue of thoughts themselves and how to manage them during practice. Thoughts come from nowhere, which is space, and they dissipate back into nowhere, which is space. It is said, "All thoughts, good and bad, vanish like the imprint of a bird in the sky." The initial object of practice is to manage the thoughts and create a gap in between them and with consistent daily practice expanding that gap. It is associated with the gap when we exhale, and for a brief second or two there is a gap before we inhale. It is empty space. The Indo-Tibetan tradition of shamatha has nine stages. When these stages are examined, they are equated with longer and longer periods of time without a thought. A daily practice at home is different than a weeklong meditation retreat where practice is done all day long—with breaks, of course. That is usually when some progression of nonthought can be observed. Nonthought is not the absence of thoughts. It is an allegiance to sitting in the awareness of the element of space—a self-knowing and nonreferential awareness that recognizes thoughts being in the background of perception and not the foreground. We become the host of our mind rather than the guest. We turn and face our thoughts for spiritual healing and self-learning as thoughts are recognized in their relentless quality, and the capacity to maintain an erect posture with placement of the breath in the abdomen is harmonized. In the long run, we practice coming alive and being complete as a human being with our upsides and downsides. It's like watching the ticker tape running at the bottom of the television screen during a business show. It is also compared to sitting inside looking out a window and simply noticing the traffic going by on the street at a distance. In both the shamatha and zazen traditions, counting breaths is a basic technique for beginning to create gaps between thoughts. Inhale, mentally count one; exhale, mentally count two; and so forth up until ten; and then start over again. However this is only used as a technique for several minutes and not the whole session. Begin gradually; try to count the entire cycle of breath as one, and then try two, and so on. These techniques are used in the early stages of learning meditation practice in order to break attention capture and create a gap.

Sometimes when we sit at home, there can be a lot of noise in the background. This can be very distracting and create a lot of judgment, which detracts from practice. In my neighborhood, lawn maintenance equipment is loud and regular during the week, so when there are loud noises, I simply concentrate on the noise and have that be the object of concentration until it dissipates. Anything can be used as the object of concentration in meditation even where our hands are located when giving a biodynamic session.

As the elements gradually harmonize through the wind element in our meditation practice, awareness is experienced. The beauty of inherently complete space is viewed. This quality of self-knowing awareness is recognized after being primed numerous times by mindfulness of attention capture of the past and future that periodically dominates the landscape of our thinking mind. We reboot the computer many times until posture, breath, and mind are synchronized by the flight simulator in the brain and body. The act and experience of recognizing how our mental attention is captured, then shifting our attention back to the earth and water of our posture and the wind of our breath, kindles an innate state of awakeness and clarity. It is a panoramic view of space. Once mindfulness delivers us back to the earth, water, and wind elements of our practice, we let go of mindfulness and its precision. This letting go is a window into awareness, the element of space. In zazen this is called shikantaza. It is choiceless awareness. Phenomena are perceived as homogenized, a background merged with a foreground in which objects are equalized in their potency and have a decreased ability to capture our attention, fantasy, or desire.

Since the elements are constantly cycling, the meditation becomes a process of stopping, observing, resting, and enjoying the view. It starts with a stop sign, and in life we roll through many stop signs; in meditation we stop our body and sit in space like a mountain. There really is no other purpose to meditation than this. It is said that there are benefits of meditation in our daily life if we are willing to practice meditation 24/7 with every experience we encounter.

Belly breathing can be done in every human encounter and is called somatic empathy. One such benefit is during the practice of manual therapy in which the therapist's hands are in contact with the client's fluid body and its essence of the water and earth elements, which are cool and clear. If we approach our body and the client's body as being constituted by the five elements, then we can literally see inside the client's body unobtrusively. The elements are pathways of vision and knowing, a light such as what Dr. Sutherland described. We are a two-person biology, and we are also deeply interconnected with all five elements. It is a practice of space awareness, perception of the element of space and the elements unfolding through continuous practice.

PLANE OF VISION: SKY GAZING

The eyes usually remain partially open during meditation. Taking a siesta for several minutes and closing the eyes periodically during practice is normal. When the eyes remain closed longer, Chögyam Trungpa said it creates too much recreation for the mind and thoughts. The eyes are open to see the element of space from which all other elements arise. There are three planes of vision during practice. The *first* is gazing on the ground six to ten feet in front. This is not a stare down but rather using a soft gaze that includes the entire peripheral vision. Objects in the field of vision are not named or "objectified" as different than the meditator. Visual elemental space is the starting point, especially when there are a lot of thoughts, sticky thoughts, or storylines happening that capture our attention for longer periods of time in the initial phases of learning how to meditate. *Secondly,* as the mind settles, the eyes can be lifted to the horizon, which synchronizes the central nervous system, brain, and its third ventricle to the wind element on the horizon. The field of vision takes in more of space below and above the horizon. *Third,* if the mind remains settled, then periodically the eyes can look above the horizon more directly into the element of space. The element of space is a container that generates the four remaining elements. This is called *sky gazing.* It is here at this angle several degrees above the horizon where all five elements are dancing, arising, and dissipating simultaneously. Buddhist literature on death and dying describes internal images of the individual elements dissolving sequentially starting with earth: appearance of mirages; water: appearance of smoke; fire: appearance of fireflies or sparks within smoke; wind: appearance of a sputtering butter-lamp about to go out; space: at first, a burning butter-lamp, then clear vacuity filled with white light. These images and metaphors are also used in the sky-gazing practice. The training is to see the elements arise and dissipate in their constant dance in space.

A preparatory practice for sky gazing taught in the shamatha-vipashyana tradition is what I call "lookin' around." Once or twice during a practice period, while having the eyes gazing on the floor in front, I gently and slowly lift my head and simply look around while rotating my head slowly to the right and then to the left, just taking in all of space. The other reason for this is to break attention capture when mindfulness needs a spark. All traditions including Zen teach the vocalization of a loud, sharp sound to break the attention capture when the mind is really locked up in a story, emotion, or concept. Bellowing out verbally in a shrine room with other practitioners is not possible, so lookin' around is. We must develop as many options as possible to break attention capture and return to the felt sense of earth, wind, water, and fire in our practice.

The Buddha did not have domed stadiums in which to teach meditation. Meditation was originally practiced outside in the natural world. Sky gazing above the horizon is usually a practice once shikantaza (choiceless awareness) is established with a felt sense of the elements as presented above in meditation. The elements of space and wind each have a primary function of carrying sound. The Tantras say that the cosmic sacred sound manifests a sacred symbol (found in the Sanskrit Om, Tibetan Ah, Chinese or Japanese alphabet symbols, or certain mudras). This sacred symbol then generates the element of space. The element of space then generates the remaining elements.

One practice I teach to facilitate self-knowing awareness is to listen to stillness in the meditation room (or anywhere for that matter). This occurs when attention is placed on the ears, the faculty of hearing. The human sense of hearing is the only sense that never turns off during life. It is always on even when we are sleeping and makes a faint sound, like background static on a radio station far away, which can be perceived.

With attention placed on any sound internally, such as the heart, or externally, like traffic, with no "I" hearing a sound, the eyes gaze at the element of space above the horizon. Without naming any object in the visual field, those objects are all sacred symbols, such as the clouds that become the water element. Then the manifestation dance of the elements can be seen. All the symbols of the sacred synchronize while listening to the sound of no sound in my inner ear. Posture and breathing are usually considered the initial objects of concentration for meditation practice. When shikantaza manifests, shikantaza becomes the object of concentration, including these components of perceiving the origin of the elements from sound and sacred symbol.

Thus, in the continuous practice of zazen, once the space element is born, everything is viewed as a sacred symbol of origin. Every perception is a perception of the sacred origin. All the senses, including the mind as a sense organ, are oriented to the origin of the elements and consequently the five lights, the clear light mind and the void or absolute ending of the previous universe. Space is the extended midline of the central channel of the subtle body. Such practice of abiding in space with the Buddhas is the essence of the practice. When the formal practice period is complete, a dedication of the merit is made. By this merit may all obtain omniscience; may it defeat the enemy wrongdoing. From the stormy waves of birth, old age, sickness, and death, from the ocean of samsara, may I free all beings.

NOTA BENE

Research indicates that as many as 25 percent of people who meditate may have an adverse reaction. At the moment one's heart rate accelerates, or waves of anxiety begin, or if physical pain increases, one must get up immediately and leave the meditation room and walk outside. If I am with a client, I may let them know I need to use the bathroom and exit the treatment room for several minutes and do a little yoga in the bathroom.

✣

Practicing the Foundations of Stillness: A Meditation

1. Sit up straight on the forward half of your chair or on a meditation cushion. Allow some curvature in your lumbar spine and a little lift in the sternum and shoulder girdle. This is the posture of stillness.

2. Relax your legs or cross the legs comfortably. Your knees must be below the plane of your hips for the pelvic and respiratory diaphragms to synchronize.

3. Find the balance in your pelvis on the chair from left to right and front to back.

4. Place your hands palms down on the legs.

5. With your eyes open, rest your gaze on the floor six feet in front of you. Avoid mentally naming objects in your visual field.

6. Relax your jaw with the tip of the tongue on the roof of the mouth, just slightly in back of the front teeth.

7. Move your ears back slightly to soften the upper neck and align the ears with the shoulders.

8. Notice the breath moving down to the Hara. Settle here for several minutes.

9. Now bring 75 percent of your awareness to your exhale and 25 percent to your inhale through your nose or mouth. Take a few minutes to settle into this level of attention on the exhale of diaphragmatic breathing. It is not a breathing "technique"—rather it is a slight shift in focus. Just experience the exhalation. I often will count twenty-one exhalations to settle into this awareness.

10. If you experience any distracting thoughts, feelings, emotions, or anything that pulls you from the awareness of the exhale, say to yourself "thinking" and come back to your exhale.

11. "Not too tight, not too loose" means do not hold your body or your mind rigidly, nor should you give in to being mentally lazy or daydreaming. When you notice yourself becoming overfocused or efforting, slumping, or closing your eyes a lot, start over at the beginning with your body alignment. Let the thoughts in your mind drain out of you as you exhale. Continually resettle back into your own body posture and breathing.

12. "Touch and go" means to experience the flavor of your thoughts, then mentally say "thinking," and then let go of them while resting your attention on your exhale. No one thought is better than another, whether it's a spiritual one or a mean one.

13. Occasionally scan your body—starting at your feet, then pelvis, then trunk, arms, head and neck, jaw, and respiratory diaphragm. Use micromovement to adjust your body alignment.

14. As you settle into the exhalation, begin to notice a slight pause at the end of your exhalation just before you inhale. You do not have to think about the inhalation. Do not hold your breath. Your body will inhale naturally for you. The point is to continually rest your attention in the pause or stillpoint at the end of the exhalation without holding your breath. All of your attention and awareness come down into that slight pause.

15. As you draw attention to the end point of your exhale, imagine that your body is dissolving out into space three-dimensionally, that all the molecules and atoms that make up your body are gracefully floating apart and away from your body as you exhale. Then on the inhale just notice the solidness of your body as the lungs fill with air.

This is one practice I do at the beginning of each cranial session and during a session. It is second nature now to consider my clinical practice a spiritual practice requiring meditation to build empathy and compassion. I have found with some clients who hold a lot of shock and trauma that I will do this practice for much of the session. Even when I feel movement in the client's body, I move my attention away from it into the stillness inside or outside my body and the therapeutic container. Eventually your attention will rest in your heartbeat as you contemplate the pain and suffering of the client. PR will reveal itself, but you must be patient. In the meantime, when applied to the client, this meditation becomes a deep stillness practice. This is how you generate empathy and begin to bear witness to the client in their totality. Then you engage in compassionate action with your hands. The four foundations of stillness ignite the therapeutic container and hold the therapeutic relationship with loving kindness.

RECOMMENDED READING

Anatomy of Breathing by Blandine Calais-Germain (Eastland Press, 2006).

Bhavanakrama (Stages of Meditation) by Kamalasila. Translated by Parmananda Sharma. Foreword by the Dalai Lama (Aditya Prakashan, 1997).

Breathing, Mudras and Meridians: Direct Experience of Embodiment by Bill Harvey. Foreword by Michael Shea (Handspring Publishing, 2021).

Essential Practice by Khenchen Thrangu Rinpoche. Translated by Jules B. Levinson (Snow Lion Publications, 2002).

Fathoming the Mind: Insight and Inquiry in Düdjom Lingpa's Vajra Essence translation and commentary by B. Alan Wallace (Wisdom Publications, 2018).

Hara, The Vital Center of Man by Karlfried Dürckheim Graf (Inner Traditions, 2004).

How to Practice Shamatha Meditation: The Cultivation of Meditative Quiescence by Gen Lamrimpa. Translated by Alan Wallace (Snow Lion Publications, 1992).

Progressive Stages of Meditation on Emptiness: Experiential Training in Meditation, Reflection and Insight (3rd ed.) by Khenpo Tsultrim Gyamsto Rinpoche. Translated and arranged by Lama Shenpen Hookam (Shrimala Trust, 2016).

Sitting: The Physical Art of Meditation by Erika Berland (Somatic Performer Press, 2017).

Stages of Meditation, Training the Mind for Wisdom by the Dalai Lama (Snow Lion Publications, 2001).

Stilling the Mind, Shamatha Teachings from Dudjom Lingpa's Vajra Essence. Translation and commentary by B. Alan Wallace (Wisdom Publications, 2011).

The Art of Just Sitting: Essential Writings on the Zen Practice of Shikantaza. Edited by John Daido Loori (Wisdom Publications, 2004).

The Attention Revolution: Unlocking the Power of the Focused Mind by B. Alan Wallace (Wisdom Publications, 2006).

The Heart of Meditation: Discovering Innermost Awareness by the Dalai Lama. Translated and edited by Jeffrey Hopkins from oral teachings (Shambhala Publications, 2016).

The Myth of Meditation: Restoring Imaginal Ground Through Embodied Buddhist Practice by Paramanada (Windhorse Publications, 2019).

The Relaxed Mind: A Seven-Step Method for Deepening Meditation Practice by Kilung Rinpoche (Shambhala Publications, 2015).

Trauma-Sensitive Mindfulness: Practices for Safe and Transformative Healing by David Treleaven (W. W. Norton & Company, 2018).

Waking Up to What You Do: A Zen Practice for Meeting Every Situation with Intelligence and Compassion by Diane Eshin Rizzetto (Shambhala, 2006).

Zen Mind, Beginner's Mind: Informal Talks on Zen Meditation and Practice by Shunryu Suzuki (Weatherhill, 1970).

Zen Meditation for Beginners: A Practical Guide to Inner Calm by Bonnie Myotai Treace (Rockridge Press, 2020).

23

A Biodynamic Cosmology

WITH ANNALIS PRENDINA

ANNALIS PRENDINA has been involved in craniosacral therapy for over thirty years. She has been studying with Michael Shea since 1996. She practiced and taught in Switzerland, Bosnia, and the United States. Studying, practicing, and teaching Buddhism for twenty-five years, she integrated her knowledge and her experience into her view and her teachings of Bodywork. Currently she is teaching in Switzerland.

> *The cosmogenic myth serves as the paradigm, the exemplary model, for every kind of making. Nothing better ensures the success of any creation (a village, a house, a child) than the fact of copying it after the greatest of all creations, the cosmogony. Nor is this all. Since in the eyes of the primitives the cosmogony primarily represents the manifestation of the creative power of the gods, and therefore a prodigious irruption of the sacred, it is periodically reiterated to regenerate the world and human society. For symbolic repetition of the creation implies a reactualization of the primordial event, hence the presence of the Gods and their creative energies. The return to beginnings finds expression in a reactivation of the sacred forces that had then been manifested for the first time. If the world was restored to the state in which it had been at the moment when it came to birth, if the gestures that the Gods had made for the first time in the beginning were reproduced, society and the entire cosmos became*

*what they had been then—pure, powerful, effectual, with all their
possibilities intact.*

MIRCEA ELIADE, *RITES AND SYMBOLS OF INITIATION:
THE MYSTERIES OF BIRTH AND REBIRTH*

WHAT IS THE VOID? AN ORIGIN STORY

In the course of development of Buddhism throughout the three Yanas—from
Sutrayana and Mahayana to Tantrayana—this dualistic shamanic view of Gods
and Creation has shifted to a view of oneness. Creation has been self-arising
from beginningless time. There is this void, the pure essence, the pure light, or
the pure wisdom, which is seen as neither eternalistic nor nihilistic. It is this
void, the pure potential that brings forth the Wisdom Wind carrying the karmic seeds from one universe to the other. And by this Wisdom Wind a whole
cascade, a display of appearance and disappearance, is set in motion constantly.
Hence all appearance throughout space and time has always been and will always
be an expression of that inherent potentiality of the pure essence. And furthermore all appearance is always experienced as this constant self-arising creation
process. We are unfolding a view of nonduality rooted in the Dzogchen and Ati
traditions associated with the Nyingma Lineage of Tibetan Buddhism for healing biodynamically in our contemporary culture.

In biodynamic practice we go to the void (see fig. 23.1). The void is the absolute ending of the previous universe in Buddhist tantra and thus pure potential.
It is both the starting point and the ending point of biodynamic practice as well
as life and death. The void is the subatomic residue of dynamic stillness representing the pure essence and the element of space at the end of the previous
universe.

The void at the end of the previous universe has no midline, as it too is finished. All is extinguished: all galaxies, all star systems, and all sentient beings.
All universes and beings dissolve at their death. The progression of dissolving
with the elements is: earth dissolves into water, water dissolves into fire, fire dissolves into wind, and wind dissolves into space. Then you arrive at the void, the
actual origin and ending as one unified state of pure essence. This is the deepest
level of the element of space.

The dynamic stillness (space) as biodynamic midline collapses into a
fulcrum consisting of a single subatomic particle, the residue of dynamic
stillness as the pure essence. This fulcrum is not the Source. It is simply a con-

tainer or vehicle, a piece of luggage that contains a homeopathic remnant of all the elements. The Wisdom Wind with its karmic seeds carries all the residual unfinished karma from the previous universe by carrying it as one infinitesimally small particle to the next universe. It is a seed of the smallest variety capable of sprouting into an entire universe of possibilities. Even this unfinished karma is perfectly pure.

There is a Wisdom Tide (wind)—using a biodynamic metaphor—still moving the karmic seeds in this barren landscape of no beginning and no ending. The Wisdom Tide is one of many variations of Primary Respiration. It moves the homeopathic particle of pure essence that includes karma, which is perfectly pure from the previous universe into the empty space and potential of the next spontaneously arising universe (see figs. 23.2–3), the potential for a new beginning. It is a total paradox because without a new beginning there was no end. The universe appears by itself in this view.

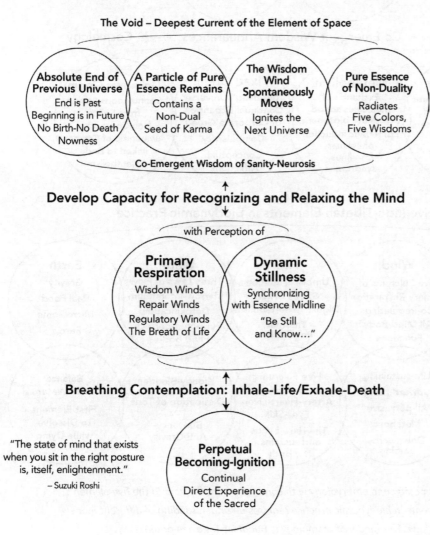

Fig. 23.1. The Definition of void in biodynamic cosmology. The void *is a term used by Dr. Jealous in his teachings on biodynamic osteopathy. In this image the void is presented as the felt sense of an absolute ending or the deepest access to dynamic stillness. "It is impossible to exaggerate the importance of this obsession with beginnings, which, in sum, is the obsession with the absolute beginning, the cosmogony. For a thing to be well done, it must be done as it was done the first time"* (Eliade 1958, xiii).

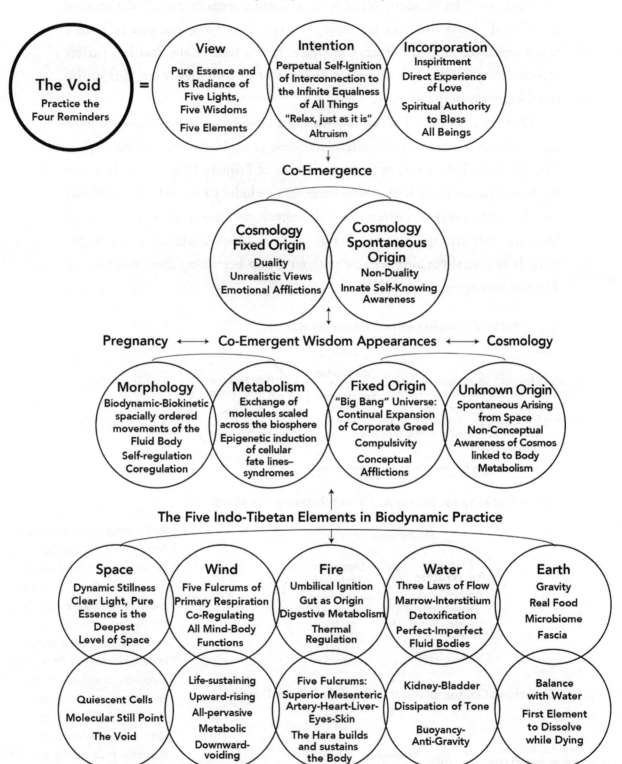

Fig. 23.2. Biodynamic cosmology and embryology with continuity from the void to the five elements.
To integrate the five elements in biodynamic practice requires an understanding of different models
of cosmology. This model of cosmology is Buddhist Tantra in origin.

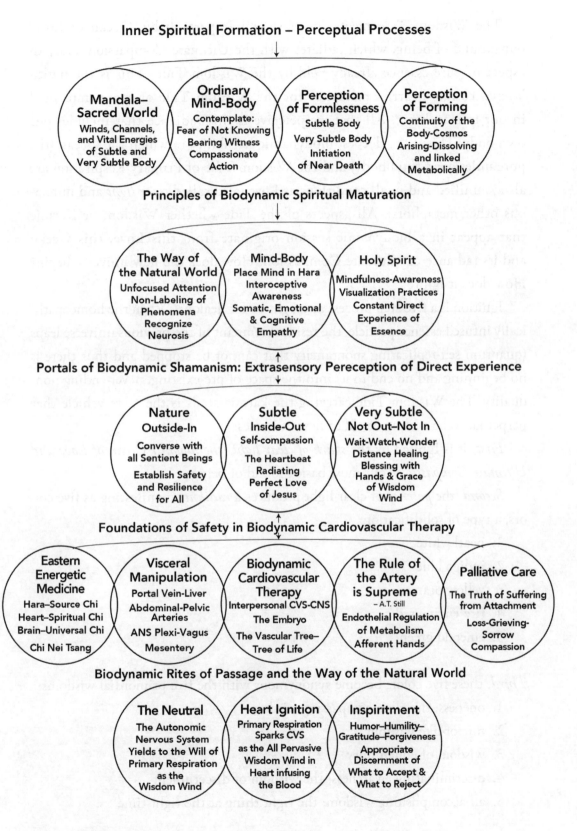

Inner Spiritual Formation – Perceptual Processes

Mandala–Sacred World
Winds, Channels, and Vital Energies of Subtle and Very Subtle Body

Ordinary Mind-Body
Contemplate:
Fear of Not Knowing
Bearing Witness
Compassionate Action

Perception of Formlessness
Subtle Body
Very Subtle Body
Initiation of Near Death

Perception of Forming
Continuity of the Body-Cosmos
Arising-Dissolving and linked Metabolically

Principles of Biodynamic Spiritual Maturation

The Way of the Natural World
Unfocused Attention
Non-Labeling of Phenomena
Recognize Neurosis

Mind-Body
Place Mind in Hara
Interoceptive Awareness
Somatic, Emotional & Cognitive Empathy

Holy Spirit
Mindfulness-Awareness
Visualization Practices
Constant Direct Experience of Essence

Portals of Biodynamic Shamanism: Extrasensory Pereception of Direct Experience

Nature
Outside-In
Converse with all Sentient Beings
Establish Safety and Resilience for All

Subtle
Inside-Out
Self-compassion
The Heartbeat Radiating Perfect Love of Jesus

Very Subtle
Not Out–Not In
Wait-Watch-Wonder
Distance Healing
Blessing with Hands & Grace of Wisdom Wind

Foundations of Safety in Biodynamic Cardiovascular Therapy

Eastern Energetic Medicine
Hara–Source Chi
Heart–Spiritual Chi
Brain–Universal Chi
Chi Nei Tsang

Visceral Manipulation
Portal Vein-Liver
Abdominal-Pelvic Arteries
ANS Plexi-Vagus
Mesentery

Biodynamic Cardiovascular Therapy
Interpersonal CVS-CNS
The Embryo
The Vascular Tree–Tree of Life

The Rule of the Artery is Supreme
– A.T. Still
Endothelial Regulation of Metabolism
Afferent Hands

Palliative Care
The Truth of Suffering from Attachment
Loss-Grieving-Sorrow
Compassion

Biodynamic Rites of Passage and the Way of the Natural World

The Neutral
The Autonomic Nervous System Yields to the Will of Primary Respiration as the Wisdom Wind

Heart Ignition
Primary Respiration Sparks CVS as the All Pervasive Wisdom Wind in Heart infusing the Blood

Inspiritment
Humor–Humility–Gratitude–Forgiveness
Appropriate Discernment of What to Accept & What to Reject

Fig. 23.3. Spiritual shamanism and the three-step rites of passage in biodynamic cardiovascular therapy. When this cosmology is integrated into biodynamic practice, biodynamics evolves to meet the needs of the contemporary client. Biodynamics is a living, evolving methodology, as is the contemporary client.

The Wisdom Tide meets the Vast and Imperturbable Ocean of Love, our ground of being, which radiates with the Ultimate Compassion Tide, an aspect of pure essence already held by the Wisdom Tide. This is the multi-layered cosmic heart, a metaphor for the Wisdom Tide of space implanted in our human heart. All that we perceive is this radiance that includes our own body. This is the deepest biodynamic sensibility in which the Ocean (the pure unlesioned fluid body) and the Wisdom Tide of Primary Respiration are always unified and in all conditions as Love (also called *clear light* and numerous other metaphors). All aspects of the Tide whether Wisdom or Karmic that appear in a biodynamic session originate from this Love, this Ocean and its radiance of Ultimate Compassion. How does the new universe begin? How does it Ignite?

Ignition is a five-step process as taught by Dr. Jealous. When the homeopathically infused essence particle, the residual remnant of the previous universe leaps (quantum self-replicating spontaneity that cannot be stopped and thus there is no beginning and no end to it) into the space of pre-existing, never-ending non-duality. The Wisdom Tide carrying the karmic seeds is the mere vehicle that perpetuates the cycling of old to new universes:

First, it is Ignited by the *spark of clear light (the moonlit Ocean of Love and Ultimate Compassion),* our most basic ground of being.

Second, the *potency* of clear light produces a *radiance* manifesting as five colors, a type of solidification:

1. pearl white
2. indigo blue
3. yellow orange
4. fire-engine red
5. emerald green

Third, these five colors become synonymous with the five primordial wisdoms:

1. oneness; the all-encompassing wisdom
2. mirror-like wisdom
3. wisdom of equanimity
4. discriminating awareness; the wisdom of discernment
5. all-accomplishing wisdom; the right thing at the right time

These five wisdoms liberate through their *sacred sound* the five elements from the essence particle and infuse them with the ground of being (clear light-pure essence). The most immediate sacred sound available to everyone's consciousness is interoceptive awareness of one's heartbeat, which leads to infinite Love found deep in the subtle body of the heart itself.

Fourth, since being carried by the Wisdom Tide all the residual karma left over from the previous universe spreads out into the new universe. The single essence particle seed multiplies. A vast field of karmic seeds permeates the five lights and the five wisdoms with duality. The five wisdoms become the five poisons (confusion, anger, pride, craving, and envy).

These poisons are then further solidified in duality with the six psychological realms of existence:

- gods
- jealous gods
- humans
- animals
- hungry ghosts
- hell beings

We are ignorant of our origin and fall prey to the cycling of the twelve nidanas, also called the Wheel of Life. *Nidana* is a Sanskrit word that means cause or motivation. The word is derived from *ni* (down, into) and *da* (to bind). These are the twelve causes that bind us down into unhappy karmic existence. The ninth nidana, compulsivity, is considered to be the main driver of karma. We separate into good and bad, this and that, then duality of me and other, then the polarization of concept and story lines that polarize groups of humans and create immense suffering as can be seen in our contemporary culture. We forget our source, our ground of being, the clear light of Love and Ultimate Compassion. We develop a documentary film of our dualistic life and try to get it on Netflix. Yet there is a continuity of our ground of being as being its own seed inside our body and mind called Buddha nature (nonduality). Like all seeds, it must be watered with the milk of loving kindness and given the fertilizer of meditation practice. The void as clear light and pure essence is beyond the innate potential of our Buddha nature and beyond duality.

Fifth, an augmentation, an expansion of so much duality spreads like a wildfire with the fire element into *three world systems* of karmic existence in the new universe. This is a map of samsara and a way to retrace our steps to the void for healing:

- The *desire world system,* where humans live a life of compulsive thinking and behaviors (I like, I don't like, I do not care) associated with sexuality, materialism, consumerism, and hedonism. These are the main drivers of karma, especially compulsivity. The Buddha called this suffering. The whole world is not suffering because there is also joy, ease, and well-being. Yet because of a seemingly bottomless pit of suffering, division into the six psychological realms occurs. These realms describe distinct styles of suffering. All human beings have their own style of suffering. The famous Sanskrit mantra of Avalokiteshvara (the Bodhisattva of Compassion; His Holiness the Dalai Lama is the reincarnation of Avalokiteshvara) *Om Mani Pad Me Hum* (Om, the jewel in the lotus) is an ancient powerful purification mantra for the beings in the six realms of suffering.

- The *form world* where desireless embodiment is achieved through meditative concentration. One's entire attention dwells uninterruptedly on a mental or physical object. The mind passes through various stages in which the currents of emotional reactivity gradually fade away. This is achieved by shamatha-vipashyana or zazen meditation. This world is accessible through meditation on the Four Immeasurables:

  1. Equanimity (absolute equalness of all phenomena)—antidote for hatred, aversion, and attachment (where attachment is based on exaggerating the good qualities of an object)
  2. Loving Kindness (to those who are equal to us)—antidote for anger and resentment
  3. Great Compassion (for those who are less fortunate than us)—antidote for fear, worry, and sorrow
  4. Sympathetic Joy (for those who have more than us)—antidote for sadness, joylessness, and a poverty-stricken mind

- The *formless world* is a purely spiritual realm consisting of four heavens. These four meditative concentration states are based on:

  1. The Limitlessness of Space
  2. The Limitlessness of Consciousness
  3. Nothing Whatever/Absolute Nothingness
  4. Beyond Awareness and Nonawareness

The five colored lights, five elements, and six psychological realms further solidify and become the Buddha Families (categories of psychological behavior from the six realms) that contain an antidote to identifying karmic blocks. The afflictive patterns of the Five Buddha Families co-emerge and convert to the Five Wisdoms. The conversion happens through spiritual practice in which the poisons transform into the wisdoms. Spiritual practice is critical for such transformation. The desire realm further hardens under the demand of the five skandhas (having a body, sensation, perception, conceptualization, and discernment). Zazen can help unwind the realms toward their originality. However, zazen is applied 24/7 in all activities. It is the self-enjoyment practice of a Buddha. This is the internal unwinding process to rest in our intrinsic Buddha nature and nurture it with zazen. There are thousands of spiritual aptitudes for the karmic unwinding process. Each of the three worlds just described are beneficial for spiritual practice. However, they do not eliminate all vestiges of consciousness that interfere with our perception of the ground of being at the core of our Buddha nature.

THE NEUTRAL, IGNITION, AND DYNAMIC STILLNESS

The residue of the essence particle as dynamic stillness takes form and function as a variety of fulcrums and midlines in and outside the body. Fulcrums arise first in development as small points of orientation. They are always present and filled with the biodynamic potency of stillness. Midlines form next with their unique potency because of their connection of the universe to the body. Thus, the midline and fulcrum as dynamic stillness are routes back to the void. The void shares its originality with the originality of our embryo. The embryo is the vehicle that gives us a body to engage in spiritual practice (experience Buddha nature) and is synchronized with the outer universe at a metabolic level. *As with out, so with in* best describes the interconnection.

Jim Jealous spoke of three levels of dynamic stillness:

- **Level One Stillness:** The Balance Point between atmospheric pressure and the body's fluids; No Breathing
- **Level Two Stillness:** The stillness through which breathing relates to the relational field of client-therapist; thoracic respiration, Primary Respiration
- **Level Three Stillness (i.e., the dynamic stillness):** No rate, renewal, void

These three levels of dynamic stillness relate to Ignition as defined by Jim Jealous. The Ignition process refreshes itself every minute without fail, another route to the void. The phase changes of Primary Respiration (Wisdom Winds,

Karmic Winds, Creation Winds, and others) are critical components of the Ignition process. We can know these routes by the perception of a Neutral where ordinary perception shifts to extraordinary perception of self and other. I, Michael, call this *shamanic perception*. The object called client unites with the subject called therapist and become Inter-Are (or Zone A and B collapse into themselves and become a *two-person biology,* as the neurological literature calls it, and an interpersonal cardiovascular system). First, pay attention to your heartbeat. That is where emotional empathy and emotional safety start. To be present for the other person and to serve them appropriately requires that the therapist perceive their own Neutral. It is a vital threshold to the void. The biodynamic therapist shows the Way, the perceptual process free from extremes (of existence and nonexistence) based on the felt sense of love.

Ordinary perception must shift to be carried by the *Tide That Returns to the Void*. The void is already present in our body and in our mind. Much of our body's cells die every moment. We are all gradually moving toward our death, and our organism knows this reality. This reality is the void. It is the boundary of the void. It is also a place of renewal if we biodynamically touch the void shamanically before death. How beneficial this can be! Being given a threshold crossing, an invitation to the return to origins, to one's originality—it is an invitation to be of service to relieve suffering.

All of these thresholds are merely mirrors of a *finger-pointing at the moon,* so to speak. But biodynamically the therapist must enter and go onto that path of extraordinary perception. It is a lot of effort, a joyful effort, to sustain the self-compassionate discipline necessary to access this extraordinary perception regularly. It is an essential component of biodynamic shamanism.

VISUALIZATION

Tantric visualizations, especially of the five lights, anything having to do with an image, or perception of the literal heart, sustain one on the path to the void (see figs. 23.1–3 on pages 245–47). It is an antidote for the ego where less dualism is involved. Visualizations are simply food for the unconscious and great dream material. At some point the visualizations come alive.

Visualizations begin by constructing an image and holding that image outside of our self—perhaps above our head or in front of us above the ground and so forth. As more clarity is gained on the externalization process, a bridge is constructed to internalize and embody the visualization. Many visualizations end up in the heart, and, as mentioned earlier, the cosmic heart becomes implanted in the human heart. The next phase of visualization involves awareness of the movement and transformation occurring internally with the configuration of light that we are visualizing. A specific form can be visualized or simply light. Gradually in this way it comes alive and the practitioner becomes informed by the embodied visualization as something that is already pre-existing within us and it becomes a direct bodily experience. My pure wisdom begins to speak to me, it teaches me and loves me as it expresses itself in relationship with my sensory and subtle body. It is at once both shamanic and extraordinarily medically adept. The training in zazen meditation, contemplative practice, and mindfulness are prerequisites that naturally awaken the healing potential of such visualizations by biodynamic therapists.

Such shamanic visualizations are not like a mechanical, static movie that keeps repeating and replaying constantly. Such repetition is ordinary mind faking enlightenment. The visualizations are a dream coming alive in our waking reality. But you need to meditate zazen before or after such practice to really pacify the mind into no attachment to ordinary mind. Nonattachment here is about allowing the mind to relax into its natural state of nonthinking. We necessarily follow our concepts and perceptions down a dead-end street and can't find the path back out without meditation. The ordinary mind is quite powerful, but it can be trained and become relaxed or subdued, as the sutras say. When we are nonattached to our thoughts, or most of them, all thoughts are of the nature of the five lights, facilitating the complete severance of compulsive thoughts and concepts. Ultimately in this view, everything we perceive is an aspect of the radiance of clear light, the five colors.

There is a broad spectrum of threshold experiences between ordinary and extraordinary perception in the biodynamic model already—Primary Respiration, dynamic stillness, Neutral, Ignition, Midline, fulcrum, potency, and so forth. These terms need to be incorporated into a living, conscious, extrasensory perception of the therapist's own body-mind first. How can we be expected to return a client to the void for the sake of healing cosmologically without fear without knowing that state of spiritual formation in ourselves first?

Taming the mind is vital and sometimes claimed to be the most important so we can see the clear light and its appearance of five colors. We have to build a relationship with our own suffering and know its relative nature. However, there are autonomic nervous system setpoints for stress-resilience cycling, which vary from person to person. There are also different metabolic parameters for interoceptive awareness. Resilience and interoception are built by meditative stabilization and become the ground for visualizations of pure essence. In other words, everyone is unique, so the *threshold experience* is available on a broad spectrum of perceptions shamanically. One's spiritual aptitude is also quite variable for the whole of the journey and its inner commitment to spiritual formation.

So multiple biodynamic and lifestyle practices must be approached with trial-and-error mind and with curiosity and nonbiased witness awareness to overcome our fears. They are used to increase the stress-resilience cycle but without crashing too deeply into the negativity of rage, polarization, and hatred. Ordinary perception (see figs. 23.2–3 on pages 216–17) can be used for problem-solving and perspective-taking, for sensing of other people empathetically, and for building a foundation of compassion. That is what it loves to be able to do best at a survival level and at best at a contemplative level.

Experientially one needs to perceive a phenomenology of each of the elements (see figs. 23.2–3). When we are working with biodynamic perception of the Tide in the attunement process with the client, our hands are on the client for long periods of time or short periods of time. That can be concurrently maintained with visualizations regarding the five lights and the application of meditation techniques, such as mindfulness, to manage a busy mind. Daily zazen is highly important. These are skills to see the world as a living dream, to see the void—rather than as a nightmare of suffering—as the absolute ending but also the absolute origin simultaneously right now in the present moment free from karma.

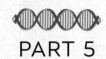

PART 5

THERAPEUTIC APPLICATIONS

Biodynamic Cardiovascular Therapy

as a Healing Cosmology

24

Attunement and the Principles of Artery Palpation

From fast to slow, different pressures generate tempos in the embryonic fluid body to establish structure and function in the embryo. The tempo of Primary Respiration is an essential factor that generates order and organization throughout the life span. Throughout this book I have constantly reminded the reader that slowing and pausing for stillness are the basic tempos by which the fluid body is optimized in growth and psychospiritual development. PR modifies the speed and heat generated by all metabolic and physiological forces moving in the embryo and adult. PR and stillness are the principal metabolic factors that provide order and organization for growth and development. They also promote self-regulation. These are the foundation of biodynamic practice.

Self-regulation is a neuro-physiological interpretation of the therapeutic relationship. It derives from attachment theory between infants and caregivers over years and years of research of how the autonomic nervous system functions in relationship. One of the first considerations of the therapeutic relationship must be the stabilization of the autonomic nervous system in both the therapist and the client, which will be discussed in more detail in chapter 25. Figures 24.1 and 24.2 provide details on self-regulation and its importance.

In this section (the marrow) of multiple manual therapy protocols, attunement to PR, and the slow, mindful movement of attention are practiced in each hand position. It begins by breathing gently into the lower abdomen. The therapist gradually moves her attention toward her heartbeat at the tempo of PR. Attention gradually becomes suspended into the environment out to the horizon and back to the heartbeat at the tempo of PR. This constitutes one basic cycle of attunement that is repeated frequently in a session. This quality

Self-Regulation – Coregulation Theory

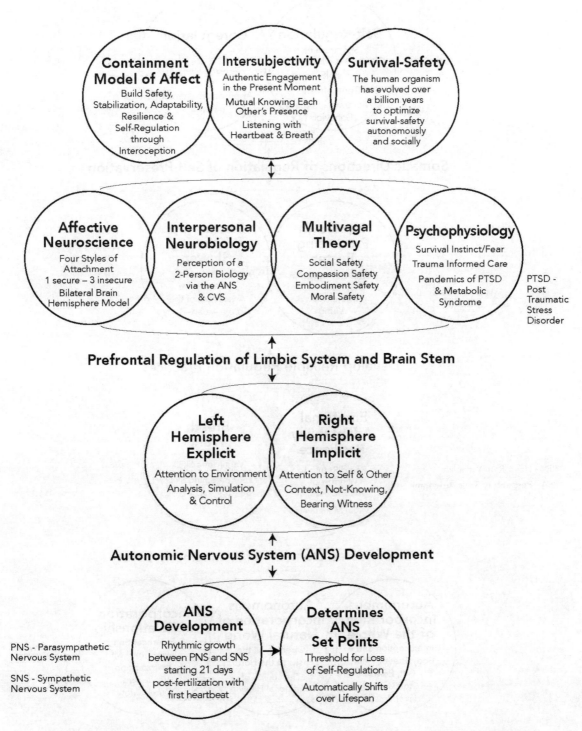

Fig. 24.1. Regulation theory and neuroscience. The prevailing paradigm of the therapeutic relationship is neurologically based. Presented in figures 24.1–2 are the roots of the neurological paradigm starting with attachment theory between the infant and caregiver. The origin of the structure and function of the autonomic nervous system must be known and its felt sense accessible to the contemporary therapist as a valid starting point in establishing safety through the felt sense of a two-person biology.

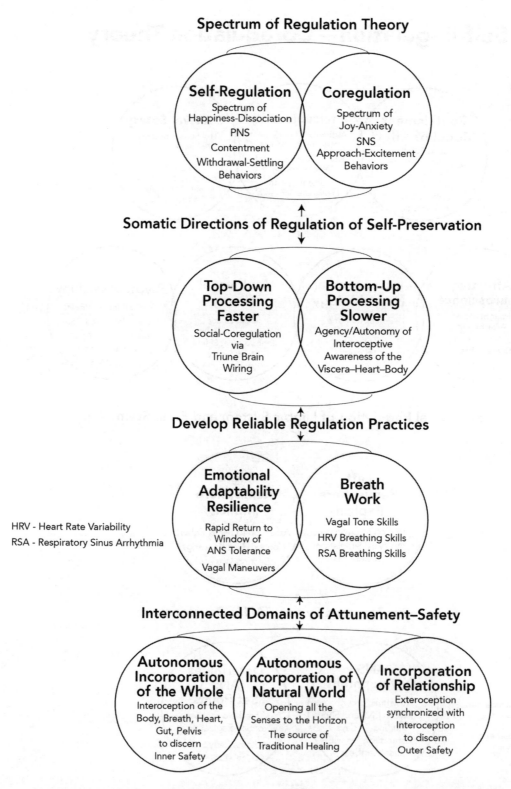

Fig. 24.2. *The world of cranial osteopathy and craniosacral therapy is dominated by descriptions of the therapeutic process in the client. The therapeutic process begins and ends in the felt sense and perceptual process of the therapist. The biodynamic therapist learns to pendulate between his or her felt sense and that which the hands, mind, and heart are perceiving in relation to the client. It is impossible to know precisely what is happening for the client or what they need.*

of attention generates a self-knowing awareness. Meditation and mindfulness were discussed earlier in this book, as a ground for biodynamic practice. Now, in this section of the book, we will put all of the words and practices into the therapeutic relationship. There are variations, especially between the therapist's hands and heart, that spontaneously come into view during a biodynamic session. These are spontaneous variations and ones that we do not need to preprogram, think about, or even anticipate. It is a gradual process in which attention is synchronized with the priorities of PR and the dynamic stillness.

The therapist still needs to deal with her mind when it becomes overactive, recreational, conceptual, or simply zoned out. That is all part of the biodynamic practice. Hitting the restart button when we are lost in thought happens frequently and does not require any judgment or interpretation. We restart with our posture and our breath, our attention, and our compassionate intention to serve the client in front of us. Gradually one's attention becomes suspended between one's heart, body, and the horizon so that very little effort is needed to move attention between those locations. Attention is gradually trained to move with the subtle Tide of PR.

A constant interchange is happening between the stillness and PR and between the office space and the natural world. The therapist is a silent but mindful observer of this rhythmic, balanced interchange. Sometimes students feel like they cannot perceive it because PR seems to fade in midcycle or the stillness is interrupted. This is a natural perception of the fluctuation of one's perception in the constant interchange of stillness and PR. The restart button in one's perception is clicked on constantly, always coming back to mindfulness of the heartbeat, sitting comfortably, and the feeling of the breath moving into the lower abdomen. Biodynamic practice is a self-enjoyment practice of compassion.

Therapist attunement in the tempo of PR can potentially naturalize imprinting (a type of stress memory) from the preverbal and postnatal time of life. Such naturalization is free of emotional distress. PR self-regulates strong emotions to the subtle emotions of kindness, empathy, gratitude, and grace. It does not release emotions, and the therapist has no intention to release the client's emotions.

The cycle of attunement builds self-regulation and resilience in the therapist. This creates resilience and self-regulation in the client through interpersonal resonance with the therapist's nervous and cardiovascular systems. It creates safety and resilience (see figs. 24.3–4). This is how coregulation works intersubjectively. It thus has the potential to change the client's nervous system through the

The Spectrum of Safety and Self-Preservation

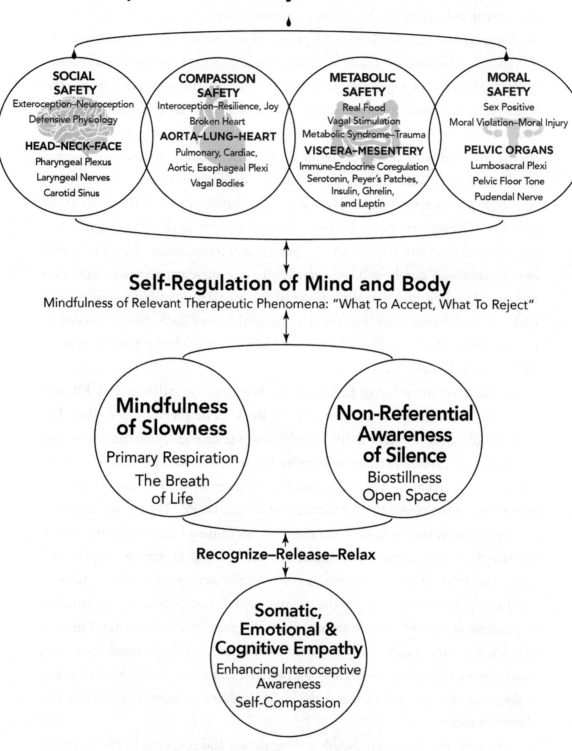

SOCIAL SAFETY
Exteroception–Neuroception
Defensive Physiology

HEAD–NECK–FACE
Pharyngeal Plexus
Laryngeal Nerves
Carotid Sinus

COMPASSION SAFETY
Interoception–Resilience, Joy
Broken Heart
AORTA–LUNG–HEART
Pulmonary, Cardiac,
Aortic, Esophageal Plexi
Vagal Bodies

METABOLIC SAFETY
Real Food
Vagal Stimulation
Metabolic Syndrome–Trauma
VISCERA–MESENTERY
Immune-Endocrine Coregulation
Serotonin, Peyer's Patches,
Insulin, Ghrelin,
and Leptin

MORAL SAFETY
Sex Positive
Moral Violation–Moral Injury
PELVIC ORGANS
Lumbosacral Plexi
Pelvic Floor Tone
Pudendal Nerve

Self-Regulation of Mind and Body
Mindfulness of Relevant Therapeutic Phenomena: "What To Accept, What To Reject"

Mindfulness of Slowness
Primary Respiration
The Breath of Life

Non-Referential Awareness of Silence
Biostillness
Open Space

Recognize–Release–Relax

Somatic, Emotional & Cognitive Empathy
Enhancing Interoceptive Awareness
Self-Compassion

Fig. 24.3. The perception of safety in biodynamic practice. The four quadrants of safety are presented and will be elaborated in figures 25.2A–B. Safety is the most critical component of the therapeutic relationship. The body and brain of the client toggles back and forth between these quadrants to activate or deactivate the survival instinct. This instinct is the most ancient instinct. Appropriate slowness and stillness are the foundations of safety.

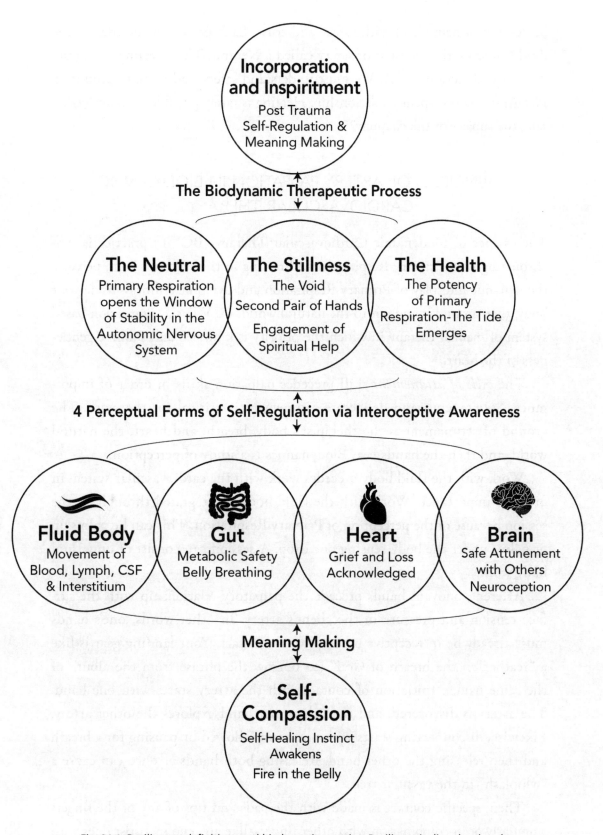

Fig. 24.4. Resilience—definitions and biodynamic practice. Resilience is directly related to self-regulation. It is the ability to prepare for, recover from, and adapt to stress, adversity, or challenge. Self-compassion builds resilience.

perception of being held with safety and trust. Each person in the therapeutic dyad can sense the moment of safety called a Neutral. Then healing can ignite under the direction of PR. We must understand safety and its role facilitating Health in the therapeutic relationship. Healing is rarely possible without feeling safe, the subject of the chapter 25.

PRINCIPLES OF ARTERY PALPATION IN BIODYNAMIC CARDIOVASCULAR THERAPY

The essence of Biodynamic Cardiovascular Therapy (BCVT) practice is synchronizing with Primary Respiration and resting in the stillness. First, perceive the dynamic interplay of Primary Respiration and dynamic stillness inside your body, then around it and out to the natural world. BCVT is a compassion-based system of manual therapy in which the priority is kindness and sublime gentleness of the heart.

The *cycle of attunement* skill precedes palpation skills in order of importance. Spontaneous and deliberate attunement is critical for the work. The ground of attunement is the therapist's body, breath, and heart, the natural world, and then the hands last. Biodynamics is a study of perception.

Work with the fluid body precedes work with the cardiovascular system in order of importance. Work with the fluid body is integrated throughout the session because of the perception of Primary Respiration. This can be palms up or palms under the body sensing one drop. A session can consist of only fluid body work.

Afferent, buoyant hands precede the palpatory relationship with the surface tension and pressure in the client's artery. In other words, one's hands must already be in receptive mode prior to contact. Your landing gear is like a "feather on the breath of God" (to borrow the phrase from the album of the same name). Initiation of contact with the artery starts with one hand. The artery is discovered, and then the other hand explores the other artery. Likewise, disconnecting starts with one hand followed by pausing for a breath and then releasing the other hand. Releasing both hands at once can cause a "whiplash" in the vascular tree.

Then, specific contact is made with the pads and tips of any of the fingers singularly or in combination with other fingers, like an acupuncturist does with the radial artery. The broadest possible finger(s) surface is preferred with each artery. The pads of the thumbs are perfectly appropriate when necessary. Avoid using your fingers as the talons of a hawk but rather like the foot pad of an elephant without the weight.

Any micropressure placed into the artery is only done in increments of milligrams and millimeters. Use a milligram of pressure, then pause for the artery to surface, and if it does not, then offer the next microgram of pressure followed by a pause, and then another microgram with a pause until the artery becomes clear. So the formula is: micropressure, pause and attune, breathe, then wait for the artery. When the artery shows itself, soften contact to its surface where the most superficial contact can rest (not rigid or static). It is called floatability, buoyancy, and afferent hands. Your hands are buoys floating on the surface of an ocean that is constantly contracting and dilating, ebbing and flowing.

Stylistically, some therapists will prefer to sit at the surface, without much use of micropressure, and wait for the artery to surface. Other therapists prefer the micropressure, pause, and release skill. It is the pause that refreshes in both styles.

Ipsilateral work is preferred over bilateral work on the arteries wherever possible. This is especially true with the arteries of the neck, specifically the subclavian and carotid arteries. Regular verbal solicitation of a client's comfort during a session is necessary, especially around the neck and shoulders.

Therapists have unique aptitudes for integrating the basic BCVT protocol. The first priority, however, is to follow the above steps. Then practice each step in the protocol from beginning to end as long as possible before moving to the next position in the sequence. On the other hand, some learners need to go through the whole protocol in a short period of time with the practice client. Remember to check in with your client. Also remember: vascular work is preceded by fluid body work with palms up or the pietà.

Without care and attention, mindfulness, and compassion regarding the above steps, it is possible to alert the protection system of the heart and recruit defensive physiology both in the brain and heart. This most frequently manifests as anxiety, rapid heart rate in the client, or a sense of deep discomfort. By practicing the above steps, the protection system of the heart, which is both a safety system and a trauma resolution system for catastrophic injuries, will not likely get recruited, awakened, or triggered. Do no harm. Start with step one above. The protection system of the heart is balanced by the pleasure system of the heart. The cycle of attunement and coherent breathing by the therapist tickles the pleasure system. Slow Down Now.

Establish a heart-to-heart connection with the following four-step process:

1. Sense the movement of your heart. Feel your heartbeat and count it up to seventy beats to build empathy.
2. Expand the geography of your chest in which the awareness of the movement is occurring. Let it spread everywhere in the body.
3. Place attention outside your body into the heart field. It is an electromagnetic globe or bubble extending up to fifteen feet around.
4. Sense PR reciprocally moving through the interconnected heart fields.

This attunement process precedes sensing Primary Respiration in the client's fluid body and their vascular system via palpation. Start with your heart, literally, and trust the Tide.

Dynamic stillness rules the artery and its endothelium. Whenever available, completely and thoroughly rest in the stillness. Hands can become rigid when searching for an artery, concentration narrows, and an inertial fulcrum can be placed into the vascular system. Be still and know. Let your hands and body melt into the stillness.

25

Palpations for Vagal Stimulation and the Role of the Safety System

Safety is associated with different environmental features when defined by bodily responses versus cognitive evaluations. In a critical sense, when it comes to identifying safety from an adaptive survival perspective, the "wisdom" resides in our body and in the structures of our nervous system that function outside the realm of awareness. In other words, our cognitive evaluations of risk in the environment, including identifying potentially dangerous relationships, play a secondary role to our visceral reactions to people and places.

STEPHEN PORGES, *THE POCKET GUIDE TO THE POLYVAGAL THEORY: THE TRANSFORMATIVE POWER OF FEELING SAFE*

As discussed in the previous chapter, attunement is a critical foundation of safety. The vagus nerve is implicated in the perception of safety both consciously and unconsciously. This chapter establishes a protocol for coming into relationship with the vagus nerve and promoting the felt sense of safety. There are four types of safety according to Sandra Bloom in her book *Creating Sanctuary: Toward the Evolution of Sane Societies*. Social safety (or "neuroception," according to Stephen Porges) is experienced in environments that are free from verbal abuse, social anxiety, gossip and rumors, bigotry and hatred, and disorganized infant attachments. Social safety allows and encourages nonviolent communication, secure interconnections, humor, clear and safe boundaries, and resolution of conflicts. A sense of agency refers to the feeling of control over actions and their consequences. It was mentioned in chapter 17 in its function of palliative care. Agency is linked to safety. A return to wholeness (see fig. 25.1) that includes mind, body, and spirit is integrated by the vagus nerve, as we will explore in this chapter.

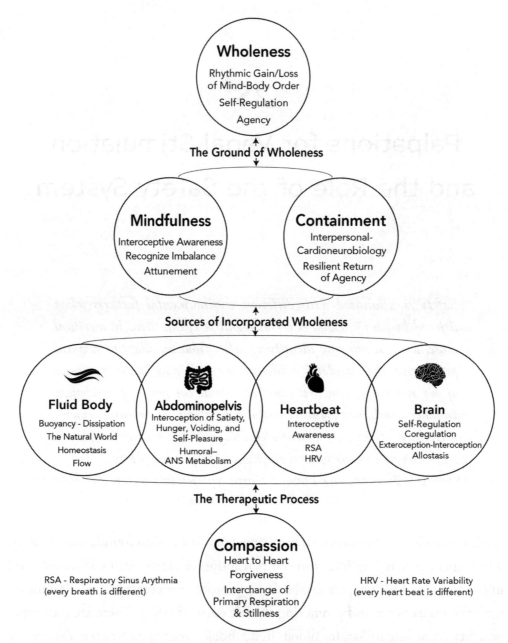

Fig. 25.1. The incorporation of wholeness in biodynamic practice. Wholeness is an old metaphor for interrelatedness and inherent connectedness. This image is a review of the neurological model of the therapeutic relationship and prepares the reader for the depth of the multivagal system forthcoming in the chapter.

POLYVAGAL NEUTRAL

To understand the Neutral it is important that the neurobiology associated with it is known as a felt sense. That is the work of the polyvagal theory of Stephen Porges. Because without safety, healing is not possible at any level, spiritually or otherwise. It is possible to come into relationship with the client's autonomic nervous system and allow it to resonate with the nervous system of the therapist while he or she is consciously practicing mental, emotional, and physical safety skills such as calm abiding meditation, visualizations, and breathing practices. The client, in their own timing and tempo, cycles through their evolutionary history of the dorsal vagus (DMNX), which is claimed to have originated five hundred million years ago in the fossil record of mammals and the history of the evolution of the human central nervous system. And it is also the older branch of the vagus system that coregulates our intestines and the organs of the pelvic floor both structurally and functionally. All of that history, if unable to be processed metabolically or physiologically, gets stored in the mesentery in the abdominal and pelvic cavities below the respiratory diaphragm. Historical overwhelm and stress are attempting to exit through the umbilicus, which is where the original consciousness came through embryonically.

The embryo and fetus show us that life is a two-way street. Waste products are designed to originally leave through the umbilicus. And since the umbilicus is closed off and there is an immune-compromised abdomen and mesentery full of inflammation, the dorsal vagus system then alerts the brain and heart, especially with pressure on the cardiovascular system in the heart itself and with the functions of breathing, swallowing, and talking. These functions and their related structures are interconnected with the dorsal vagus, the ventral vagus, and the sympathetic nervous system. Once that cycling through the DMNX settles, the client and her nervous system will then do a search of their sympathetic nervous system (SNS) memories.

The SNS is said to be a quarter of a million years old, so it's a bit younger than the DMNX. It was originally built to experience joy and happiness, as we know, in the infant-caregiver bonding experience. It was also built with the dual function of fighting and fleeing. So it is likely that the birth experience and the first year or two of neonatal existence will cycle through the SNS for memories regarding safety. There may already be a set point preverbally in which the threshold of stimulation is set as far back as millions of years ago. It is not only reviewing memories of safety, but also reviewing experiences of pleasure, joy, and happiness. It is the SNS that provides the dilation of the arterial wall called the endothelium. The SNS knows the joy of openness and expansion at the metabolic level in the cardiovascular system. Once again there is no particular timing, and it could happen in minutes or after a number of sessions where that SNS cycle is finished, albeit temporarily.

Finally the client will cycle through the processes associated with the new vagus nerve, the ventral vagus. The ventral vagus is the new vagus and only several million years old. Its primary function is to manage the heartbeat and keep it at 70 beats a minute as well as monitor the metabolic saturation of the oxygen molecule with specialized structures at the top of the aorta and another cluster of cells in the carotid sinus. It also has interconnections through the trunk, neck, and head with the dorsal vagus and SNS. This is where the evolution of the human central nervous system regarding the management of pleasure—and particularly sexual pleasure and sexual orgasm—is interconnected (see fig. 25.2A–B). The dorsal vagus carries the neurotransmitter for the female orgasm. So both branches of the vagus are obviously associated with procreation in terms of evolution, and it was the sexual aspect, especially orgasm, that was elevated to a spiritual practice by numerous religions and spiritual traditions to sacralize the event and prevent sexual abuse and sexual misconduct in the small villages and communities in ancient India and the far East. Just like Europe had traveling bands of actors and musicians performing roadshows during

---

4 TYPES OF SAFETY

Social safety (neuroception according to Stephen Porges) is experienced in environments that are free from verbal abuse, social anxiety, gossip and rumors, bigotry and hatred, and disorganized infant attachments. Social safety allows and encourages non-violent communication, secure interconnections, humor, clear and safe boundaries, and resolution of conflicts. Mindfulness is a foundation of safety. "I love my fellow man, because I see God in his face and in his form." A. T. Still, D.O.

Compassion (emotional) safety is experienced in environments that are free from unnecessary fear, being harassed, being shamed or humiliated, and betrayal trauma. Compassion safety allows and encourages light-heartedness, humor, joy, self-regulation, vulnerability, curiosity, tolerance for diversity and empathy. The heart is willing to take great risks in the pursuit of love at every level.

Embodiment (metabolic) safety is experienced in environments such as compassionate kitchens and homes in which one maintains interoceptive awareness of embodied safety from eating real food. The gut is the source of metabolic syndromes that are now pandemic.

Moral safety is experienced in environments that are free from cruelty especially around toilet training, private bathroom use, clergy abuse, sexual abuse, injustice, racism, and hatred which are moral violations and may result in moral injury. Moral safety allows and encourages being sex positive, nonviolent reproduction and birth, embodiment of consensual and self-pleasure, and gratefulness for a safe bedroom and bathroom.

Adapted from Sandra Bloom: *Creating Sanctuary, Toward the Evolution of Sane Societies*. Routledge; 2 ed. (2013)

Fig. 25.2A. The multivagal safety system defines the four types of safety and footnotes. These four types of safety were previewed in figure 24.3. A Neutral cannot occur without the felt sense of safety. It is critically important.

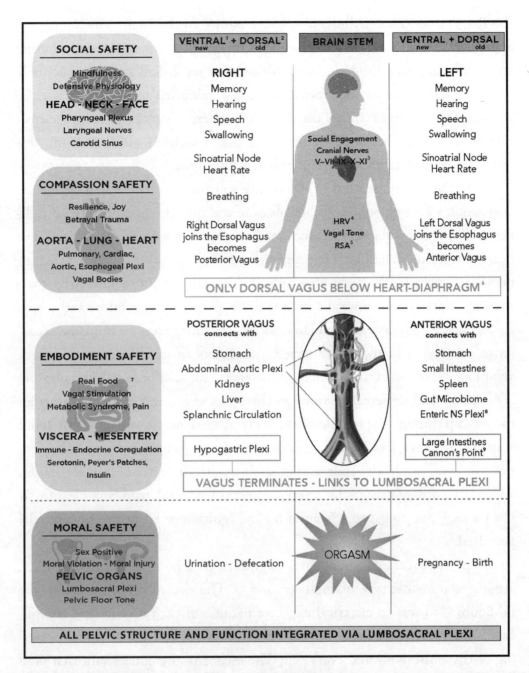

Fig. 25.2B. The multivagal safety system. The four quadrants of safety are explored through the lens of the vagus nerve. The vagus nerve does not innervate the organs of the pelvis; rather it synapses with the sacral outflow of the parasympathetic nervous system at Cannon's point in the large intestine and the hypogastric plexi.

1. Nucleus Ambiguus (New Vagus)
2. Dorsal Motor Nucleus (Old Vagus)
3. Trigeminal - Facial - Glossopharyngeal-Vagus (old & new) - Spinal Accessory
4. Heart Rate Variability - A Critical Marker for Mortality
5. Respiratory Sinus Arrhythmia - Breathing and Autonomic NS Balance
6. Posterior & Anterior Vagus partially separates from the Left & Right Dorsal Vagus
7. The Vagus carries inflammation information to the brain and returns anti-inflammatory signals to the liver and spleen
8. Auerbach's (Myenteric) and Meissner's (submucosal)
9. Anterior Vagus & Superior Mesenteric A ends & Inferior Mesenteric A begins, Sacral PNS begins

the Renaissance, ancient India also had a tantric roadshow in which ethically appropriate sexual practices were taught to small village communities, including teenagers and young children. I don't doubt that these demonstrations actually happened due to the spiritual focus on the man not ejaculating while inside the woman. She learned to control the man's level of excitement to prolong the erection by employing the various spiritual practices associated with kundalini yoga and the chakra system that were prevalent at that time.

Here there is a historical bridge to the spirituality of the vagus. It has an association with immobilization for pleasure and the felt sense of spiritual well-being. The client will give different names to their felt sense of the Neutral. I've heard my clients describe their experience of the Neutral differently when all nervous systems in the body, especially the central and autonomic, drop their tone and start moving toward a self-regulated frequency of comfort and safety. As Stephen Porges once told me, to defecate or urinate requires the same capacity to immobilize safely via the same vagal centers associated with sexuality. A voluntary relaxation of the internal sphincters for the sake of release and pleasure is necessary, and those connections go through the gut and brain and heart all the way up through the middle of the body. A biodynamic session is not about sexuality, however, and it must be remembered that to lie down on a treatment table and receive a biodynamic session safely requires a degree of immobilization and cycling through the evolutionary instincts of survival, pain, and pleasure. It is a package deal to get to a Neutral for the Ignition of Health to be mutually perceived.

There is a great joke about three engineers, on a break at a big conference, arguing about what type of engineer God is. The electrical engineer said that no doubt God was an electrical engineer because of the exquisite and complicated beauty of the human central nervous system and its electrical powering of the entire body and every cell. The mechanical engineer said that God was no doubt a mechanical engineer because of the ability to move and the way joints are constructed for the most meaningful activity of all life. The civil engineer replied that he thought that God was a civil engineer, because who else but a genius, a divine genius, a God, would place a sewer line in a recreational area.

Keep these four types of safety in mind, body, and spirituality. I will now proceed to describe a comprehensive set of hand positions to facilitate safety and vagal stimulation for anti-inflammation and to balance the client's autonomic nervous system.

Heart Fulcrum

1. Sit at the head of the table.

2. Negotiate permission for contact.

3. Place the hands palm up, fingertips touching under the spinous processes between C3–C6. This is the location of the cardiac and vagal neural crest cells that move through the arch arteries of the embryo to the entrance of the developing right atrium to become the sino-atrial node. They contribute to other structures in the neck as they move through to the heart.

4. Primary Respiration lifts the fingers toward the embryonic pathways to the embryonic heart in the anterior neck and then reverses.

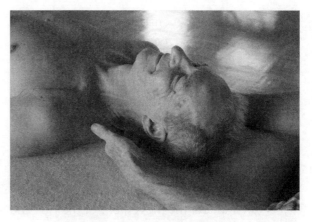

Fig. 25.3. Heart fulcrum

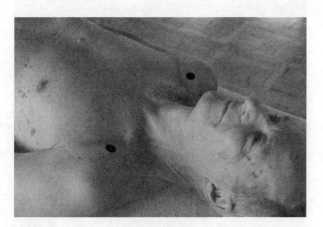

Fig. 25.4. Coracoid processes

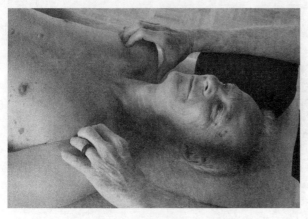

Fig. 25.5. Axillary artery

Bilateral Axillary Artery

1. Sit at the head of the table. Place hands palm up over the client's shoulders and tune into the fluid body.

2. Negotiate contact one side at a time and gently palpate the coracoid process bilaterally with a finger.

3. Place finger pads and tips of one hand on the anterior-inferior border of the deltoid muscle as if trying to get under it.

4. Listen for the artery under the deltoid and pectoralis minor muscles and then contact the other side. Shift the client's arms from by their side to overhead slightly to gain greater access to the artery if necessary. This is Heart meridian I, called "the point of all possibilities." It is an important channel in the subtle body of the heart chakra.

5. Sense PR heart to heart.

Cardiac-Pulmonary Plexi

The cardiac and pulmonary plexi are where part of the vagus nerve (DMNX) joins the sympathetic nervous system. It is a critical fulcrum for the heart-lung relationship both structurally and functionally.

1. Place the fingers of one hand palm up between TI–T3.
2. Wait and feel the movement of the ribs and breathing of the client.
3. Then place the other hand palm down with the finger pads of the opposite hand over the sternal angle between the manubrium and sternum. The palm can also be used to contact the sternal angle.
4. Stay focused on sensing the client's breathing and the PR expanding between the two hands and gradually filling the lungs and thorax in a slow, reciprocal breathing motion.
5. Light pressure and release can gently invite balance in the heart and lungs.

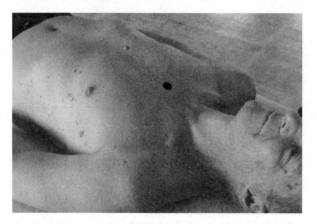

Fig. 25.6. Sternal angle

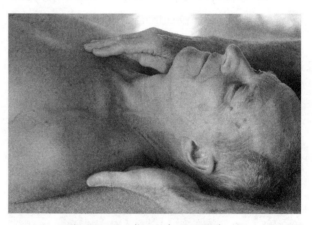

Fig. 25.7. Cardiac-Pulmonary plexi 1

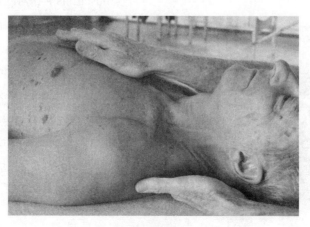

Fig. 25.8. Cardiac-Pulmonary plexi 2

Carotid Sinus-Vagal Bodies

1. While sitting at the head of the table, make gentle finger pad contact with the right carotid sinus.

2. Wait and contact the vagal bodies (aortic bodies) posterior to the sternoclavicular notch with a finger of the left hand.

3. Synchronize with PR to breathe between the hands.

4. Then reverse the hand positions. This is a treatment for both cranial nerves: IX, the glossopharyngeal, and X, the vagus nerve. They function together especially in the pharyngeal plexus and in the metabolism of the carotid sinus and vagal cell bodies called chemoreceptors.

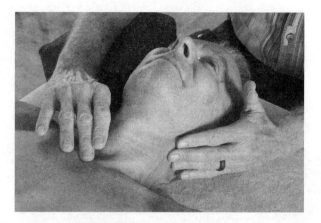

Fig. 25.9. Carotid sinus-Vagal bodies 1

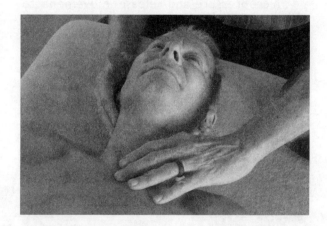

Fig. 25.10. Carotid sinus-Vagal bodies 2

Tragus

The tragus of the ear is richly innervated by the vagus nerve and used in research to stimulate the anti-inflammatory component of the vagus.

1. Sit at the head of the table and negotiate permission to contact the tragus of the client's right ear with the thumb and index finger.
2. Wait and then contact the left tragus.
3. This is a very gentle (micrograms), slow micropressure-and-release movement to stimulate the vagus nerve.
4. Periodically stop and listen for PR heart to heart, the motion of the temporal bones, or pulsation in the maxillary artery if they come into awareness.

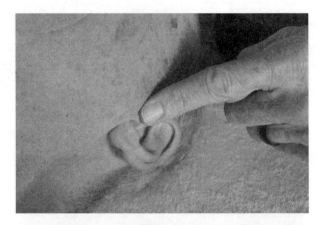

Fig. 25.11. Tragus

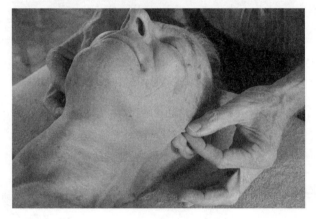

Fig. 25.12. Bilateral tragus

❧

Occipital Mastoid Suture-Styloid Process

1. Sit at the head of the table and allow a finger or two to contact the occipital mastoid suture on the right side of the client's cranium.

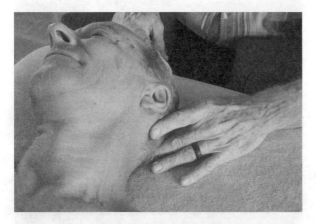
Fig. 25.13. Occipital mastoid suture 1

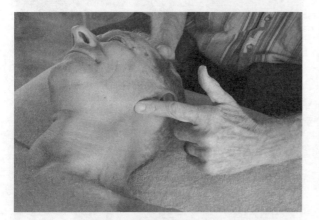
Fig. 25.14. Styloid process 2

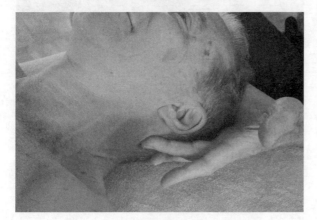
Fig. 25.16. Occipital mastoid suture 4

2. Wait, then place a fingertip on the left styloid process of the client.

3. Synchronize with PR to breathe within the fluid fields of the face and neck. Then reverse hands. The palms of the hands are open to sense the fluid fields of the cranium.

4. Let PR breathe between your two hands or the fluid body begins to decompress. The occipital mastoid suture is a transition zone between the vagus and other cranial nerves innervating the dura mater. Dr. Becker said the occipital mastoid suture was the most important suture in the cranium.

5. Our hands are asymmetrical to "come in under the radar" of the autonomic nervous system.

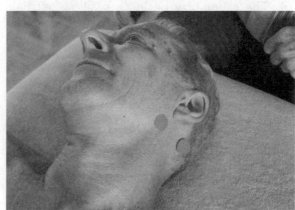
Fig. 25.15. Occipital mastoid suture-styloid 3

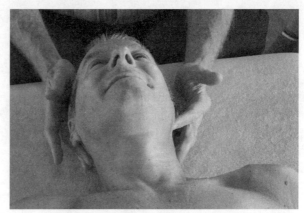
Fig. 25.17. Occipital mastoid suture-styloid 5

⚬

Pharyngeal Plexus

The pharyngeal plexus is where the vagus nerve joins the sympathetic nervous system to coordinate swallowing.

1. Sit at the head of the table.
2. Contact the atlanto-occipital joint space with several fingers of each hand in the most familiar way.
3. Allow the muscles of the suboccipital triangle to soften. Sense the head relax more into your hands. When the client's head releases toward you, that indicates that the esophagus has softened and the pharyngeal plexus has come into balance.
4. The client may begin to swallow as their vagus nerve is stimulated.

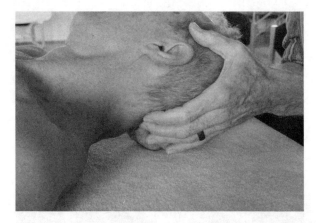

Fig. 25.18. Atlanto-occipital joint 1

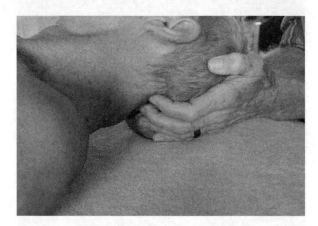

Fig. 25.19. Atlanto-occipital joint 2

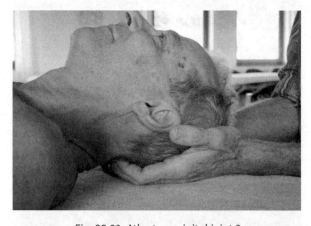

Fig. 25.20. Atlanto-occipital joint 3

The Voice and the Vagus

1. The therapist sits at the side of the table and uses the thumb and pad of the index finger to make gentle contact with the hyoid bone.

2. Depending on the size of the client's anterior neck, the pad of the thumb and forefinger of the other hand contact the laryngeal prominence or cricoid cartilage superior to the thyroid gland.

3. If only one hand fits on the client's anterior neck, then place the other hand either on the parietal bones, with the edge of the hand resting on the table, or under the neck contacting the heart fulcrum.

4. The anterior neck is very delicate and richly innervated by the ANS. The vagus nerve innervates the muscles controlling the voice. In the previous pharyngeal plexus skill, the esophagus itself was explored via the atlanto-occipital joint in relation to swallowing in the posterior neck. Now the hands move to the anterior neck for the voice.

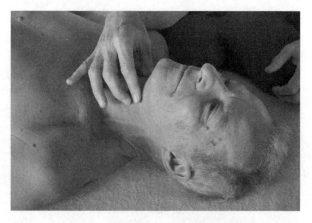

Fig. 25.21. Hyoid-pharyngeal plexus

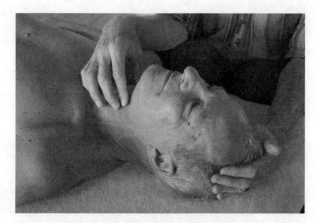

Fig. 25.22. Hyoid-parietal bones

Sternal Notch–Xiphoid Process

1. Place the pads of one or two fingers by the client's sternal notch to access the vagal bodies.
2. The pads of one or two fingers of the other hand contact the inferior border of the xiphoid process.
3. Listen to the client's breathing. Synchronize with PR.

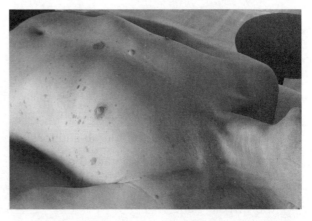

Fig. 25.23. Sternal notch-Vagal bodies

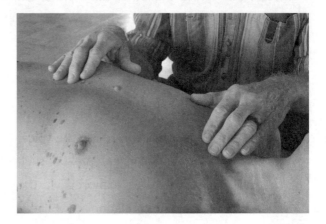

Fig. 25.24. Xiphoid process

Umbilicus Sequence:
Part I

The umbilicus is the center of the abdominal ANS plexi where the DMNX portion of the vagus nerve joins the SNS (see fig. 25.25).

1. Place the tip of the middle finger in the umbilicus and the other hand palm down or with pads of fingers over the xiphoid process.
2. Synchronize with PR to breathe between the two hands.
3. Then keep the one finger in the umbilicus and shift the hand from over the xiphoid process to the costal arch anterior to the inferior vena cava (IVC). Sense the space of stillness in the IVC.
4. Synchronize with PR.

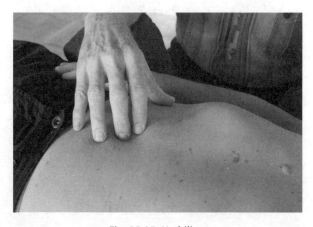

Fig. 25.25. Umbilicus

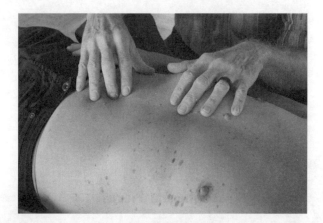

Fig. 25.26. Umbilicus–Xiphoid

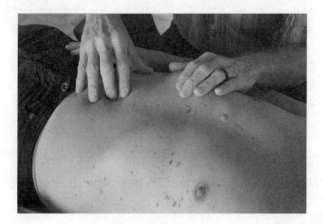

Fig. 25.27. Umbilicus–Inferior vena cava

Umbilicus Sequence: Part 2

1. Depending on which side of the client you are sitting, place one finger in the umbilicus and the other finger at the coccyx. The coccyx accesses the sacral outflow of the parasympathetic nervous system.

2. Synchronize with PR to breathe between the two hands.

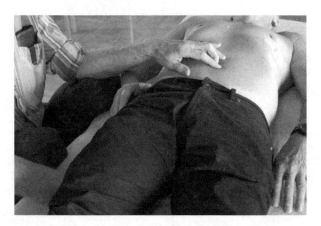

Fig. 25.28. Umbilicus-Coccyx

Esophageal Plexus

1. Place one hand under the client between T8–T12 and place the other hand palm down over the lower sternum such that the heel of the hand or pads of the fingers are over the xiphoid process.

2. The fingers of the top hand are pointing superiorly or toward the client's head on the sternum.

3. Sense a deep sheering motion in the esophagus, a settling and PR beginning to breathe through the esophagus as a gentle wind blows through a tunnel.

4. Then the plexus may begin to expand and contract between the two hands in the tempo of PR.

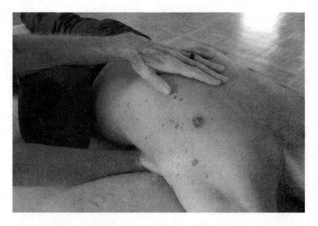

Fig. 25.29. Esophageal plexus

Umbilicus Sequence: Part 3

1. Place the tip of the middle finger in the umbilicus and the tip of the middle finger of the other hand toward the bifurcation of the abdominal aorta into the common iliac arteries.
2. Synchronize with the client's breath to contact the tips of your fingers three times.
3. Notice if the client's exhalation allows your fingers to sink a little deeper. Take up any slack given during the exhale and do not go beyond the tissue barrier.
4. Synchronize with PR.

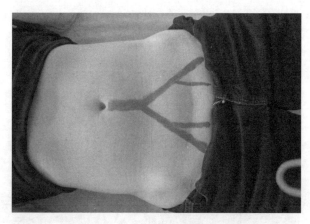

Fig. 25.30. Bifurcation of common iliac arteries

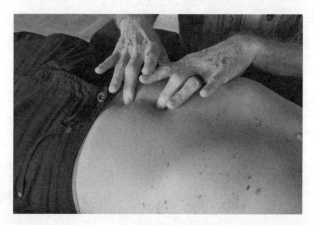

Fig. 25.31. Umbilicus bifurcation 1

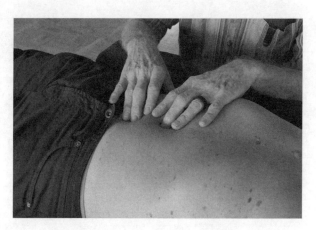

Fig. 25.32. Umbilicus bifurcation 2

✄

Celiac Plexus and Artery

1. Place one hand over the other with the pads of the fingers contacting the celiac artery/plexus.

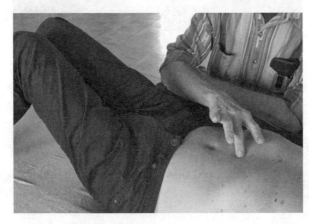

Fig. 25.33. Celiac artery

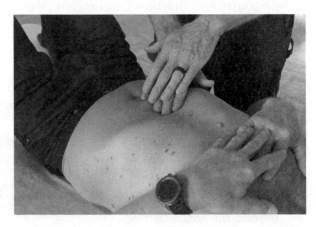

Fig. 25.34. Celiac plexus

✄

Superior Mesenteric Artery

1. Similar to the celiac artery palpation, place one hand over the other and allow the finger pads of the bottom hand to contact the superior mesenteric artery/plexus.

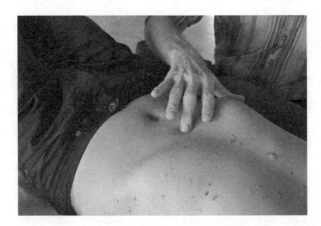

Fig. 25.35. Superior mesenteric artery 2

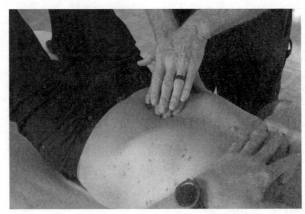

Fig. 25.36. Superior mesenteric artery 3

Stomach-Cannon's Point

1. While seated of the right side of the client, use as many finger pads of the left hand as possible to contact the gastric body of the client's stomach.

2. The other hand is contacting Cannon's point on the transverse colon. The stomach is attached to the transverse colon and the hands will be close to each other.

3. Both the anterior and posterior branches of the vagus nerve innervate the stomach and pylorus. The anterior vagus then terminates at Cannon's point.

4. Synchronize with PR between your two hands.

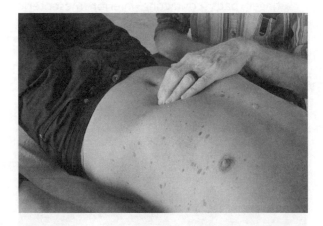

Fig. 25.37. Stomach

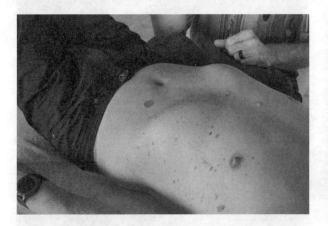

Fig. 25.38. Cannon's point

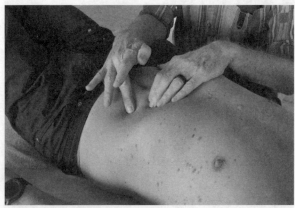

Fig. 25.39. Stomach-Cannon's point

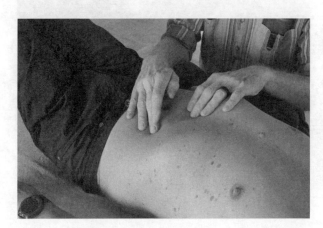

Fig. 25.40. Pylorus–Cannon's point 1

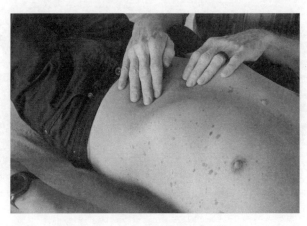

Fig. 25.41. Pylorus–Cannon's point 2

❧

Inferior Mesenteric Artery

1. Repeat the same stacked hands process with finger pads contacting inferior mesenteric artery/plexus. As an alternative, contact both the inferior mesenteric artery and the left colic artery of the Large Intestine. This is innervated by the sacral outflow of the parasympathetic system and is coupled to the anterior vagus that terminates at Cannon's point.

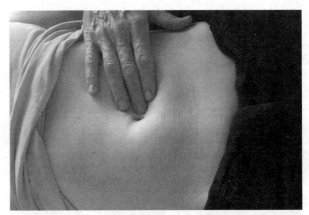

Fig. 25.43. Inferior mesenteric artery

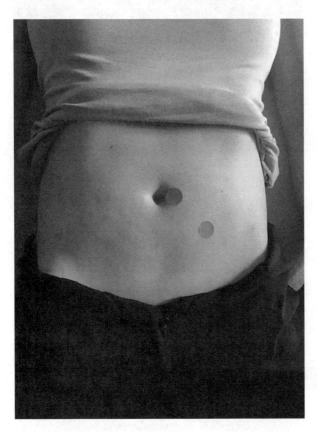

Fig. 25.42. Inferior mesenteric-Left colic arteries 1

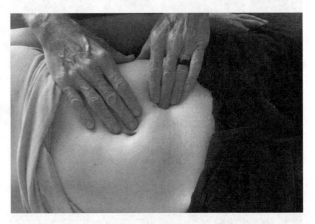

Fig. 25.44. Inferior mesenteric-Left colic arteries 2

∞

Hypogastric Plexi

1. Use the same stacked hands skill as above to contact the lower abdominal aorta where it bifurcates into the common iliac arteries/superior. This is where the superior and inferior hypogastric plexus is located (see fig. 25.30 on page 281).

2. These Abdominal ANS plexi skills require careful listening for the client's breath to contact the pads of the fingers at least three times in each position. During the exhalation allow the fingers to sink more deeply if that space opens. Keep attuning to PR.

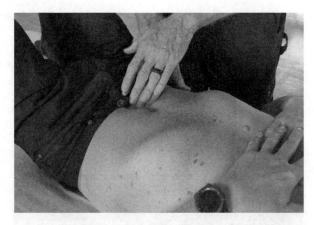

Fig. 25.45. Hypogastric plexi

≫

Renal Arteries

1. Gently contact the client's renal artery on the right side. This is approximately above the umbilicus.

2. Then with the finger pads of the other hand contact the renal artery on the client's left side.

3. The left kidney is slightly more superior than the right. Make sure the fingers are slightly more superior than the other side.

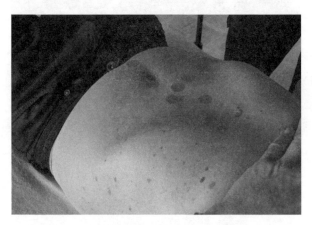

Fig. 25.47. ANS plexi-renal arteries

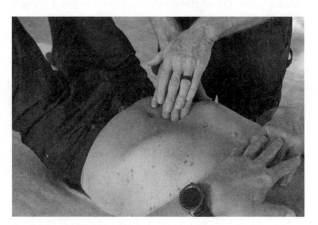

Fig. 25.48. Left renal artery

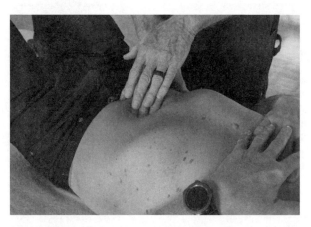

Fig. 25.49. Right renal artery

These are very delicate palpations. It is not wise to attempt to do all of them in one session with a client. In general, I recommend choosing a quadrant of the body based on the four levels and anatomical locations of the vagus nerve detailed in figures 25.2A–B on pages 268–69. This graphic of the vagus nerve needs to be studied to understand its function and especially when it goes below the level of the respiratory diaphragm. Metabolic syndrome starts in the gut and radiates throughout the body from there via the endothelium of the cardiovascular system. When choosing which of these segments to use with a client, it is best to place them in the middle of the treatment. Stay on familiar ground with the beginning and end of the treatment.

26

Harmonizing the Five Elements
with Primary Respiration

The Star Trek *Protocol*

Classical Eastern systems of medical theory state that the body is composed of five elements—space, wind, fire, water, and earth—as they guide the metabolic function of the human body and harmonize us with nature. This chapter is derived from Tibetan medicine. To perceive the body being made of five elements, it is necessary to hold the body as a mandala. A mandala is a sacred space with a center and a well-defined boundary. In biodynamic cardiovascular therapy, the heart is the center of the mandala. A mandala is a template for wholeness and a container for the ultimate spiritual essence of compassion. The boundary of the mandala has five layers or directions—east, south, west, and north plus the center, which is always the heart. These directions are established through the therapist's perception when palpating the elements. The mandala represents the container of the universe, and healing rituals, whether biodynamic or traditional, must establish the container and its boundaries for the forces of transformation (such as Primary Respiration) to manifest without emotional triggers or unnecessary side effects.

The *Star Trek* protocol—named by my wife after receiving it for the first time—is based on PR and its potency being a spiritual principle. She said that she felt she was on the Starship *Enterprise* riding through the universe. Primary Respiration constantly guides and balances the other elements in the body. In this way PR is the wind element, space is dynamic stillness, fire can properly ignite, water can properly flow, and earth can properly ground the body in Health. Biodynamics is a contemplative practice with a focus on the element of space (dynamic stillness). The nature of the therapist's mind is a sense organ itself. Non-thinking meditation is taught to produce clear perception when practicing with the elements internally and in the natural world.

The hand positions detailed below are based on the location of the five Vayus (Sanskrit for source locations/fulcrums) in the body associated with the element of wind in Tibetan medicine and ayurvedic medicine (see fig. 26.1). The acupuncture meridian points associated with the contacts are for harmonizing the elements from classical Chinese medicine in conjunction with the five Vayus.

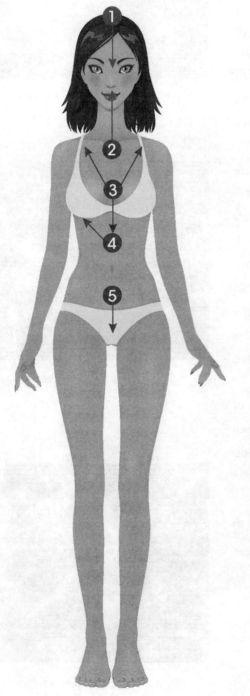

Fig. 26.1. The five embodied fulcrums of the wind element. This configuration of the five fulcrums of the wind element derives from Ayurvedic and Tibetan Medicine. Primary Respiration is sensed in the direction of the arrows. © TME—Tibetan Medicine Education Center (www.tibetanmedicine-edu.org), reprinted with permission.

∞

The *Star Trek* Protocol Basics

1. Begin the whole sequence with several minutes of sitting meditation as detailed in chapter 22. The first level is belly breathing on the inhale into Ren 6 below the umbilicus. Exhale and imagine your mind emptying its thoughts and let any discomfort in your body dissolve out into the element of space. (In the next chapter we will use a different visualization.) Repeat this belly breathing briefly with each contact in the protocol, inhaling into your lower dantian (the space between your umbilicus and pubic bone) and exhaling slowly, dissolving out into space your attention, your body, and your mind of thoughts.

2. Beginning at the feet, make bilateral contact using the thumbs on or around Kidney 1. This point is located on the sole of the foot between the second and third metatarsal bones. It is approximately one-third of the distance between the base of the second toe and the heel in a depression formed when the foot is plantar flexed.

3. The pads of the index and middle fingers of each hand are contacting the space between Liver 2 and Liver 3 on the dorsalis pedis artery as close to the big toe as possible while still feeling the artery.

4. Attune to PR with your heart. In general, all wind from the five Vayus exits the feet.

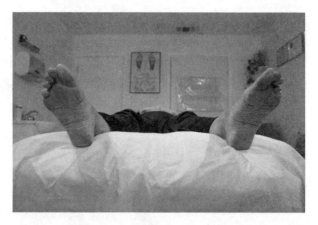

Fig. 26.2. Kidney 1

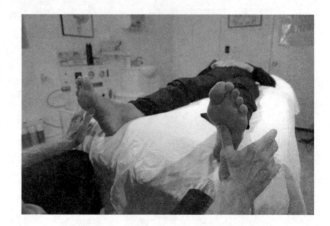

Fig. 26.3. Kidney 1

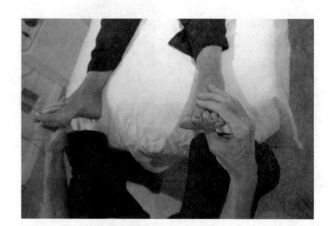

Fig. 26.4. Kidney 1–Liver 2–3

5. Then proceed to either the right or left arm. If it is the right arm, sitting heart to heart, contact Heart 8 and Pericardium 8 in the palm of the client's hand. Use all three finger pads of index, middle, and ring fingers. The index, middle, and ring finger pads of the left hand are contacting Lung I and 2.

6. Heart 8 is located on the palm in the depression between the fourth and fifth metacarpal bones, where the tip of the little finger rests when a fist is made. Pericardium 8 is between the second and third metacarpal bones, in a depression at the radial side of the third metacarpal bone.

7. Lung I is located inferior to the coracoid process medial to the crease formed by the deltoid and pectoralis muscles. Lung 2 is on the inferior border of the clavicle again in the septum between the deltoid and pectoralis muscles. It is enough to feel the axillary artery near that location. The channel formed between the two contacts is like a tunnel in which PR moves the elements.

8. Attune to PR heart to heart until the channel manifests its quality of movement. The All-Pervasive Wind Vayu of the heart moves out through these points.

9. Now repeat on the other arm.

10. Sitting at the head of the table, use your thumbs either overlapping each other or with the tips of the thumbs touching to contact Du 20. This point is approximately five centimeters superior of the lambdoidal suture on the midline of the sagittal suture. It is a very powerful energetic spot. This is the meeting point of the Governing vessel with the Bladder, Gall Bladder, Sanjiao

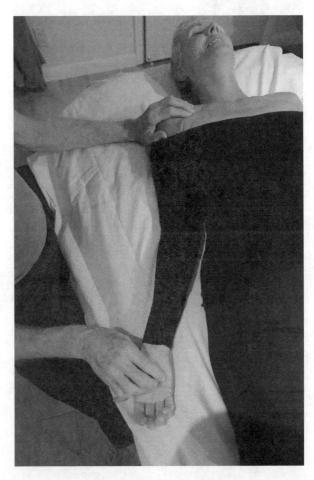

Fig. 26.5. Heart 8-Pericardium 8–Lung 1–2a

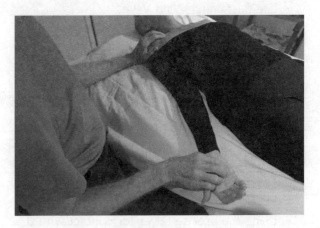

Fig. 26.6. Heart 8-Pericardium 8–Lung 1–2b

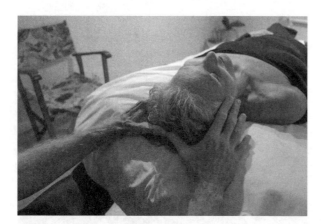

Fig. 26.7. Du 20

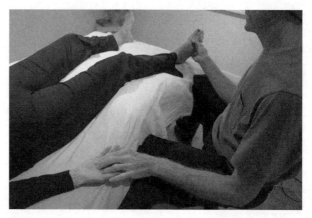

Fig. 26.8. Palm–Sole 1

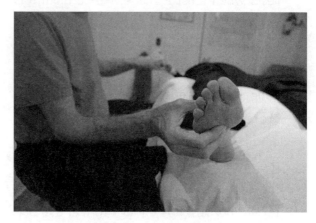

Fig. 26.9. Palm–Sole 2

(Triple Warmer), and Liver channels. It is called the Point of the Sea of Marrow in traditional Chinese medicine.

11. Sit at the side for contact with the hands and feet. If you start with the right side, the left hand contacts Heart 8 and Pericardium 8 as in number 5. Use the pads of the index, middle, and ring fingers. The right hand contacts Kidney 1 by using the pads of the index, middle, and ring fingers.

12. Sense the tunnel of PR moving the sea of elements within it. Periodically attune to PR heart to heart. This is the location of the Life Sustaining Wind Vayu.

13. Repeat on the other hand and foot.

14. Sit at the side of the table facing the abdomen of the client. It is your choice on which side to begin. I will describe starting on the right side with the pads of my right index, middle, and ring fingers making contact on and around Ren 6. The finger pads are lined up on the midline with the middle finger being the precise finger for contact with the point itself. It is located approximately two or three finger widths below the umbilicus on the midline. It is the lower dantian, the bottom of the central channel of the subtle body in the Taoist tradition.

15. The pads of my left index, middle, and ring fingers are spread in, above, and below the umbilicus. This is the geography of Ren 8. Use the tip of your middle finger in the umbilicus while the pads of the index and ring finger are above and below the umbilicus. Tune into PR heart to heart and begin to sense the elements spiraling under your hands. These are the meridian acupuncture point locations of the Downward Voiding Wind Vayu and the Fire Accompanying Wind Vayu.

16. Shift your position from whichever side of the table you are located to opposite your client's heart. I will describe continuing with the right side of the client's trunk. Contact Ren 17 with the right hand. This point is located directly on the sternum between a man's nipples. Otherwise, locate the costal cartilage of the second rib which is at the level of the sternal angle where the sternum meets the manubrium. Then locate the second intercostal space below it and count down to the fourth intercostal space. As usual, the pad of the middle finger will make the contact, with the pads of the ring and index fingers below and above the point.

17. The left hand contacts Ren 22. This point is just a millimeter above the sternoclavicular notch right over the thyroid gland. Be as delicate as possible with the pad of the middle finger in contact while the pads of the index and ring fingers are gently above and below the point. This is also known as the anterior midline of the heart. The focus is on attunement to PR heart to heart. This is the location of Ascending Wind Vayu.

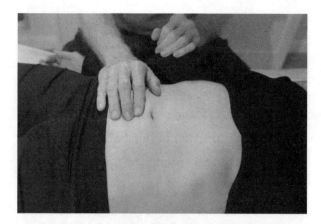

Fig. 26.10. Ren 6

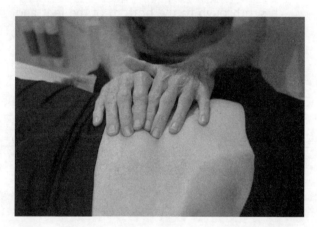

Fig. 26.11. Ren 6–8

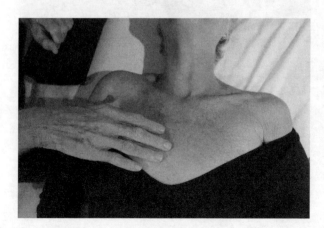

Fig. 26.12. Ren 17

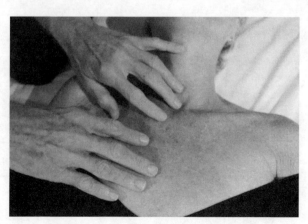

Fig. 26.13. Ren 17–22

18. Now move to the sacrum on your preferred side of working. I usually work from the right side with the pads of my right index, middle, and ring fingers on or close to the coccyx and sacral sulcus. My left hand repeats a portion of number 15 above with contact in and around the umbilicus (Ren 8; figs. 26.14–15).

19. Now finish as we began with bilateral contact on the feet with Kidney 1, Liver 2, and Liver 3, and the dorsalis pedis artery. Notice any shift or change if PR has balanced the flow of the elements from the top of the head through to the bottom of the feet and out the palms of the hands in the client. Please proceed to the next chapter for a detailed explanation of this protocol.

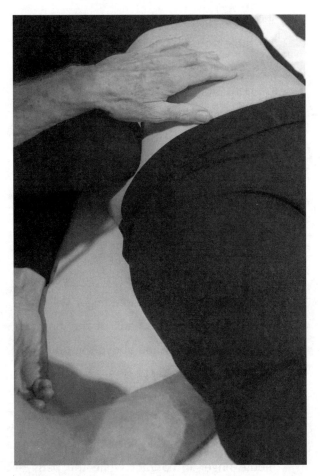

Fig. 26.14. Coccyx-Ren 8a

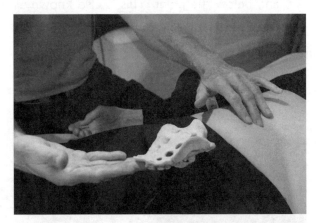

Fig. 26.15. Coccyx-Ren 8b

27

The Color of the Elements

Advanced Star Trek *Protocol*

INTENTION

Medical anthropology suggests that there are two basic types of healing rituals for a patient stricken with disease. The first is a symbolic regression to one's embryonic time when each of us was a single-celled, whole human being. In that ritual, the undifferentiated wholeness of the fertilized ovum symbolizes order and restoration from illness being recovered and brought forward into a differentiated wholeness via Primary Respiration. (See figures 12.1–3 on pages 135–37 for a detailed map of embryonic geography.) The second ritual is a symbolic regression to the beginning of the universe, the cosmos, or even into a previous universe. So it is with the second ritual of integrating a cosmological narrative into biodynamic practice that this protocol is offered. Both rituals suggest that such an originality is necessary for healing to take place. Both rituals maintain the essence of Primary Respiration and its association with the wind element. (See figures 23.1–3 on page 245–47 for a detailed map of the cosmological terrain.)

It is a return to origins symbolically while staying in the present moment with the client that facilitates a reconnection with the cosmos. As is said in tantra, "as with out, so with in." Thus, the intention of the cosmological ritual is to realign the microcosm of our body with the macrocosm of the cosmos. This is a necessary ritual emerging from the consciousness of our current plague time. The ritual includes a narrative from the Buddhist perspective of how the universe began and how to integrate that information into clinical practice. It is also based on the interchange of Primary Respiration and dynamic stillness. As biodynamic therapists we already have those fundamental skills in place.

THE ORIGIN OF THE UNIVERSE

At the end of the previous universe, when all its galaxies were burned out and all its suns extinguished, the only thing left was a particle of the element of space no bigger than an atom. This *space particle* contained the seeds for all five of the elements: space, wind, fire, water, and earth. This space particle is the remnant of all the unresolved karma from the previous universe and its inhabitants. Consequently, this seed gets moved into a new universe, the one we are now in. This transfer from one universe to another is accomplished by Primary Respiration transforming into two types of potency winds called *karmic winds*. One is *moving* and one is *stationary*. Both winds carry the space particle forward into the new universe.

Our ground of being is called *clear light mind*. It is enlightened mind itself, ultimate compassion. Clear light mind *radiates five wisdom colors* that make up the basis of all appearances in the universe: white, blue, red, yellow, and green. These five colors potentize the space particle, and the five elements of duality manifest to form a universe. The unresolved karma co-emerges with clear light mind.

To continue forming a universe with a hundred billion galaxies, Primary Respiration then manifests as *ten potency winds*. The ten potency winds are classified into three groups according to their functions: *holding* potency winds, *churning* potency winds, and *shaping* potency winds.

Holding Winds: The potency winds related to the *water* element gather the subtle particles that remain in space following the destruction of the previous universe and its galaxies. The potency winds related to the *earth* element solidify this conglomerate of particles. These are the holding winds.

Churning Winds: The churning winds are related to the fire element. They enhance the conglomeration of particles by their churning action.

Shaping Winds: Following the churning and enhancement of the conglomeration of particles, the shaping potency winds related to the *wind* element, shape the galaxies, planets, and sentient beings while developing and placing them in various locations in the space of the universe.

THE MICROCOSM

Human conception contains these exact same winds scaled to our biology (see fig. 27.1). The sperm and the egg, the sun and the moon, the five elements, and nada (the sacred sound carried by the wind of space and the wind of wind) coalesce at conception. Karmic winds carry one's consciousness forward after death, like a space particle through the intermediate state or bardo of becoming until conception and incarnation in the next human form. These three types of what I prefer to call biodynamic cosmological winds are mimicked in the dynamic morphology of a human embryo regarding biokinetic differentiations known as: positioning, shaping, and structuring (see the color insert and figures 12.1–3 on pages 135–37 for details):

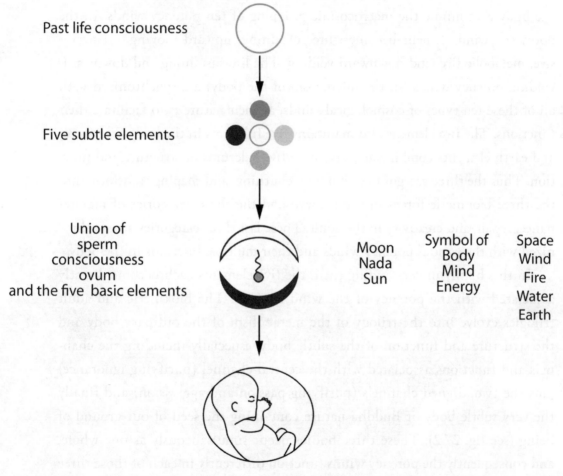

Past life consciousness

Five subtle elements

Union of
sperm
consciousness
ovum
and the five basic elements

Moon
Nada
Sun

Symbol of
Body
Mind
Energy

Space
Wind
Fire
Water
Earth

Fig. 27.1. The five elements at conception. At conception wind unfolds from space as the uterine environment. This creates the context for the earth element sperm to mix with water element female egg (oocyte). During the first week with internal compression via the multiplication of cells, the spark of Igniting the fire element begins. That is the spark that begins the Ignition process. During the second week this droplet of earth and water reaches into the uterus for the fire element of the mother's blood. A strong connection is made to the hearth, the fire and the source of external nurturing. The third week begins when the exchange of fire moved by the wind comes through the umbilicus and establishes the heart as center. During the third week, the fire is contained within the three coelomic cavities: peritoneum, pericardium, and pleura. The circuit of chi that manages the heat in the three cavities is the Triple Warmer meridian, the radiator of the fire element in the core of the body.

1. Topokinetics—Differential rates and direction of pressure based on position or location in the embryo
2. Morphokinetics—Shaping of cell groups as pressure differential determines cleavage plane of the cell and thus its differentiation toward its final fate
3. Tectokinetics—Gelled scaffolding, a prestructuring, occurs for all organs prior to their end function

These three biokinetic processes are generated by the ten potency winds in the body that mimic the macrocosmic grouping of ten potency winds. In the body, the wind element becomes: life sustaining, upward moving, all pervasive, metabolic fire, and downward voiding. The life-sustaining and downward-voiding potency winds (in the microcosm of the body) are synchronized with all of these ten types of cosmological winds, as their nature is to facilitate their functions. The fire element also maintains five fulcrums in the body. The water and earth elements combine and also have five fulcrums of structure and function. Thus the three categories of holding, churning, and shaping transform into the three biokinetic forces in the embryo and the three categories of maintenance, repair, and creativity in the adult. These last three categories are synchronized with the various potency winds and their multiple fulcrums in the body.

In this bodily understanding then, the five elements each become directly associated with the potency of the wind element. The biokinetic and adult trilogies evolve into the trilogy of the metabolism of the ordinary body and the structure and function of the subtle body, especially including the channels and functions associated with the central channel (purifying ignorance) plus the two aligned channels (purifying passion and aggression) and finally the very subtle body or Buddha nature containing the seed of our ground of being (see fig. 27.2). These three bodies occur simultaneously as one whole, and consequently the potency winds function differently in each of those three structural levels.

At this level of the united triune body, the potency winds are called *elemental winds:* the wind of space, the wind of wind, the wind of fire, the wind of water, and the wind of earth. This makes for a total of ten potency winds (the elements/five lights and elemental winds) in the microcosm as in the macrocosm. Nothing moves without the wind. Our perception of the element of space cannot happen without the wind facilitating that perception or of any other element. Thus, the perception of Primary Respiration is synchronized with the

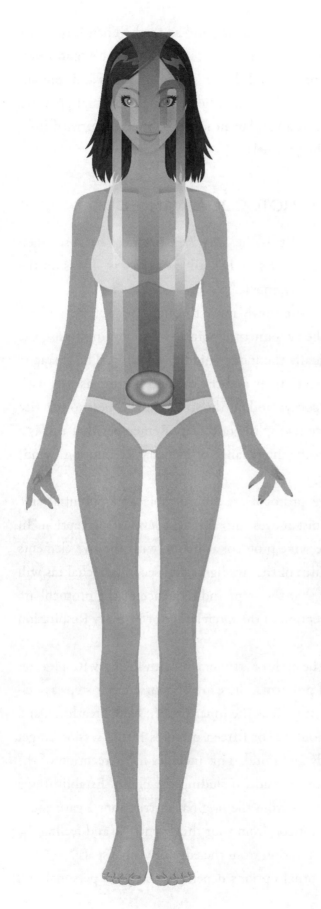

Fig. 27.2. The central channel of the subtle body and its two associated lateral channels and colors in Tibetan medicine. The bottom of the central channel is the lower dantian. The top exit is the acupuncture point Du 20. (See fig. 26.7 on page 292 for physical location on the cranium.) It is the meeting point of the Governing meridian with the Bladder, Gall Bladder, Triple Warmer, and Liver meridians. Sometimes called the Hundred Meetings, it is known as the Point of the Sea of Marrow. The lateral channels also start at the lower dantian and exit at each nostril.

subjectivity of openness, buoyancy, heat, density, and so forth. Then it becomes synchronized with the subtle movement of love, compassion, grace, and kindness. The perceptual process becomes clouded with strong emotions and compulsive thoughts that need to be purified or detoxified through spiritual practices adapted to each individual. Such residue thus needs to be further purified from the subtle body and especially the channels.

THE *STAR TREK* PROTOCOL ADVANCED

As mentioned in chapter 26, I call this the *Star Trek* protocol because when my wife stood up after the treatment I gave her, all she said was "I was on the Starship *Enterprise* during a *Star Trek* movie."

The first part of the practice is to slowly move through the protocol and get familiar with the locations of the acupuncture points by attempting to use the pads or tips of three fingers, usually the index, middle, and ring. The therapist moves to all four sides of the client's body and the top and bottom as well with the hand placements under the coccyx and on the sternum. It is best to practice this protocol several times before taking the next step. Remember that this is a potency-wind protocol based on the interchange of Primary Respiration (wind) and the dynamic stillness (space).

Once the mechanics of the protocol are comfortable and potential side effects are stabilized, the therapist moves into the next level of perception. In this next practice and using the same protocol as before with the five elements and acupuncture points, the source of the five lights and secondary chakras will be integrated. Please remember that the steps and sequence of the protocol are always determined by one's perception of the interchange of Primary Respiration and dynamic stillness.

The *first* step is to establish the cycle of attunement with Primary Respiration heart to heart as in the original protocol. There are of course other steps associated with the cycle of attunement such as the inner breath, belly breathing, and the slow breath. It takes me about ten or fifteen minutes into a session to get synchronized with my own body and mind. This includes my perception of the five elements inside of myself and outside, including the client. Establishing a sense of the elements outside comes from the original instructions I gave about letting your attention go to the horizon from your third ventricle and feeling the reciprocal nature of Primary Respiration from the edge of visible space.

So there are different perceptual options depending on your personal and *unique to you* biodynamic aptitude. Remember that the elements are constantly forming and dissolving, forming and dissolving. They come into appearance and disappear. This is simply the dance that the elements do with the five wisdom colors and their source of clear light mind.

The *second* step involves starting the protocol and the specific hand positions considering that the specific acupuncture points are clustered in discs called secondary chakras. These secondary chakras are about the diameter of the therapist's three finger pads or fingertips. The finger pads and tips thus assume a configuration of a mudra placed within the disc of the secondary chakra. The secondary chakra contains the acupuncture points.

Gradually there is a synchronization of the five elements under the direction of the wind as mentioned earlier. In a treatment I did on my wife, it was not until the fourth or fifth segment of the protocol that I felt all five elements in her body become synchronized under the direction of Primary Respiration (the one single original wind element emerging as a formless color from clear, light mind).

Then the *third* step is the visualization of my heart, sequencing through five colors very slowly and gradually from a pearl white, a dark blue, a yellow orange, a deep red, and finally an emerald green. Each of those colors represent the original source and state of the elements and their wisdom aspects.

There must be a few moments, a few minutes or longer, to notice a reflection of your color visualization from the client's elemental body. You can either do one visualization of your whole heart being the specific color or the color being generated from a light source, such as a bulb inside of your heart and radiating throughout your own body, out the pores of your skin, and filling the universe. Practice one color at a time and wait for feedback from the client's elements before visualizing the next color. It is not directly linked to the hand positions but rather to one's perception of the elements rebalancing.

In a practice session, I might not be able to visualize all five colors in one hand position, or it would be too much. Consequently, I may only do one or two colors within the remaining hand positions based on the feedback I receive with my hands and observation of my client. Sometimes one color becomes dominant for the whole session based on your perception. As a basic guideline, you can do one color per session if you plan on seeing the client for five sessions.

With the next client that comes in, it will be a different experience. If I follow these three basic steps and wait for feedback in the sense that the five elements are maintaining their integrity in the client and constantly rebalancing, then it is no problem how many of the steps in the protocol that you do. I do recommend following the sequence until you feel there is a completion, a balancing, or some indication of completion, which could be on the first hand position or on the last. In the Primary Respiration model, Health is defined as the potency of Primary Respiration (potency winds). You can trust the Tide in this regard with all five elements.

SACRED SOUND

So again, it all depends on your perception, and of course this will take some practice. But the basic skill is already in place: the perception of Primary Respiration and dynamic stillness. This is the dance between the element of space and the element of wind that builds potency through friction between the elements. Remember that the wind is the primary focus of this protocol because it is the wind that needs to be balanced first and last. The elements carry the sacred sound, and *finally* we must listen for this sacredness while being centered in our heart of compassion. The heartbeat is the sacred sound.

RECOMMENDED READING

A Manual of Acupuncture by Peter Deadman and Mazin Al-Khafaji (Journal of Chinese Medicine Publications, 2016).

Birth, Life and Death: According to Tibetan Medicine and the Dzogchen Teaching by Namkhai Norbu (Shang Shung Publications, 2016).

Bø & Bön: Ancient Shamanic Traditions of Siberia and Tibet in Their Relation to the Teachings of a Central Asian Buddha by Dmitry Ermakov (Vajra Publications, 2008).

First International Conference on Tibetan Medicine, Man-Medicine-Society (1983). Several Tibetan Physicians, including Namkhai Norbu and Trogawa Rinpoche, have chapters (Shang Shung Publications 2018).

Health Through Balance: An Introduction to Tibetan Medicine by Yeshi Döndon. Translated and edited by Jeffrey Hopkins (Snow Lion, 1986).

Medicine Buddha Teachings by Khenchen Thrangu Rinpoche. Introduced, edited, and annotated by Lama Tashi Namgyal (Snow Lion Publications, 2004).

Mirror of Beryl: A Historical Introduction to Tibetan Medicine. Dangye Desi Gyatso. The Library of Tibetan Classics translated by Gavin Kilty (Wisdom Publications, 2010).

Sowa Rigpa Points: Point Study in Traditional Tibetan Medicine by Nida Chenagtsang (Sky Press, 2017).

The Healing Buddha (revised ed.) by Raoul Birnbaum (Shambhala, 1989).

The Secret Map of the Body: Visions of the Human Energy Structure by Gyalwa Yangönpa. Translated from the Tibetan and Annotated by Elio Guarisco (Shang Shung Publications, 2015).

The Spiritual Medicine of Tibet: Heal Your Spirit, Heal Yourself by Pema Dorjee. Foreword by His Holiness the Dalai Lama (Watkins Publishing, 2005).

The Tibetan Book of Health: Sowa Rigpa, the Science of Healing by Nida Chenagtsang (Tibet House, 2018).

Tibetan Medical Paintings, Illustrations to the Blue Beryl Treatise of Sangye Gyamtso (1653–1705). Edited by Yuri Parfionovitch, Gyurme Dorje, and Ferdinand Meyer. Foreword by the fourteenth Dalai Lama (Harry N. Abrams, 1992).

Tibetan Medical Seminar, Third Tibetan Cultural Event on Birth, Life, and Death (Shang Shung Publications, 2013).

28

The Three-Generation
Model of Immune Function

The Original Marrow Part 1

The three-generation model of immune function is embryonic in origin (see fig. 28.1). Part 2 of this book on the fluid body provides detail on embryological development that I recommend reviewing as a supplement to these next four chapters on treating the immune system. How does bone marrow learn to produce blood cells and immune cells and a host of other complementary cells? It starts with the extra embryonic mesoderm in the second week of development. This is our original blood that forms outside of our very young body at that time. It is the interface between our young embryonic body and the placenta that will be delivering nutrients ultimately through the umbilical cord. This early blood is filled with connective tissue cells and surrounds the early embryo to help form a connecting stock to the placenta. This is first-generation blood developing any inner lining of the chorion, the membrane adhering to the placenta and thus closest to the mother's blood, which will be filtered into small enough molecules to pass through and feed the growing embryo. Several weeks later the yolk sac attached to the undeveloped abdominal cavity will take over production of blood cells thus making it easier for the blood cells to flow into the embryo and directly to the heart.

The second generation of blood development begins with the liver at about the fifth week of embryonic development. The metaphor of seeding is valuable because the blood cells from the chorion seed the yolk sac, and those cells seed the liver.

Finally, there is a third generation starting at the eighth week, where the matrix deep inside the bone marrow—especially of the long bones and clavicle—begin to generate blood cells. At the same time the lymphatic system unfolds

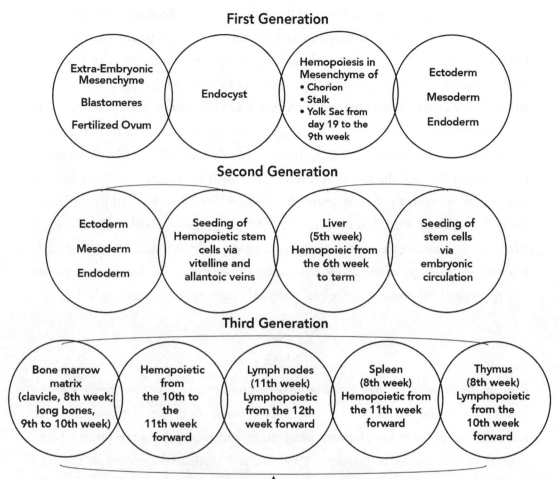

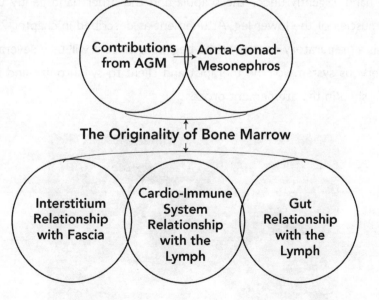

Fig. 28.1. The three-generation model of embryonic immune system development. The importance of the bone marrow, the third generation, must be stressed. I consider the bone marrow to be analogous with the first generation and therefore the marrow is our embryo metaphorically and metabolically. It expresses originality at the deepest level of healing in the body.

from this third generation of blood cells, including the spleen and thymus.

Based on this three-generation model, I reviewed several traditional and contemporary osteopathic practices with my own study and clinical practice into four biodynamic protocols to optimize the function of the blood, lymph, related fascia, and immune system in the contemporary post-COVID-era client. In general, as discussed throughout this book, the contemporary client is metabolically dysregulated and needs to be understood through the lens of body metabolism. The client needs to be treated through the lens of spirituality in which the therapist forms a perceptual bridge between the four domains of spiritual disease as detailed in the introduction and chapter 16. I am calling the following four protocols "The Original Marrow". Contacting the marrow is contacting the embryo that lives in all of us. It is a source and origin of metabolic well-being. Gradually by the fourth protocol we will go beyond the embryo to the cosmological origin of the human body.

∞

Pietà

I usually begin with all my clients by making contact with the fluid body. I called this the pietà (see fig. 28.2). The fluid body is made up of the elements of water and earth. It is made up of every living atom and molecule in the human body. Everything that makes us human is dissolved and dissipated throughout the fluid body. Thus, we are contacting the totality of the human body and its metabolic level. One hand is gently under the scapula and the other hand gently under the hamstring muscles of the lower leg. Attunement as described in chapter 24 is practiced. This is a preparatory contact at the beginning since it will take several minutes for both nervous systems of the therapist and client to synchronize and for safety to be established in the attunement process.

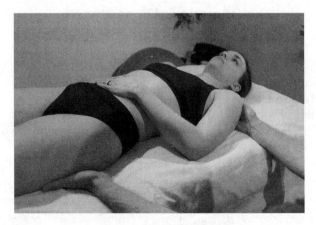

Fig. 28.2. Fluid body pietà

❧

Vascular Tree

Once a settling is experienced (the Neutral) in the motion of the fluid body, the vascular tree is approached with contact on the radial and tibialis arteries (see fig. 28.3). The metaphor of a tree is very valuable as the element of wind via Primary Respiration is constantly moving the tree, just like any great tree in the world of nature. Wait until the tree bends and shimmies or contracts and expands in a slow tempo with PR.

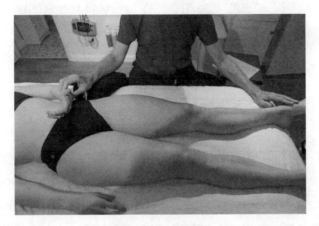

Fig. 28.3. Vascular tree

❧

Embryonic Kidneys

The next contact is with the embryonic kidneys. The embryonic kidneys go through three phases of development and, initially in the embryo, extend all the way to the shoulders (see figs. 28.4–5). This is a template also for the lymphatic system, especially the thoracic ducts, where one hand is located. Simply sense PR moving between your two hands.

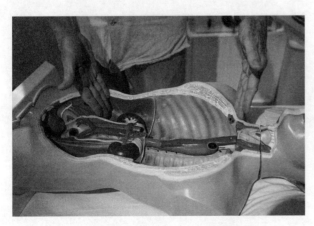

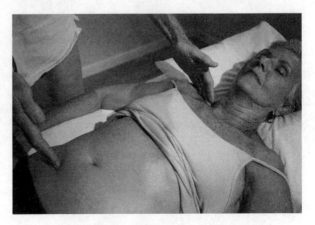

Fig. 28.4. Embryonic kidney 1   *Fig. 28.5. Embryonic kidney 2*

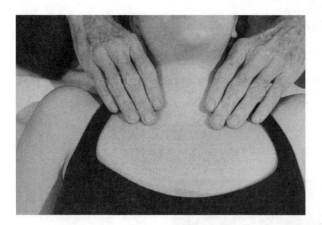

Fig. 28.6. Clavicles

Clavicles

The next contact is with the clavicles because the clavicles are where the marrow begins in the embryo. This is also an excellent preparatory contact for optimizing the movement of the lymph through the thoracic ducts with the traditional Sutherland thoracic wave pump.

Sutherland Thoracic Pump

This wave pump (see figs. 28.7–8) is a vibratory movement with a vector from the anterior to posterior plane of the body. The vibration starts slowly, and gradually the fluid body and lymphatic system will begin to rebound back into your fingers as if in a constant communication. It is a wave, and it is reciprocal. Dr. Sutherland frequently ended all of his sessions with this technique. But we begin here because in osteopathy it is felt that the thoracic ducts should be optimized first. It is important to honor the osteopathic lineage, which has several centuries of knowledge and skill. In addition, it is important to consider the location of the lower dantian just anterior to the bifurcation of the abdominal aorta into the common iliac arteries. It is posterior to Ren 6 as shown in chapters 26. The lower dantian is the center of the Hara, which in Taoism is the creative center of the body located in the abdomen. It is visualized as a glowing, moonlit pearl the size of a golf ball. In the case of the different lymphatic pumps in these immune system protocols, I ultimately aim for sensing or visually observing the vibration of the pumping motion that I am offering to the client's body by going through and moving the pearl.

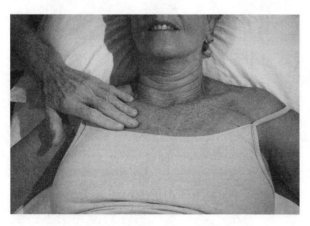

Fig. 28.7. Sutherland thoracic pump 1

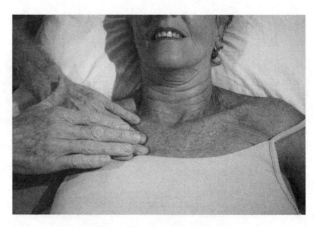

Fig. 28.8. Sutherland thoracic pump 2

❧

Cisterna Chyli

Next move to the cisterna chyli in the abdomen (see figs. 28.9–14). The cisterna chyli sits deep, close to the spine and approximately posterior to the stomach on the midline. Remember that it collects all the lymph coming from the lower

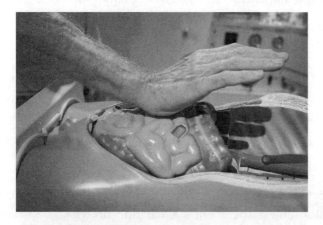

Fig. 28.9. Mesentery-Cisterna chyli 1

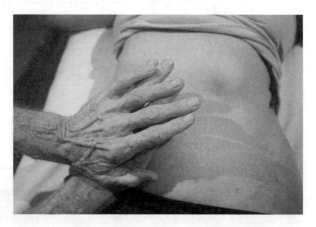

Fig. 28.10. Mesentery-Cisterna chyli 2

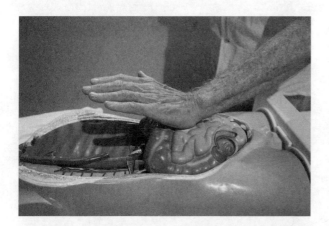

Fig. 28.11. Mesentery-Cisterna chyli 3

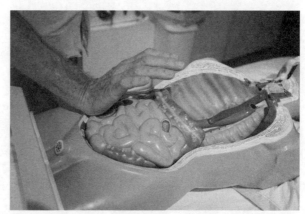

Fig. 28.12. Mesentery-Cisterna chyli 4

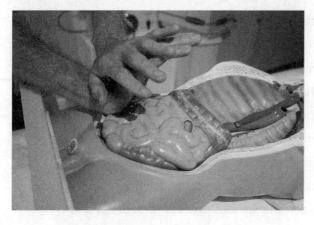

Fig. 28.13. Mesentery-Cisterna chyli 5

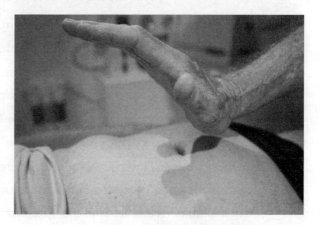

Fig. 28.14. Mesentery-Cisterna chyli 6

extremities, pelvis, and abdomen before shunting it up to the left thoracic duct in the shoulders. The right thoracic duct drains the right shoulder, arm, and neck. I use the heel of my hand to gather the mesentery (or the sides of my hands as shown). The mesentery itself is rich with lymph nodes all draining into the cisterna chyli. Once the mesentery is gathered, a slight vibration with the hand on a vector aiming for the location of the cisterna chyli is employed. As always, the vibration begins slowly, and there is a necessary period of waiting until the movement is reciprocal and reverberates into my body.

At the same time, it is very important to sense the client breathing into the point of contact before you begin any vibratory motion. If the client's breath is not felt at the point of contact, ask the client to breathe directly into your hand. Usually sensing three cycles of breathing and while the client is exhaling, the therapist may explore taking up the slack and sinking more deeply into the mesentery on a vector toward the spine. This permission is with the exhale. Do not go beyond any barrier of tissue tension unless the client's exhalation brings you deeper.

∞

Intervertebral Notochordal Stillness

This is a wonderful skill that I learned from the work of Dr. Jealous. Figures 28.15–17 show an anatomical model in prone position. Red dots were placed over the spinous processes. The skill is practiced, however, while the client is supine and not prone. It does not make much sense to show a photograph of my hands under the client. Consequently, this skill is about using the fingers to contact the spaces between the spinous processes. The remnants of the embryonic notochord are in the nucleus pulposus of each intervertebral disc. There is a structural quiescence, a dynamic still-ness that can be perceived in these fulcrums. Simply place both hands under the client's lumbar vertebrae. Find the space between the spinous processes. Settle in and attune to PR until the dynamic stillness becomes the prominent perception.

❧
Spinous Processes of Lumbar Vertebrae

Proper anatomical breathing is vital to the movement of lymphatic fluid in the human body. The cisterna chyli is embedded in the fascia of the crura of the diaphragm itself. A very important way to support the client's breathing and lymphatic flow is to place the pads of your fingers directly on the spinous processes of the lumbar vertebrae. A very slight pressure, perhaps several grams of lifting pressure, is used (see figs. 28.15–17). Begin to sense how the breath moves the vertebrae if at all. Play with different types of lifting/relaxing pressure, but not as if you were fixing a flat tire and jacking up the frame of a car. Gradually, the lumbar vertebrae will start to soften and the entire respiratory diaphragm breathing function and lymphatic flow through the cisterna chyli can be optimized. This is a very elegant and simple skill of playing with the lumbar vertebrae gently until the breath moves them.

Observe the function of the transversus abdominus muscle while the hands are supporting the lumbar vertebrae posteriorly. The transversus abdominus muscle covers most of the abdomen and interdigitates with the respiratory diaphragm in such a way that when inhalation occurs the transversus abdominus muscle inflates like a balloon and the umbilicus moves out. During exhalation the muscle relaxes, and the abdomen falls back naturally. Thus, it is important that the client be able to breathe into the point of contact with your hand wherever it is located on the abdomen, as we shall see in chapter 31.

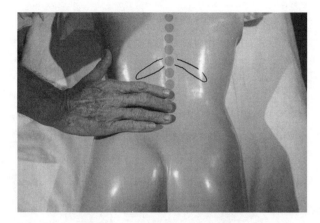

Fig. 28.15. Spinous processes 1

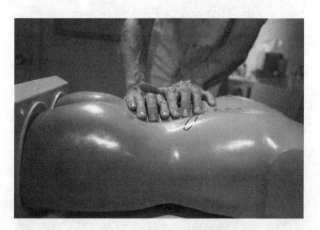

Fig. 28.16. Spinous processes 2

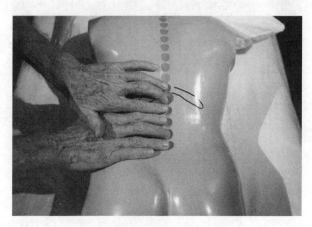

Fig. 28.17. Spinous processes 3

Spleen–Thymus

The spleen and thymus are critical in the coregulation of the immune system. Figure 28.18 shows a contact with my finger pads over the thymus and the palm of my other hand surrounding the spleen over the costal arch. The therapist can be standing or seated. In this image, I approach from the opposite side of the spleen for my own comfort. Any of these skills can be adapted depending on the territory you encounter, with the basic rule of thumb being maximum comfort and ease for the therapist. I synchronize with PR, and I wait until I feel our relationship between my two hands. That can be PR simply expanding my hands away from each other and back together with micromovement, or it can be a sense of the fluid body making waves between my two hands, or any number of other possibilities. The key point is making a heart-to-heart connection with PR.

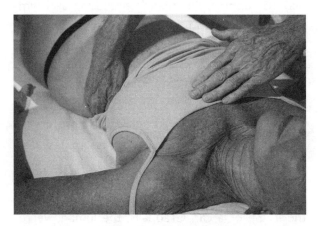

Fig. 28.18. Spleen–thymus

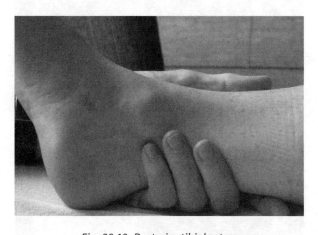

Fig. 28.19. Posterior tibial artery

Posterior Tibial Arteries

Next, move to the feet and contact the posterior tibial arteries as shown in figure 28.19. This is an important acupuncture point called Kidney 3. From this point the downward voiding wind can be sensed by the therapist not only through the hands but also through the trunk of the therapist's body. This area around the medial malleolus can have a buildup of connective tissue from a history of sprains and breaks in either or both ankles. The pulsation of the posterior tibial artery is underneath the tendons and fascia approximately where the pad of my middle finger is located. If the fascia is thick, a slight amount of pressure can be used to help melt the fascia and allow the pulsation of the artery to reach your consciousness.

∝

Seated Respiratory Diaphragm

Finally, I have the client sit on the edge of the table and contact the client's costal arch as shown in figure 28.20–22. I gently roll my fingers around the costal arch and under it to sense the movement of the respiratory diaphragm. Again, ask the client to breathe directly and gently into the point of contact. During the exhalation explore any areas that need stretch or lift.

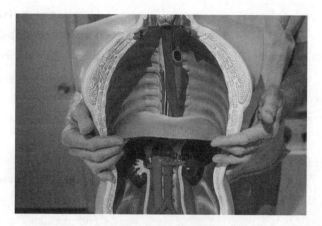

Fig. 28.20. Diaphragm 1

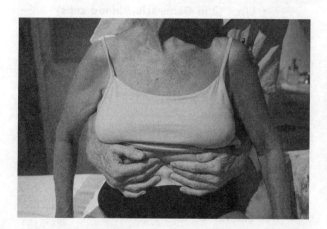

Fig. 28.21. Diaphragm 2

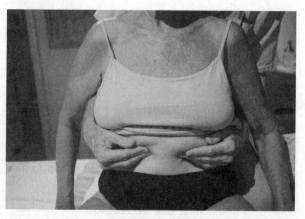

Fig. 28.22. Diaphragm 3

This completes the first protocol in supporting and optimizing the immune system. It is a basic generic protocol. I recommend practicing with it numerous times until moving forward to the next protocol in chapter 29. Finally I link the Three-Generation Model to the fluid body as explored in part 2 of this book. Please review the key embryonic structures (see figs. 28.23A–B) to be clear on the progression of clinical skills associated with the four protocols on the marrow.

The Fluid Body in the Age of the Immune System

I. Biodynamic (growth of the whole over time) and Biokinetic (local development) Laws:
  I. Containment:
   - Three cavities formation (amnion, yolk, chorion)
   - Bilamination of membranes (fascial system)
   - Interstitium – intermediate space
 II. Resistance:
  2. Rooting in periphery (dorsal amnion – placenta)
   - Centralization: radial – axial symmetry
   - Restraining function
   - Spectrum of stillness and slowness
  3. Flow:
   - Perpendicular, horizontal, permeating
   - Canalization zones – heart field – diaphragm (breathing)
II. Three Cavities:
  I. Amnion Cavity:
   - Rooting in periphery
   - Connecting stalk – umbilical cord **(2nd Generation seeding of blood cells to Liver)**
   - Primitive streak – Notochord
  2. Chorion – Placenta
   - Vasculogenesis – Angiogenesis
   - Extraembryonic mesoderm
   - Remodeling

  3. Umbilical Vesical (yolk sac)
   - Hematopoiesis **(1st Generation blood cells)**
   - Vitelline vein **(2nd Generation seeding of blood cells to liver)**
   - Allantois (bladder)
   - AGM – aorta, gonads, mesonephros (seeding of blood cells)
   - Septic system
III. Internalization – Coelomic Sacs:
  I. Cardiogenesis – Vasculogenesis:
   - Dorsal – ventral pericardium
   - Endothelium
   - Respiratory diaphragm
   - Liver **(2nd Generation blood cells)**
   - Seeding of stem cells
  2. Pleura:
   - Parietal – visceral
   - Root of the lungs
  3. Peritoneum:
   - Mesentery – stomach – spleen **(3rd Generation blood cells, lymph)**
   - AGM – aorta – gonad – mesonephros region
  4. Vagal Neural Crest Cells
   - Enteric Nervous System
IV. Germ layers:
   - Endoderm
   - Ectoderm
   - Mesoderm

Fig. 28.23A–B. Biodynamic laws, early cavities, coelomic sacs, and developmental metabolism of the immune system (see also fig. 28.1, p. 305).

This is an important review of embryology related to these biodynamic cardiovascular therapy explorations and the illustrations by Friedrich Wolf in the color insert.

The Fluid Body in the Age of the Immune System (*cont.*)

V. Craniocervical Region – Pharyngeal Arches:
- Face/tongue – thyroid
- 4th arch – thymus, 6th arch – clavicle

  (3rd Generation bone marrow, lymph)
- Lymphatic system

VI. Retroperitoneum – Canalization Zones:
1. Kidneys – mesonephros, metanephros, final kidneys serve as template for lymphatic ducts and azygos veins
2. Lymph vessels, cisterna chyli
3. Brown and white fat
4. Adrenals
5. Abdominal musculature (transversus abdominus)
6. Aorta, inferior vena cava
7. Esophagus above diaphragm
8. Lower third of rectum

VII. Hematopoiesis sequence of development:
1. Yolk sac **(1st Generation)**
2. umbilical vein/vitelline vein: liver

   (2nd Generation)
3. spleen – bone marrow – thymus – lymph vessels **(3rd Generation)**

VIII. Endocrine Pathways:
1. Pituitary – thyroid – thymus – adrenals – gonads
2. Stomach, small intestine, large intestine, liver, pancreas
3. Microbiome

IX. Detoxification Pathways:
1. Fascia – interstitium – lymph
2. Venous return
3. Liver
4. Kidneys
5. Lungs – large intestine

Fig. 28.23A–B (cont.). Biodynamic laws, early cavities, coelomic sacs, and developmental metabolism of the immune system. This is an important review of embryology related to these biodynamic cardiovascular therapy explorations and the illustrations by Friedrich Wolf in the color insert.

29

Palpating the Abdomen, Pelvis, and Lower Extremities

The Original Marrow Part 2

This protocol will now take us a step deeper into the bone marrow directly. We will trace the vascular tree in its branches through the lower extremities, the pelvis, and abdomen.

The Innominate Bones

The innominate bones are the largest reservoir of bone marrow in the human body. They are located at the juncture of the lymphatic system and transition from the lower extremities to the superficial vessels of the abdomen and the deep lymphatic vessels of the pelvis. That access point or line is the inguinal ligament as we will see in a future protocol. As can be seen in figures 29.1–4, contact was made with the anterior superior iliac spine and the other hand the ischial tuberosity. In this way

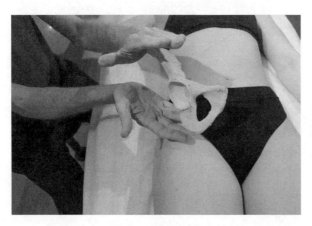

Fig. 29.1. Innominate bones 1

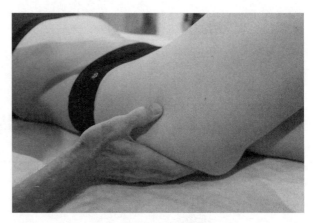

Fig. 29.2. Innominate bones 2

the entire innominate bone is held. Once the hands and arms are supported with proper cushions, the intraosseous motion of the bones can be sensed with Primary Respiration. Of course, the interosseous motion associated with the sacrum and femurs can also be sensed. The bones themselves may rotate if they are out of alignment. All of this can be taking place waiting for PR to breathe the bone from inside its marrow.

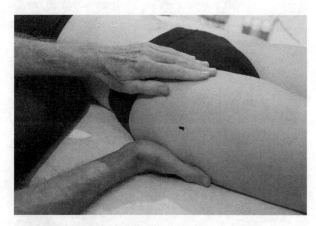

Fig. 29.3. Innominate bones 3

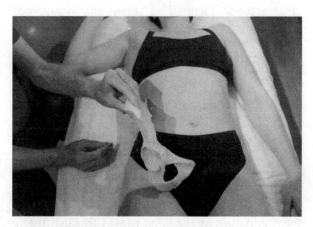

Fig. 29.4. Innominate bones 4

∾

Vascular Tree Branch:
Popliteal–Ulnar Arteries

Following this we move down into the lower extremity. As you can see in figures 29.5–7, contact is going to be made with the popliteal and ulnar arteries. Figure 29.5 shows the location of the artery in prone position. Figure 29.6 shows the contact in supine position, which is the optimal position to use. This branch of the vascular tree also involves contact with the ulnar artery as is shown. As was practiced in the second protocol in the previous chapter, all parts of the vascular tree bend, shake, and shimmy in relation to Primary Respiration. It is very helpful to observe trees in nature as the wind moves through them. This is the most helpful perceptual practice you can do for these skills involving the vascular tree.

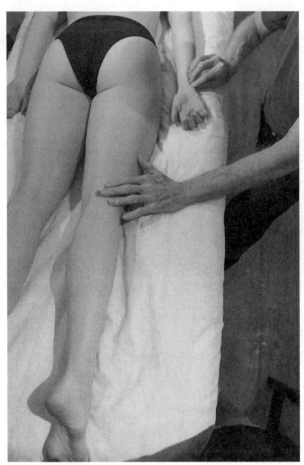

Fig. 29.5. Ulnar–Popliteal arteries 1

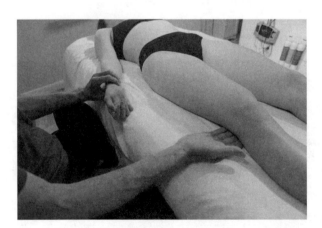

Fig. 29.6. Ulnar–Popliteal arteries 2

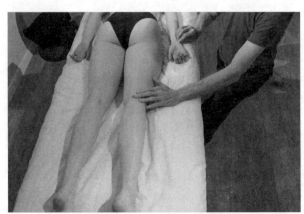

Fig. 29.7. Ulnar–Popliteal arteries 3

❧

Umbilicus–Liver

Once the tree settles, move to the contact for the umbilicus and liver (see figs. 29.8–10). Place the tip of the middle finger in the umbilicus with the client's permission. If there is discomfort this can certainly be done through the clothing of the client. If it remains uncomfortable, ask the client to place their hand on top of your hand.

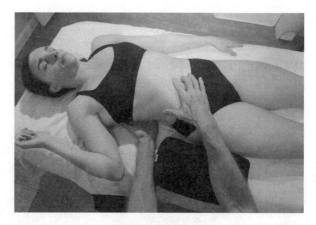

Fig. 29.8. Umbilicus–Liver 1

The other hand is over the costal arch approximating the location of the liver. The attunement process involves making a heart-to-heart connection with PR and gradually sensing the vector of PR between the umbilicus and the liver. This is a very deep embryonic connection and a second-generation blood development skill. There are numerous ways to approach the liver manually and affect its structure and function. Any of those visceral manipulation skills can be practiced at this point in conjunction with beginning and ending with the umbilicus. This will become clearer in the fourth protocol.

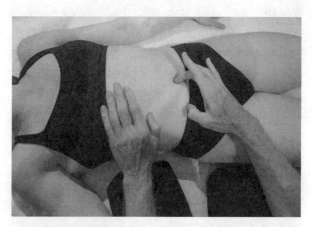

Fig. 29.9. Umbilicus–Liver 2

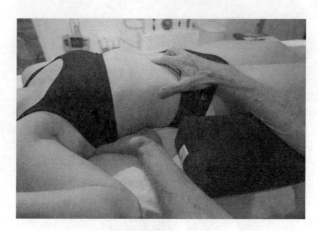

Fig. 29.10. Umbilicus–Liver 3

⨯

Spleen–Mesentery

The next skill involves contacting the spleen with two hands (see figs. 29.11–12). This can be a mechanical but gentle lifting and rolling of the rib cage around the spleen or simply settling with both hands and feeling PR breathing the spleen. Remember that the spleen is third-generation blood development. Figures 29.13–15 show one of my hands over the client's spleen and my other hand slightly below the umbilicus on its edge to gently contact the mesentery as was done in the first marrow protocol. Both hands begin to sense PR and the embryonic suction field as if the hands were pulling taffy, stretching and shortening a substance between the two of them. The spleen forms embryonically in the mesentery, and here we are making a contact to feel the originality of the spleen.

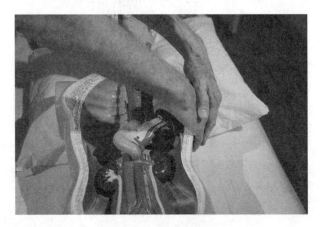

Fig. 29.11. Spleen 1

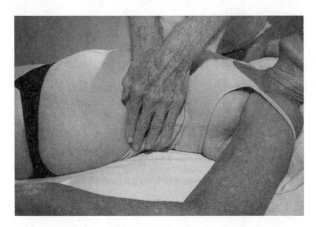

Fig. 29.12. Spleen 2

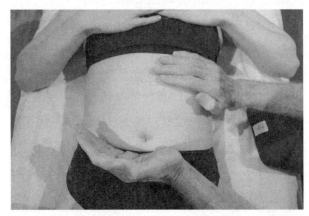

Fig. 29.13. Spleen–Mesentery 1

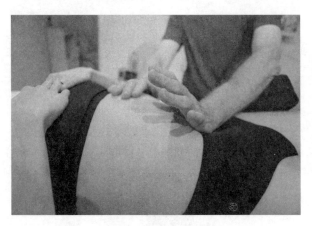

Fig. 29.14. Spleen–Mesentery 2

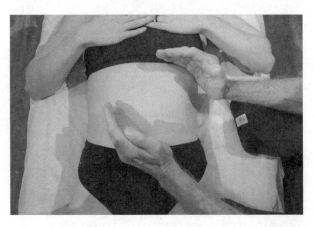

Fig. 29.15. Spleen–Mesentery 3

Twelfth Rib

Next, contact is made with the twelfth rib (see figs. 29.16–17). As mentioned previously, breathing is such a critical component of moving the lymphatic fluid and especially freedom of the twelfth rib. I usually align my fingers with my middle finger approximating the location of the twelfth rib while my other hand is underneath it or to the side depending on the comfort level not only of myself but also the client. The rib will rotate, and because it contains so many attachments of all the different tissues associated with the diaphragm and breathing, it will tend to latchkey in the sense of it compressing toward the spine and then reversing directions and floating back out laterally. But this is not the goal, per se; rather it is sensing the breath coming into the point of contact and the quality of movement in the rib itself. Bones also breathe autonomously with PR. They simply expand and contract within their matrix. This is called intraosseous motion.

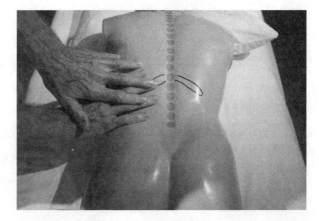

Fig. 29.16. Twelfth rib 1

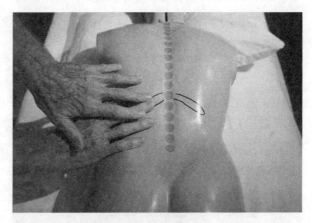

Fig. 29.17. Twelfth rib 2

External Iliac–Femoral Arteries

Next, contact is made with the external iliac artery and femoral artery on one side as shown in figure 29.18. This is a vital connection of the cardiovascular and lymphatic system between the lower extremities, abdomen, and pelvis. Stay with the arterial pulse and dance with it while attuning to PR.

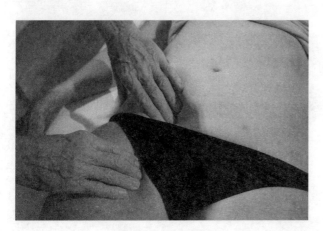

Fig. 29.18. Iliac–Femoral arteries

⚬

Popliteal–Posterior Tibial Arteries

Next move to the popliteal artery and posterior tibial artery (see figs. 29.19–20).
This skill, like the preceding one, is a fantastic setup for the foot and knee lymphatic
pumps that follow. I like to palpate the popliteal artery as it goes over the posterior
part of the tibial plateau. As with many arteries and their palpation, I will frequently
need to move my fingers several times, a millimeter here and there, until clear contact is made with the popliteal artery. The posterior tibial artery is underneath the
fascia and ligaments, and if there is a history of ankle sprains, breaks, or fractures
in a client's foot, the connective tissue will be thicker and will need more time to
soften and give way to sensing the artery. Consequently, it is important to simply
wait as the tissue melts and the artery recognizes a friendly hand. The artery will
find you if you cannot find it. Calm abiding is required to invite the artery into your
fingers and perception. These are very important pathways in the whole vascular
lymphatic structure and function.

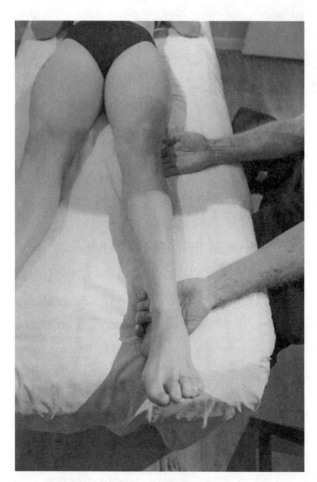

Fig. 29.19. Popliteal–Posterior tibial arteries 1

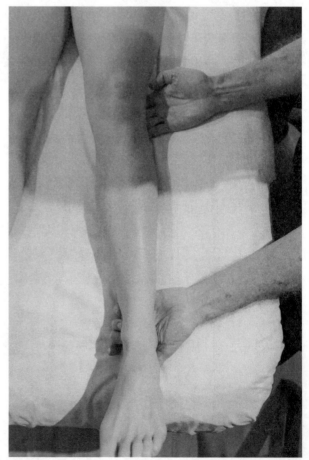

Fig. 29.20. Popliteal–Posterior tibial arteries 2

∝

Dorsal Lymphatic Foot Pump

Now start with the dorsal lymphatic foot pump (see figs. 29.21–22). I like to gently dorsi flex the feet with the heels of my hands by making contact around the balls of the client's feet. This is also the location of an important acupuncture point, Kidney 1, which is important for the chi of the body to ground through to the earth. Begin to explore a gentle vibration into the feet bilaterally with a vector through the spine and out the top of the head.

Palpation and Exploration of the Lymphatic Pumps

All of the lymphatic pumps, including the Sutherland thoracic duct pump practiced in chapter 28, involve three levels of palpation and exploration:

1. First, set the hands comfortably and induce a gentle vibratory motion along the vectors indicated such as through the spine and out the top of the head to begin this foot pump.

2. Secondly, when a reciprocal wave-like motion from the fluid body responds into your hands, the vector can be changed to include the whole body or the whole fluid body or the whole vascular tree. This is the time to explore a different tempo with the vibration until the therapist can observe the entire body of the client vibrating, especially the pearl in the lower dantian as described in the previous chapter.

3. At the third level the bones containing the marrow, especially in the lower extremities, are channels within the fluid body that provide the blueprint for all endothelial vessels. The bones and the marrow become like a garden hose that is full and flexible or like a snake making a serpentine movement. To experience the originality of the marrow is to experience the embryo, and the therapist needs to be noncognitive for such a perception of originality.

4. Imagine you are vibrating a container of Jell-O but at the center of the Jell-O is a dense core that is still part of the fluid body. At this point the marrow and the bone start to move as if they were a flexible hose or snake. Stay with this wave-like phenomenon at least three to five minutes. Then gently move to the side of the body toward the knee that might be most affected in the client.

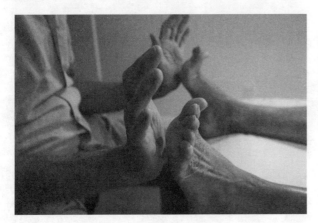

Fig. 29.21. Foot marrow pump 1

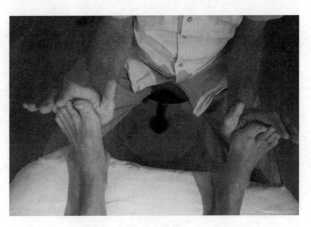

Fig. 29.22. Foot marrow pump 2

Knee Lymphatic Pump

Figures 29.23–24 show contact with the client's knee flexed. I am simply jiggling very gently along the knee, medial to lateral, exploring the three-level palpation skill for the marrow just mentioned above. In this case the femur and its connection into the innominate bone will gradually open and allow more length to flow. These last two lymphatic pump skills are so important for the contemporary client because of the proliferation of knee and hip problems requiring surgical interventions. And of course, postoperatively these are excellent skills. If there is any doubt, always get medical clearance from the client's physician.

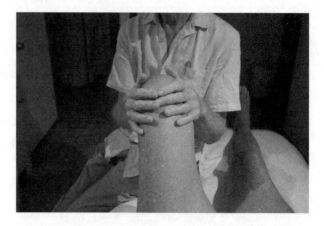

Fig. 29.23. Knee-Inguinal pump 1

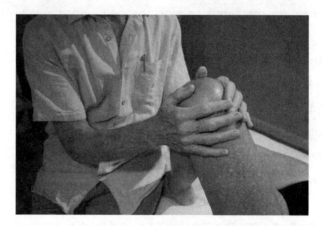

Fig. 29.24. Knee-Inguinal pump 2

Bilateral Anterior Tibial Arteries

There are several ways to finish a biodynamics session. One of my favorite ways is to simply place a hand under the coccyx with my other hand under the twelfth rib to balance the respiratory diaphragm and pelvic diaphragm at the end of a session. This is particularly valuable to stabilize the autonomic nervous system through the organization of breathing in the trunk abdomen and pelvis. The breath needs to return to the abdomen.

My other favorite way to end a session is to make bilateral contact with the anterior tibial arteries (see figs. 29.25–26) which change name around the middorsal part of the foot to the dorsalis pedis arteries. There is a lot of wiggle room in finding an easy placement of the finger pads to contact any part of the anterior tibial artery. I synchronize my attention with the downward-voiding wind coming from the client's pelvis via my heart. PR is good at the beginning of a session; it is good at the middle of a session, and it is magnificent at the end of a session when the Health manifests and the vascular tree has a beautiful breeze blowing through it.

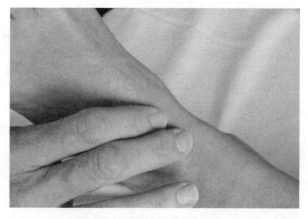

Fig. 29.25. Anterior tibial artery

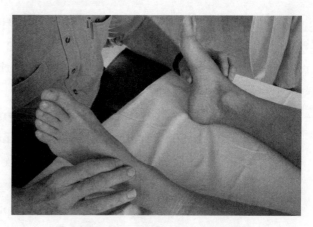

Fig. 29.26. Bilateral anterior tibial arteries

30
Palpating the Head, Neck, and Shoulders
The Original Marrow Part 3

This protocol is a series of contacts around the shoulders, neck, and head and details the embryonic unfolding of that area of the body. The contacts range from traditional osteopathic work with the lymphatic system to include contemporary biodynamic approaches based on the embryology of the pharyngeal arches. This is all blended into the slowness of Primary Respiration and the quiet of the dynamic stillness. Always the dance begins with the element of wind and the element of space. It is important to bridge between the marrow, the fascia, the interstitium, the capillaries, and the lymphatic vessels themselves. It all starts in the embryo. Figure 30.1 shows the pharyngeal arches, their embryonic development, and their structural derivations.

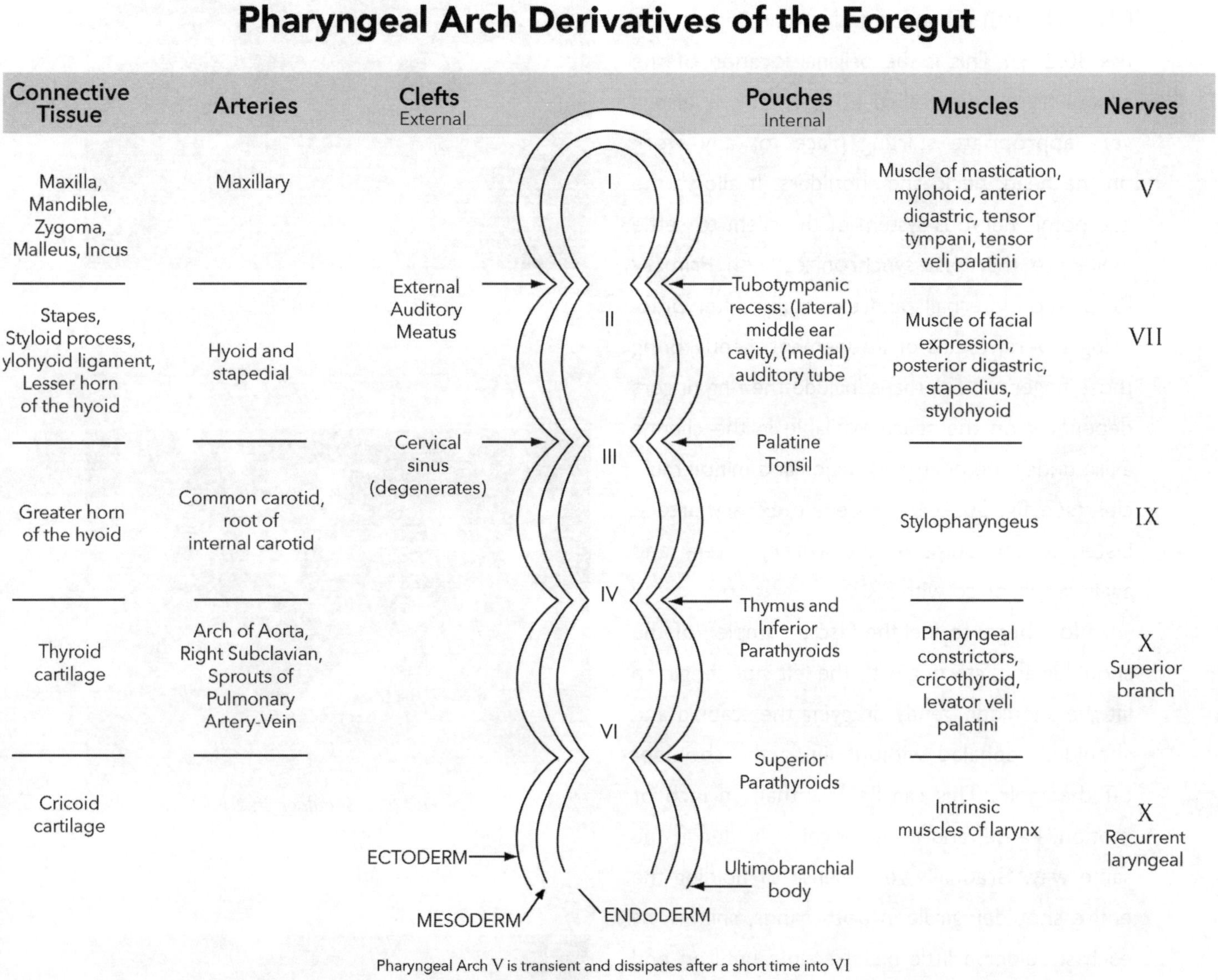

Pharyngeal Arch Derivatives of the Foregut

Connective Tissue	Arteries	Clefts External	Pouches Internal	Muscles	Nerves
Maxilla, Mandible, Zygoma, Malleus, Incus	Maxillary			Muscle of mastication, mylohoid, anterior digastric, tensor tympani, tensor veli palatini	V
Stapes, Styloid process, ylohyoid ligament, Lesser horn of the hyoid	Hyoid and stapedial	External Auditory Meatus	Tubotympanic recess: (lateral) middle ear cavity, (medial) auditory tube	Muscle of facial expression, posterior digastric, stapedius, stylohyoid	VII
Greater horn of the hyoid	Common carotid, root of internal carotid	Cervical sinus (degenerates)	Palatine Tonsil	Stylopharyngeus	IX
Thyroid cartilage	Arch of Aorta, Right Subclavian, Sprouts of Pulmonary Artery-Vein		Thymus and Inferior Parathyroids	Pharyngeal constrictors, cricothyroid, levator veli palatini	X Superior branch
Cricoid cartilage			Superior Parathyroids	Intrinsic muscles of larynx	X Recurrent laryngeal

ECTODERM

MESODERM   ENDODERM

Ultimobranchial body

Pharyngeal Arch V is transient and dissipates after a short time into VI

Fig. 30.1. The pharyngeal arches and their structural derivatives. Biodynamic skills associated with the face, neck, and cranium must consider the pharyngeal arches, especially their relationship with the arch arteries and the vagus nerve as detailed in chapter 25. The arches are an essential component of the fluid body.

Axillary Artery–Shoulder Lift

Sitting at the head of the table, gently contact the space between the coracoid process and clavicles bilaterally with the index and middle fingers (see figs 30.2–3). This is the original location of the acupuncture point called Lung 1. This is also a very appropriate starting place for any work on the head, neck, and shoulders. It allows the autonomic nervous system of the client to settle while the therapist synchronizes with Primary Respiration internally and externally. After practicing several cycles of attunement, gently bring those fingers and perhaps include the ring fingers depending on the space available in the client's axilla under the pectoralis major and minor muscles (see fig. 30.4) to sense the axillary artery. Listen to the pulse of the axillary artery and again synchronize with PR.

Now begin to feel the fascial complex of the shoulder and, starting with the left side, begin to lift the shoulder, gently dragging the scapula and shoulder cephalad without lifting the shoulder off the table. This can be less than an inch of motion. Pause, and lift the right shoulder in the same way. Gradually get a sense of holding the entire shoulder girdle in both hands, shimmying each shoulder a little bit at a time until an end point is reached or a barrier. Do not go beyond the tissue barrier. This allows the thoracic ducts of the lymphatic system to drain more fully and opens the entire vascular system in the thoracic inlet/outlet area. Wait several minutes and practice attunement. Notice any shifts in the client's breathing, particularly movement in the upper three ribs of the client's trunk.

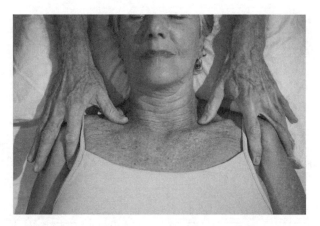

Fig. 30.2. Shoulder lift 1

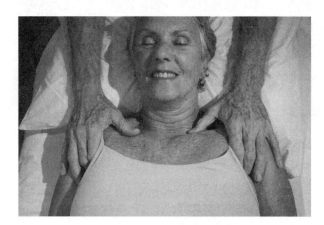

Fig. 30.3. Shoulder lift 2

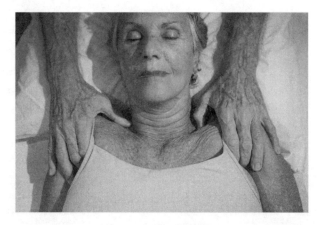

Fig. 30.4. Shoulder lift 3

Arm Pump–Marrow Spiral

This next process with the arms is like the foot and knee lymphatic pump. Choose the side of the body that seems in most need. Support the elbow in the palm of one hand and make palm-to-palm contact with your other hand and that of the client. Gently start a lateral-medial oscillating motion with the client's elbow going one direction and the client's hand in the opposite direction. This is a very slow and intentional movement. Please review the three-step process for freeing the marrow in the previous chapter.

Play with different motions, such as wiggling the arm from the palm only, to get to the third stage, like feeling a flexible garden hose or a swimming pool noodle filled with marrow. This is such excellent work for the axillary lymphatic vessels for anyone who has had surgery in the arms or shoulders and especially women who have experienced mastectomies. This is very gentle and loving contact.

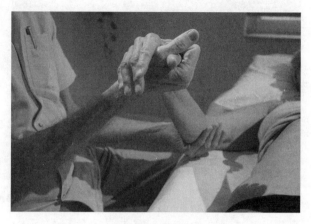

Fig. 30.5. Arm pump

Atlanto-Occipital Joint

Figures 30.6 and 30.7 on page 330 show a traditional atlanto-occipital joint exploration contact (AOJ). As Dr. Becker said, "The AOJ is the gateway to the cranium." I particularly like this skill because it also helps the therapist evaluate lymphedema in the upper neck, especially if the client has a neck injury from a motor vehicle accident or a mild traumatic brain injury (concussion). There are numerous schools of lymphatic drainage, and all of those techniques are valuable because if the therapist senses lymphedema in the atlanto-occipital joint area, attention must shift toward proper drainage of the lymphedema from the head and neck into the thoracic ducts. It must be remembered that the original lymphatic vessels first arise in the neck along the current track of the jugular vein. When biodynamic practice is applied to the neck area in general, it has such a deep influence on the lymphatic system since the left thoracic duct drains 75 percent of the body's lymphatic fluid. The right lymphatic duct drains 25 percent of the body's lymphatic fluid particularly from the right arm or right side of the shoulder, head, and neck.

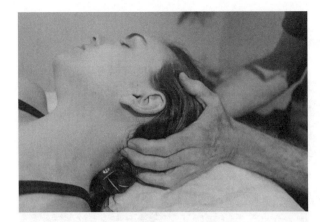

Fig. 30.6. Atlanto-occipital joint 1

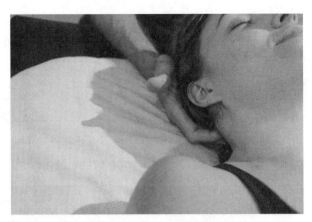

Fig. 30.7. Atlanto-occipital joint 2

⁂

Mandible-Arch I

This sequence attempts to follow the embryonic formation of the pharyngeal arches starting with arch number one in its adult form, the mandible (see fig. 30.8). Notice that the contact is bilateral, and I am using the pads of my fingers close to the ramus of the mandible, as this will influence the fascia related to the temporal mandibular joint (TMJ). It is important in the attunement process that the remaining surface areas of the palms and hands used to sense the fluid fields of the cranium extending be on the surface of the skin. The hands toggle back and forth between the mandible and the fluid fields of the cranium. The mandible was originally two bones embryonically, and when the therapist is synchronized with Primary Respiration, various mandibular motions can be perceived. Wait until all motion comes to a stillpoint and settles.

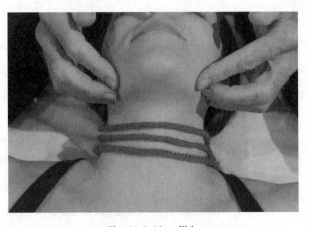

Fig. 30.8. Mandible

Digastric Muscle: Origination of the Thyroid

Figure 30.9 shows a contact with the digastric muscle at the base of the tongue. The thyroid gland arises embryonically from the tongue. This is an excellent skill to practice starting with sensing the tension in the digastric muscle and simply waiting for the tension to soften with slight pressure from the pads of the therapist's fingers. This will improve masticating and swallowing food as well as speaking.

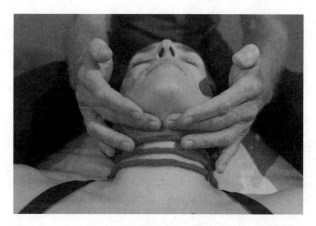

Fig. 30.9. Digastric muscle

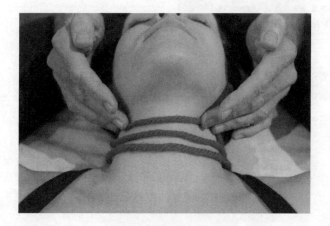

Fig. 30.10. Hyoid bone

Hyoid-Arch 2

Figure 30.10 shows bilateral contact with the hyoid bone. This bone is suspended from the cervical fascia and ligaments especially to the styloid process of the temporal bone and thus reflexing into the TMJ. All of these skills are vital to the structure and function of the neck, including swallowing and breathing as coregulated by the vagus nerve, which was covered in detail in chapter 25. All these contacts require the therapist to be attentive to their whole hand and whole body breathing with the fluid fields as they are moved in the tempo of PR. Sometimes PR can be ignited with heart-to-heart attunement or third ventricle–horizon attunement.

⨳

Cricoid Cartilage-Arch 3

Notice that figures 30.8–11 and 30.13 have three lines around the neck. These are indications of the pharyngeal arches and the pharyngeal arch arteries prior to turning vertical and becoming the carotid arteries (see fig. 30.1 on page 327). However, these lines give a sense of the location quite close together between the arches and their derivatives. By gently moving your fingers from the bilateral contact with the hyoid perhaps only a half inch or so, you can locate the cricoid cartilage. It is small and connected to the Adam's apple, which is the more prominent part of the thyroid cartilage. This requires a very delicate palpation skill by moving the pads of your fingers bilaterally millimeter by millimeter inferiorly from the hyoid bone.

When the Adam's apple is differentiated because of its prominence, simply move into the space between it and the hyoid bone, and this is the smaller cricoid cartilage. Special care is taken to observe any activation of the autonomic nervous system of the client. It is not necessary to make all of these contacts, but rather starting at the top with the mandible, always check in verbally with the client and find out if they are comfortable with each contact. If at any time the skin color of their face flushes red or their eyes glaze over or their respiration changes, it's time to move somewhere else.

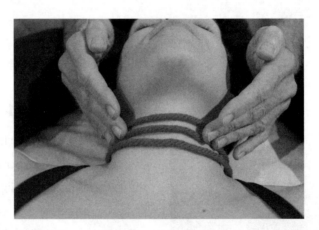

Fig. 30.11. Cricoid cartilage

❦
The Thyroid Arteries

The thyroid gland is quite beautiful. It is shaped like a butterfly and rests anterior to the esophagus close to the vagal bodies of the aorta, and its inferior portion lies directly posterior to the sternoclavicular notch. The inferior thyroid arteries come directly from the subclavian arteries. The superior thyroid arteries come from the carotid arteries. Figures 30.12–13 show a very gentle contact bilaterally with the index fingers or more laterally with other fingers depending on the comfort level of the client for this palpation. It is important to get a sense of the pulse of both the superior thyroid artery that comes from the carotid artery and inferior thyroid artery that comes from the subclavian artery. If you start with the superior thyroid artery, then shift your fingers inferiorly for the inferior thyroid artery. You can also begin with the inferior thyroid artery and work superiorly. This is a very deep, contemplative practice; sense PR heart to heart while contacting the thyroid arteries. You can also begin and end this step by contacting the digastric muscle as done above.

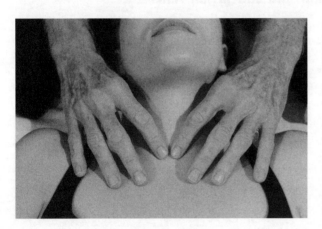

Fig. 30.12. Thyroid 1

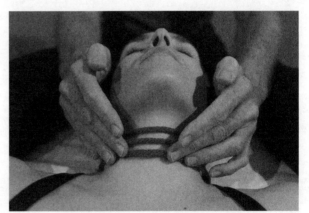

Fig. 30.13. Thyroid 2

❦
The Clavicles-Arch 6

Figure 30.14 on page 334 shows my fingers contacting the clavicle. I begin with the index fingers contacting the proximal end of the clavicular head. As much as possible the pads of my other fingers are gently and buoyantly contacting the clavicles. This is really getting close to the heart of the third generation of blood development, as some texts say that the marrow initially begins in the clavicles as they are formed from the sixth pharyngeal arch embryonically. It is important to differentiate intraosseous motion originating from the wide variety of stem cells in the marrow breathing with the potency of PR and interosseous motion regarding the various attachments and connections that the clavicles have to the surrounding structures. This is an excellent preparatory palpation prior to the next exploration.

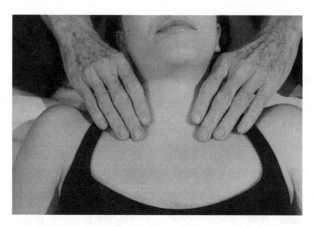

Fig. 30.14. Clavicles

The Thoracic Ducts:
The Junction of the Jugular and Subclavian Veins

I prefer to palpate the subclavian artery superior to the midpoint of the clavicles and gently sense my way mediately along the subclavian artery until the pulsation of the carotid arteries meets my fingers. I wait and pause and shift the intention of my fingers as if going underneath this junction of power arteries into the stillpoint and still place of the jugular and subclavian veins. Gently wait in the stillness of the veins and observe how the client's breath may begin to change and especially if there is a spontaneous deep breath that mobilizes the upper three ribs.

This is an indication that the thoracic ducts are working more optimally.

In addition, the palms of the hands can be sensing the motion of the notochordal midline of the embryo as if an elevator shaft filled with PR is lifting the palms of your hands, and about a minute later in the phase change of PR, the palms of the hands feel as if they are being gently sucked down toward the pelvis through the center and core of the body. This palpation has a dual intention of optimizing lymphatic flow and normalizing PR in the notochord midline of the central nervous system.

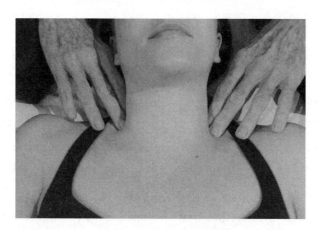

Fig. 30.15. Thoracic ducts

∽
The Thymus-Arch 4

The thymus is the University of the Immune System. It is where immune cells—especially T cells—undergo their final maturation processes and graduate. Figures 30.16–17 show a bilateral contact with my index and middle fingers over the manubrium. I like to gently sense from the manubrium inferiorly down the sternum as far as the junction of the fourth rib. Somewhere in that vicinity the pads of your fingers will be magnetically attracted to the thymus. This is where the fingers will rest for the balance of this skill. Remember: in a previous protocol contact was made with both the thymus and the spleen, which can be considered here as an adjunct or complement to this skill.

This protocol can be completed with any contact around the sacrum and/or feet. Always bring the earth element back into the session when ending.

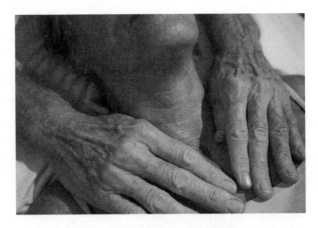

Fig. 30.16. Thyroid–Thymus 1

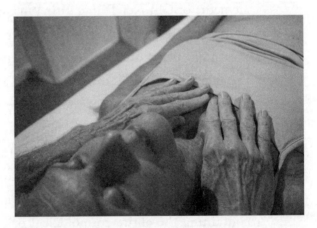

Fig. 30.17. Thyroid–Thymus 2

31
Palpating the Abdomen
The Original Marrow Part 4

This is a very special protocol derived from Taoist manual therapy. It combines elements of Chi Nei Tsang, Tuina massage, osteopathy for the viscera, and biodynamic perception of Primary Respiration. It includes recent research on the mesentery being a unique organ system. This protocol is woven together into the fabric of a biodynamic practice. Taoist manual therapy is oriented around the cosmological origin of the universe being correlated with the abdomen and specifically the umbilicus. This special cosmology of a body representation of the external universe is said to have originated from the first Chinese emperor in 2500 BCE. The emperor was said to be walking in his garden and noticed a tortoise turned upside down. He had a vision of the underbelly of the tortoise containing the entire cosmological origin of the universe. The Taoist manual therapy called Chi Nei Tsang popularized by Mantak Chia was born from this cosmology as it focuses on internal organ chi massage. The origins of the methods presented in this chapter derive from my study of Chi Nei Tsang from the master Jörg Schürpf.

Nota Bene

If the client prefers to cover their abdomen with their shirt, all of the following skills can be explored through the clothing.

⨯

Abdominal Breathing

Either standing or sitting at the side of the table, place one hand palm down between the xiphoid and the umbilicus and the other hand palm down over the umbilicus. Ask the client to breathe into the areas of contact for at least three cycles of breathing. Then place one hand palm down between umbilicus and pubis. The other hand will be over the umbilicus again. Ask the client to breath into the areas of contact for at least three cycles of breathing.

⨯

Yolk Sac Umbilical Spiral

Figures 31.1–4 show the gradual relationship of my top hand to the yolk sac. At the same time, I am practicing a heart spiral meditation from chapter 14. I actively sense my heart and pericardium suspended from the neck where the heart originated embryonically. Tuning into the tempo of Primary Respiration and the fluid nature of the heart and blood, I sense the entire pericardial sac moving circularly around the lower ribs for about a minute, pausing and reversing direction, thus making a spiral. Tuning into this heart spiral allows a much deeper contact with the umbilical spiral starting three to four feet off the body directly above the client's umbilicus. The Physioball in figure 31.1 is a rough approximation of the location of the top hand as if it were contacting an actual yolk sac (umbilical vesicle).

In Taoism, the source of that spiraling energy would be the center point of the universe, which in some texts is the North Star in the constellation Ursa Major and in other sources it is other stars in Ursa Major and the universe. I like the North Star because it gets us in the ballpark of what the ancient teachings refer to. Begin with a very small diameter and then enlarge the diameter of the spiral motion of

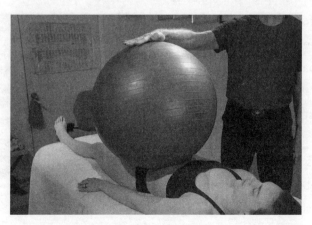

Fig. 31.1. Yolk sac

the hand until the hand is synchronized with the umbilical spiral at that height above the client. Sometimes the hand will go slow in the tempo of PR, and sometimes the hand will speed up as the spiral becomes smaller in diameter closer to the umbilicus.

It is appropriate to pause periodically so as not to compress the spiral into the client's umbilicus, which can create discomfort. After a couple of minutes, as the top hand gets closer to the umbilicus, the middle finger bends and the tip of the middle finger is placed very gently at the entrance to the umbilicus.

The opposite hand contacts the spinous process of the second lumbar vertebra. The same spiral that is moving in a clockwise direction through the umbilicus anteriorly is moving counterclockwise through the second lumbar vertebra posteriorly. It takes some time to sense those opposite directions.

Upon contact with the umbilicus, direct the client to breathe directly into the point of contact. This is the three-level belly breathing mentioned in previous chapters. With each inhalation and resulting abdominal undulation, continue to allow the finger and wrist to make a slow, spiraling micromovement. With each exhalation, notice if there is an invitation for the tip of the finger to go deeper but not with force or going beyond a tissue barrier. It is a sense of taking up slack but not challenging or going past a tissue barrier.

An end point is reached when the spiral settles into a dynamic stillness. Frequently the strong pulse of the abdominal aorta will simply begin to dominate one's perception. If it feels that the finger in the umbilicus is stuck, begin to wiggle it very gently and slowly extract the finger from the client's umbilicus.

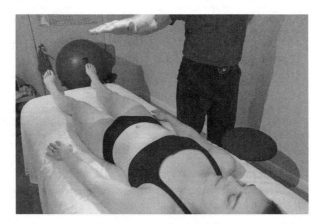

Fig. 31.2. Umbilical spiral 1

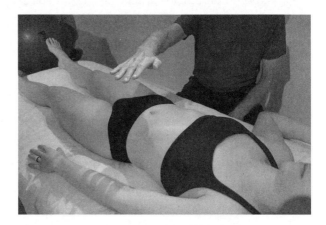

Fig. 31.3. Umbilical spiral 2

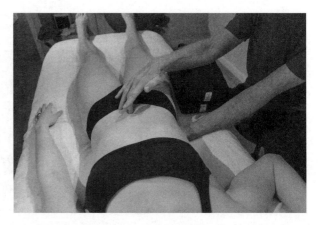

Fig. 31.4. Umbilical spiral 3

Abdominal Autonomic Plexi

Take a moment to review figures 25.2A–B on pages 268–69 in chapter 25 to see the beauty of the entire complex of abdominal autonomic plexi. Figures 31.5–7 show contact with all my fingertips and pads lined up as if they were going to play the piano. Start with the midline just inferior to the xiphoid process. Most likely your tenth finger will end up somewhere around the umbilicus. Listen for the abdominal breathing in three cycles. It is always key for there to be an invitation for the fingers to sink more deeply during the exhalation.

In addition, if the client's abdomen is very tense or tight or the client is overweight, have the client flex both of their knees together and make sure the knees are supported with the client's feet more laterally than the knees so they can rest together without muscle tension holding them up.

Next, shift your piano hands to that same midline superior of the pubic synthesis up through the umbilicus. Please note how similar the contact is with the *Star Trek* protocol in chapter 26. All of the autonomic plexi are being impacted by this contact, especially when the therapist is synchronized with PR and working internally with their heart spiral. The internal heart spiral translates to the hands and fingers, inducing a small spiral in each contact. This second part of the abdominal plexi contact is focused on the lower dantian, which is approximately midway between the umbilicus and pubic synthesis (Ren 6). I typically will wait much longer than three breaths in this position because of the importance of the lower dantian in managing the elements and channels of the subtle and physiological body.

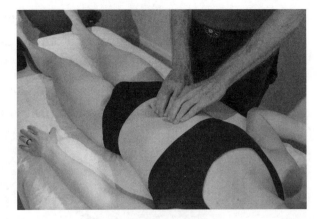

Fig. 31.5. ANS plexi 1

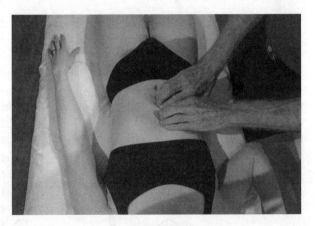

Fig. 31.6. ANS plexi 2

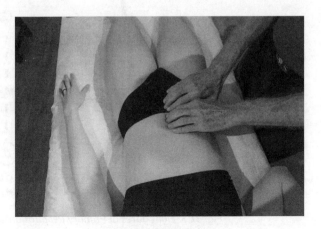

Fig. 31.7. ANS plexi 3

∾

The Eight Gates of Primary Respiration

Figure 31.8 shows the map of the eight gates of Primary Respiration. This is a compass in which the vector from the umbilicus up the midline is the heart vector. Going clockwise the next vector is the spleen, then the left kidney, then the left ovary and sigmoid colon. The vector going inferiorly down the midline toward the pubic synthesis is for the uterus and prostate. Continuing clockwise the lower quadrant is the ascending colon and right ovary, then the right kidney, and finally the liver. These are the eight gates.

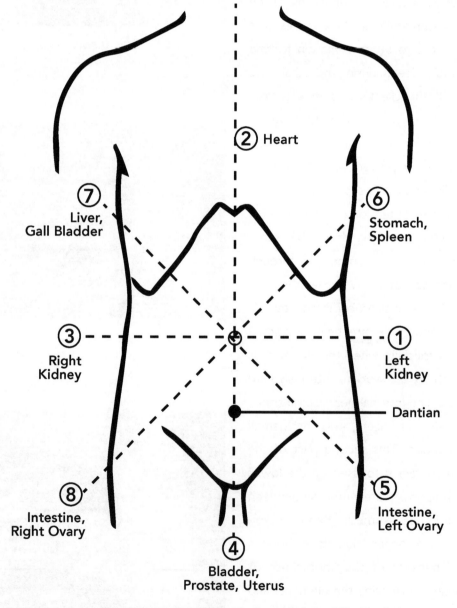

Fig. 31.8. Eight gates of Primary Respiration. As directed, the umbilical fascia is connected to all the organs indicated. This is a classical Chi Nei Tsang exploration.

My middle finger is in the client's umbilicus (see figs. 31.9–10). Following three breaths and until the middle finger is seated comfortably yet relatively deep in the umbilicus, a very gentle and minimal circular motion is started with the finger that engages the umbilical fascia, the transversalis fascia, and the peritoneum. All these fasciae, including the mesentery, hold and support these eight gates and their respective organs.

Gradually as more experience is gained, the therapist will sense what feels like a taut ring of fascia, the umbilical opening, and it is this ring of fascia that the middle finger contacts and stretches gently with not much more than several millimeters of initial motion. Synchronize with the heart spiral internally until sensing the spiral translate through the fingers. When the circular motion is not smooth in a particular vector, wait and see if the fascia will soften along that vector. If not, place your other hand on the opposite vector for a counter stretch. Slowly work your way around all eight vectors, pausing and offering openness or very gentle counterstretching.

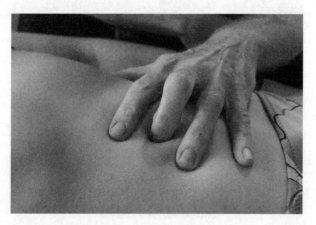

Fig. 31.9. Umbilicus 1

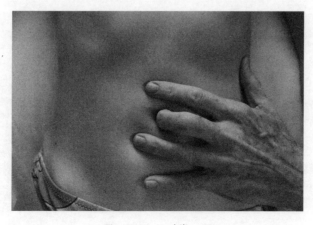

Fig. 31.10. Umbilicus 2

⚘

Mesentery

Once again, we will visit the mesentery like that shown in chapter 28. The mesentery is such an important organ, and I like to use the heel of my hand above the umbilicus to gather the mesentery (see figs. 31.11–13). In this skill, the therapist works their way around the loop of the peritoneum between the anterior superior iliac spines and pubic bone. Using the palm of the hand or the edge of the hand sinking down, lift and gently stretch the mesentery superiorly. At the same time while listening for the breath coming into the point of contact, a gentle spiral motion can be made with your dominant hand on the mesentery. It is a very simple undulating pattern that your hand makes with the mesentery. This facilitates the movement of the lymph and blood. Now the internal heart spiral becomes integrated through the therapist's body and hands such that all movement perceived is a spiral.

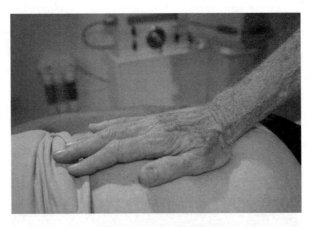

Fig. 31.11. Mesentery 1

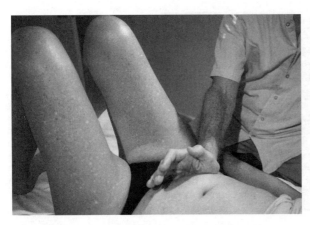

Fig. 31.12. Mesentery 2

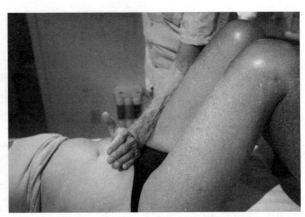

Fig. 31.13. Mesentery 3

Peritoneal Fascia
Wedge–Lower Abdomen

This skill will once again employ all the tips of the fingers as if playing the piano. As you can see in figures 31.14–16, I have all my fingertips lined up in a straight line on a flat plane. Now we are set to interact with the deep lymph nodes and vessels in the pelvic floor. In this exploration we are following the inferior loop of the anterior superior iliac spine around the superior border of the pubic symphysis, along the border of inguinal ligaments and finishing at the opposite anterior superior iliac spine.

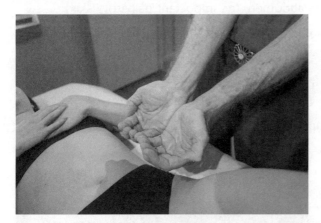

Fig. 31.14. Inguinal lymph 1

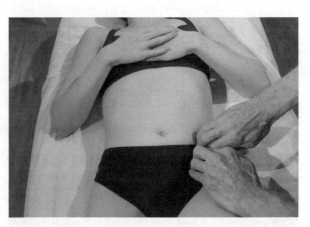

Fig. 31.15. Inguinal lymph 2

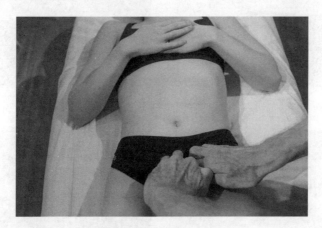

Fig. 31.16. Pubic lymph 3

❦

Costal Arch

Now continue with the same wedge formation of your fingers along the costal arch. Moving from one side of the costal arch (see figs. 31.17–20) to the xiphoid process and then to the other side in perhaps two or three locations (depending on the size of your hands and the client's costal arch), covering most of the costal arch and the associated fascia. The compressional movement is directly inferior without any vector or angle. The pressure is not on the bone itself but just inferior to the costal arch into the soft tissue of the abdomen. Again, it may be valuable to have the client flex their knees to make the abdomen more accessible and the lymph flow better.

As with all the skills associated with the abdomen, the important palpatory skill here is the three-cycle abdominal breathing with a focus on the exhalation inviting the hands deeper. Remember to keep the fingers on a flat plane to avoid one or two of your longer fingers poking or going too deeply in one area.

I like to end this protocol by holding the sacrum and diaphragm from underneath and finish holding the anterior or superior iliac arteries.

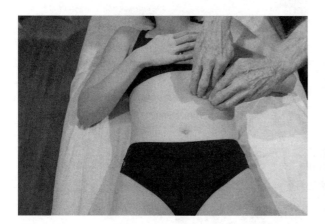

Fig. 31.17. Costal arch lymph 1

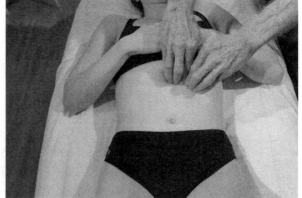

Fig. 31.18. Costal arch lymph 2

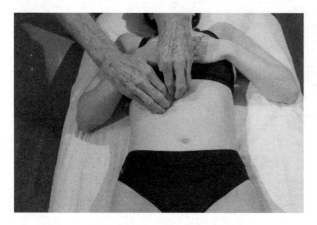

Fig. 31.19. Costal arch lymph 3

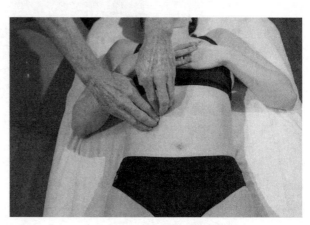

Fig. 31.20. Costal arch lymph 4

Although this abdominal work can appear to be vigorous or mechanical, it is practiced biodynamically. Focus on the client's breathing at the point of contact. The therapist's hands are always thinking and sensing spiral. The therapist's heart is always thinking and feeling spiral. The dance of PR and the dynamic stillness is always the core of the perceptual process. We slow down. We stop. We wait.

32

Neonatal Cardiometabolic Palpation
A New Paradigm in Biodynamic Practice

The most spiritual service I do is with babies. The field of love between the caregiver and the child is one of the most powerful I know and experience. I acknowledge by letting the love permeate my mind and body as deeply as possible before putting on my therapist hat. An infant's first year is the *most metabolically active time* in the entire human life span. Extensive remodeling of the brain, lungs, heart, and gut begin moments after birth. This happens intensively on many levels, from microcirculation and lipid/glucose conversion to the proper filling of diapers. The heart must adjust to a dramatic shift in oxygen intake and remodeling of its cellular reproduction (see fig. 32.1). Microcirculation increases in the brain as the endothelium changes to accommodate the intensive growth of neurons. A vast network of capillaries expand throughout the body. High levels of cortisol and catecholamines are necessary for internal combustion of living on the land (see fig. 32.2).

The lungs begin bringing oxygen into the blood and removing carbon dioxide from the blood at the level of the alveoli. The heart goes through extensive remodeling, not only in how endocardial cells function, but especially in the way that glucose is converted. Glucose is no longer stored in the heart as it was in utero, therefore the heart's energy production must switch from glycolysis to lipid conversion. Intensive microcirculation occurs in the gut to accommodate oral nutrition.

The metabolic engine of life *starts with the gut microbiome,* acquired first from the mother's body during pregnancy and birth and then through breastfeeding and skin-to-skin contact. It takes approximately three days after birth

---

This chapter was reprinted with permission from *Somatic Psychotherapy Today,* 9, no. 1 (Spring 2019).

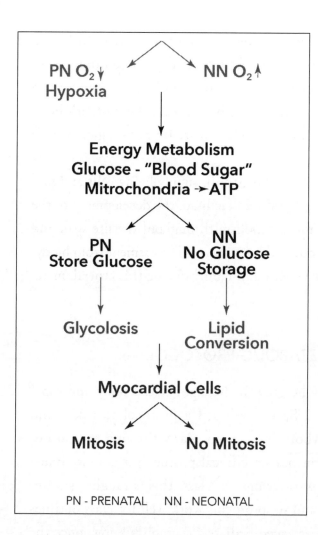

Fig. 32.1. Neonatal heart metabolism. The heart undergoes significant structural and metabolic remodeling after birth. This is especially true of the onset of lipid conversion of the infant's brown fat on which the baby can live for several days.

Fig. 32.2. Neonatal transition metabolism. The entire cardiovascular metabolism undergoes major shifts especially in the lungs, brain, and intestines.

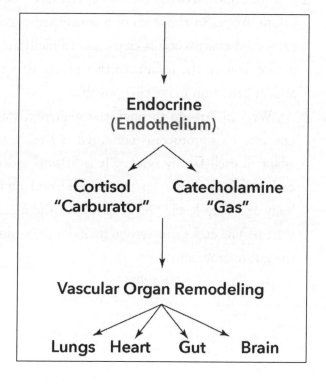

for a mother's milk to come in. Human babies are born with extra fluid and fat, and the baby utilizes these stores in its first three days. The infant relies upon its stored water for hydration and its copious brown fat for energy and lipid conversion. Prior to the arrival of mature breastmilk, the mother's body provides tiny amounts of colostrum, a thick, sweet, immunologically rich substance.

First colostrum and several days later breastmilk supply living cells and prebiotics such as human milk oligosaccharides to facilitate the development of the infant's gut microbiome, the base for metabolism throughout the life span and normal cognitive development. Gentle and knowledgeable treatment from biodynamic therapists can support the newborn and family during this crucial, metabolically active time.

A CARDIOMETABOLIC PROTOCOL

To support such dramatic metabolic growth throughout the body and especially these four organ systems, I have developed a protocol to assess and support the metabolism of a newborn baby, particularly through the cardiovascular system. This is not so much a set clinical protocol; it is more like a smorgasbord with many delightful offerings. In class, this is taught as a linear sequence. Linear progression and set protocols work well for class outlines and published articles. But as experienced pediatric therapists know, once the infant arrives in the arms of a concerned parent, adaptation is necessary, and embodied compassion is essential. To facilitate this, I usually treat the mother before or with the infant. In this protocol, simple changes in hand placement and/or attention make this possible.

We will now go through the sequence, starting with the feet and moving upward. This protocol is presented as I teach it in class knowing that you will adapt to each family system. It is helpful to know the metabolic logic behind each palpation skill. Also, let yourself wonder what is happening inside the baby's body at a deep level. The deep level is the metabolic level: the entire endocrine system. The endocrine system includes the endothelium of the blood vessels and the gut microbiome.

The Extremities

The most basic principle in biodynamic cardiovascular work is to *work from periphery to center*. When possible, begin contact with an infant with one or both anterior and posterior tibial arteries. This is especially valuable with infants who have had their umbilical cord cut prematurely, a common obstetrical procedure (versus the evidence-based and physiologically sound practice of delayed cord clamping). With early cord clamping, there is an estimated 20 to 60 percent decrease in blood transfer from cord and placenta to the infant's cardiovascular system. This may lead to hypovolemic shock. Immediate cord clamping is also directly related to anemia in the first year of life, which is a huge stressor on the infant's metabolism. Gentle contact with the *tibial arteries and the brachial arteries* supports the resolution of hypovolemic shock and relaxation of the vascular tree (see figs. 32.3–5).

Since there is extensive circulatory and metabolic remodeling happening in the heart and lungs, the infant's extremities experience a loss of blood volume. *Peripheral acrocyanosis*, or blueish-purple hands and feet, is a normal (albeit colorful) finding in the newborn. The central core metabolism of the infant is hard at work with a heart rate often twice that of an adult.

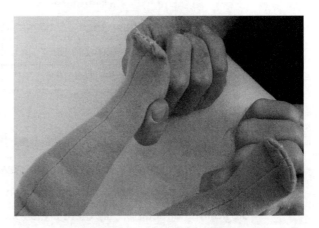
Fig. 32.3. Bilateral posterior tibial artery

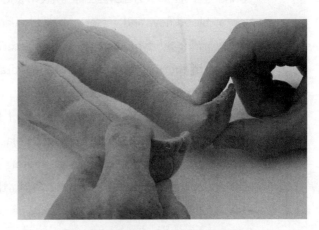
Fig. 32.4. Bilateral anterior tibial artery

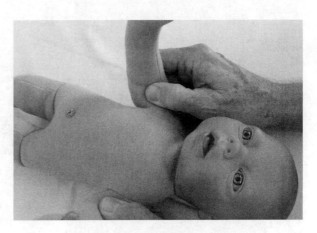
Fig. 32.5. Brachial arteries

TABLE 32.1. NORMAL INFANT HEART RATE

	Neonate (less than 28 days)	Infant (1 month–1 year)	Toddler (1–2 year)
Awake	100–205 BPM	100–190 BPM	98–140 BPM
Asleep	90–160 BPM	90–160 BPM	80–120 BPM

✄

Thermal Regulation

Another crucial metabolic function in a newborn is *thermal regulation*. Skin-to-skin contact with a caregiver supports this function. When a baby is held by a caregiver, physiologically and metabolically there are two interconnected thermal systems: the parent's and the child's. Within the baby's body, there are also two interconnected thermal systems. One is in the core of the body and the other is in the extremities. These are connected via the cardiovascular system and the sympathetic nervous system by regulation of blood flow and vessel wall dilation and contraction, especially in the capillaries.

Working biodynamically with the arteries of a newborn supports proper development of thermal regulation and the metabolism of the autonomic nervous system. Utilizing these contacts, the biodynamic therapist supports thermal regulation as the infant learns to integrate its two levels of thermal regulation, core and extremities.

After you have worked with the tibial and brachial arteries, bilateral contact is made with the *femoral arteries* at midthigh in the septum between the quadriceps and abductor muscles (see fig. 32.6). In the adult I usually work ipsilaterally. This location is a traditional Chinese medicine pulse location that supports proper blood flow to the pelvic floor for the function of urinating and defecating. Remember that a full diaper in an infant is usually a good thing. Gently using the thumbs, bilateral contact with the femoral arteries is quite easy to do on the infant's body.

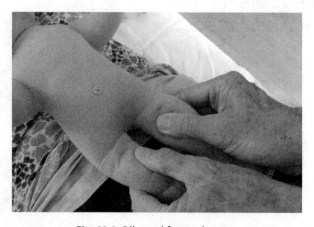

Fig. 32.6. Bilateral femoral artery

The Gut

Regarding the unconditional Health and disease, the gut is the *center of the body* from micro-circulation and neurohormone production to microbiome diversity; gut vitality and well-being is essential. Seventy percent of the metabolism of the gut is run by the microbiome, whereas the remaining 30 percent is run by the human genome. To support microcirculation in the small and large intestines, I place one hand palm up over the infant's *umbilicus* to feel the infant breathing. This hand placement continues until the slow breath of Primary Respiration is sensed through both my hand and the infant at the level of the umbilicus. Besides supporting microcirculation and respiratory integration, this also aids the wound healing of the umbilicus.

Next, I make gentle contact with one finger on the *superior mesenteric artery* (slightly above the umbilicus) and with another finger from the same hand, contact the *inferior mesenteric artery* (just to the side of the umbilicus). The mesenteric arteries are linked to the SNS and are especially helpful for thermal regulation in the newborn (see fig. 32.7). Thermal regulation in the abdomen is *core thermal regulation*. By supporting the microcirculation of the superior and inferior mesenteric arteries, two separate metabolic functions are being supported. One is core thermal regulation. The other is remodeling of the small and large intestine: substantial amounts of blood are being redirected into a vast endothelium forming in the center of this newly born body.

Then I contact the *right and left colic arteries* using the index fingers of both hands (see fig. 32.8).

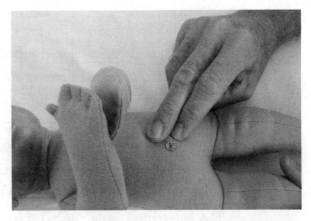

Fig. 32.7. Superior–inferior mesenteric arteries

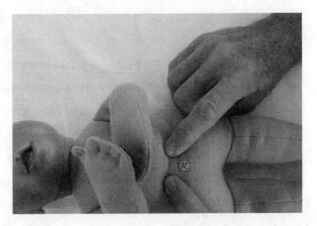

Fig. 32.8. Colic arteries

The right colic artery is a main conduit of blood to the ascending and transverse colon. It derives from the superior mesenteric artery. The left colic artery is a main conduit of blood to the descending and sigmoid colon, including the rectum. This simple contact is valuable in blending the function of these two arteries. In the distal portion of the transverse colon, where the two mesenteric arteries overlap, is the overlap of the terminating point of the subdiaphragmatic vagus and the beginning of the sacral outflow of the parasympathetic nervous system. Therapeutically, this arterial contact offers a deep relaxing balance to the ANS. It supports the function of the subdiaphragmatic vagus that is monitoring blood glucose levels in the portal vein and liver.

Along with microcirculation, the gut microbiome of the baby is being constructed. Beginning in utero, ignited at birth, then fueled with breastfeeding, snuggles, and playtime, the process of human microbiome acquisition takes approximately two years. The parasympathetic function of vagal immobilization has an essential role in bladder and bowel function, especially in the newborn. The subdiaphragmatic vagus initiates communication between the gut microbiome with its immune and endocrine functions, the brain, and heart. The vagus monitors gut inflammation and sends these signals to the heart and brain.

This gut–central–vagal communication is foundational to an internal sense of safety while the brain of the newborn is oriented to an external sense of safety via the multivagal system that includes both the vagus nerve and the facial nerve (see fig. 25.2B on page 269). Such safety is an integral part of the formation of one's body image and whether the infant loves their body or struggles within it as if eternally flawed. The rapidly developing heart mediates these responses via its heart rate variability and respiratory sinus arrhythmia. Thus the heart juggles the internal and external safety in its basic function of vulnerability and openness to the environment. The heart can be easily imprinted in this intense metabolic remodeling. The house of the body is developed on a poor foundation.

※

The Neck

The next suggested contact is with the *subclavian arteries* (see fig. 32.9). In our current culture, incredibly high levels of stress are endemic. Because of this it is important to approach the subclavian, a highly ANS innervated area of the body, gently and with great kindness. Since a baby's body is small, it is possible to make bilateral contact with just thumb and index finger. However, in my experience, babies are very particular about contact around their heads and necks. At the beginning of a session, I introduce myself to the infant and figure out a communication style where I can negotiate permission to make contact and receive a "yes" or "no." This could be anything from a nod of the head to a facial expression. At this point in the session, upon reaching the neck, reestablishing permission is important. With infants, as with most adults, I contact the subclavian arteries *ipsilaterally* and approach one side at a time. The ipsilateral approach offers a sense of safety to the wary contemporary client of any age.

Then I approach the carotid arteries (see fig. 32.10). Once again contact is ipsilateral. Remember that the left carotid artery arises directly from the aorta, and the right carotid artery arises from the subclavian artery. Each artery has a very different sensibility and responsiveness to the slow breath of Primary Respiration. I like to differentiate the middle of the carotid artery. This is the *carotid sinus* where the carotid artery bifurcates into its external and internal branches. Located here is the carotid sinus baroreceptor, an important regulator of the ANS that is innervated by the glossopharyngeal nerve. This baroreceptor is important in the regulation of blood pressure to the entire body, including the carotid arteries' provision of 80 percent of the total blood volume going to the brain and face. In the infant, the baroreceptors are doing crucial work: stabilizing peripheral and central blood pressures, regulating heart rate and variability, and coordinating cardiovascular functions with sleep and wake cycles.

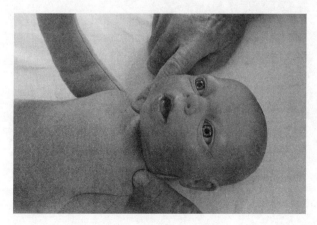
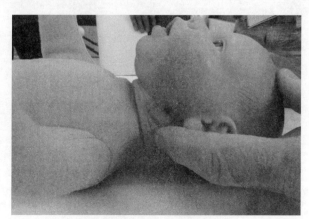

Fig. 32.9. Subclavian arteries   *Fig. 32.10. Carotid arteries*

◦⊱

The Cranium

On the rare occasion that I approach an infant at their head and face, it will be for contact with the *temporal artery*. This artery goes over the temporomandibular joint space and branches up into the temporalis muscle (see fig. 32.11). This contact is supportive of the suck-swallow-breathe reflex. Optimal functioning of this reflex is crucial for an effective, efficient, and enjoyable breast-feeding experience. The TMJ of a newborn is not a hinge joint. Suckling, whether at breast or bottle, requires that the mandible be able to glide forward, not just hinge down.

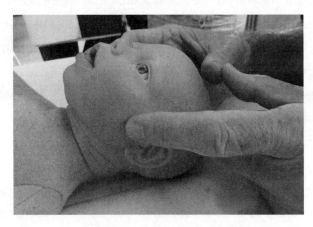

Fig. 32.11. Temporomandibular joint

∞

The Heart

Last in this teaching protocol, but never least, is the heart. The most common contact I make with any baby is centering my palm around the fifth thoracic (T5) vertebra on the child's back. Never have I had a child refuse this contact; it seems to be both welcomed and deeply appreciated. I hold the child's heart with the slow breath of Primary Respiration until I feel myself, my heart, the infant's heart, and their myocardium all breathing with Primary Respiration.

If an infant is being held by his mother (or is playing on the floor or lying supine) I may place my hand palm up over the central portion of the sternum to feel the fluid body breathing. Often, while making this contact, I notice the feeling of a blessing being offered. Using my finger pads, I connect with the valves of the heart, starting with the costosternal margin on the left third rib (R3) and finishing with the right costosternal margin of the fifth rib (R5). With fingers on the sternum in this diagonal line, the palm of the other hand can be placed at T5, supporting the back of the child's heart (see figs. 32.12–14). This contact is intended to synchronize the pulmonary valve, aortic valve, bicuspid (mitral) valve, and tricuspid valve.

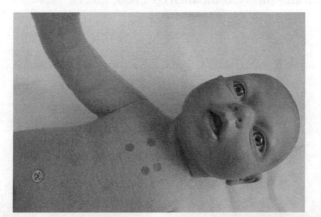

Fig. 32.12. Heart valves 1

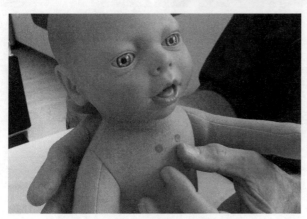

Fig. 32.13. Heart valves 2

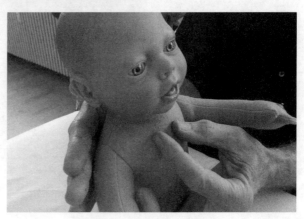

Fig. 32.14. Heart valves 3

In conclusion, I will mention that if the mother or caregiver hands the baby to me and if the baby is comfortable being held by me, I will receive the infant with one hand under its sacrum and my other hand supporting the baby's occiput. With this contact on what is commonly called the core link in osteopathy, I sense the infant's entire central nervous system breathing with Primary Respiration. This contact is especially lovely after treating the infant's abdominal arteries. Through this contact, and the entire neonatal cardiometabolic protocol as presented in this chapter, BCVT is applied to both the metabolic and physiological systems of the baby. With these invitations, balance, stabilization, relaxation, and normalization are offered nonverbally to the newborn baby and mom after their enormous work of gestating, birth, and transitioning to extrauterine life.

RECOMMENDED READING

Spirit into Form: Exploring Embryological Potential and Prenatal Psychology by Cherionna Menzam-Sills (Cosmoanelixis Press, 2021).

33

The Five Elements of Tibetan Medicine in Biodynamic Practice

How did we end up with a food system that can feed the world but makes us so ill? One that destroys wildlife, pollutes our rivers and air, and produces almost a third of our greenhouse gases?
Robert Lustig, M.D., Twitter, July 16, 2021, 7:50 a.m.

Metabolic syndrome is now considered a global epidemic. "With the successful conquest of communicable infectious diseases in most of the world, this new non-communicable disease has become the major life hazard of the modern world." Though it started in the Western world, with the spread of the Western lifestyle across the globe, it has become now a truly global problem as detailed in the first section of this book.

A 2018 study at the University of North Carolina revealed that only 12.2 percent of American adults are metabolically flexible between their innate and adaptive immune systems. This carries serious implications for public health, since a malfunctioning metabolism leaves people more vulnerable to developing type 2 diabetes, cardiovascular disease, and an inability for the body's immune system to fight a virus, leading to COVID deaths. Americans are dying at a faster rate than European counterparts, even taking COVID mortality into account, according to a 2021 study. Clearly, what is required is a new understanding of the human body for healing at a spiritual and elemental level. The health care system is not able to treat this problem because it is focused on symptoms and not the metabolic source according to Robert Lustig in his 2021 book, *Metabolical*. Metabolic disorders caused by diet need to be repaired through a Real Food diet according to Lustig.

The worldwide pandemic of metabolic syndromes requires a fresh approach to healing. In biodynamic practice we work with the embryonic forces of origin via Primary Respiration and stillness. Here we will deepen our understanding of origins to include the beginning of the universe. This is called the cosmological origin story such as the big bang and many others. This origin provides a deeper healing in traditional cultural ritual. This origin that we will learn requires seeing, hearing, and feeling the *five elements* of Tibetan medicine. Their sequence of unfolding originally is from space to wind to fire to water and finally to earth. Primary Respiration is equated with the wind and dynamic stillness with space. However, we will reverse the perceptual process and begin with space and stillness and wait for the Tide of PR to manifest. This requires *extrasensory* perception to connect with all the elements as they were in their origin.

To enter this subtle world outside and its mirror on the inside of the body, we will explore a classical Chinese medicine holistic practice called balancing Heaven–Earth–Human on three sets of arteries in the feet, hands, and face. Heaven–Earth–Human is an aesthetic view of the totality of the universe expressed in the cardiovascular system as a flower unfolding.

We will then explore the role of the veins in their reciprocal relationship to the arteries. In embryology, it is the umbilical vein that brings the incarnating consciousness into form through the umbilicus directly to the heart of the embryo. The element of space with the wind comes through first directly to the heart. In Tibetan medicine, the larger veins are associated with what are called channels like canalization zones in embryology. These channels are formally known as the central channel and two side channels (see fig. 27.2 on page 299). We will consider them as the large blood vessels of the two umbilical veins and the remnants of the heart in its tubular form early in development.

THE FIVE WINDS

PR has five specific locations or fulcrums (*vayus* in Sanskrit) in the body, and now I will add in the elements that are associated with those five winds for PR (see fig. 26.1 on page 289).

1. The crown of the head is the fulcrum for the *life-sustaining* wind.
2. The heart is the fulcrum for the *all-pervasive* wind and is associated with the element of space.
3. The throat is the fulcrum for the *upward-rising* wind and is associated with the element of earth.

4. The superior mesenteric artery of the abdomen is the fulcrum for the *fire-metabolism* wind. It is associated with the element of fire.

5. The kidneys are the fulcrum for the *downward-voiding* wind. They are associated with element of water. The element of water is said to have eight qualities: cool, sweet, light, soft, clear, soothing, pleasant, and wholesome.

Each time we sense PR in the body and its potency associated with the five winds, we can connect with the elements. PR is the mover of all the elements. There are five guiding principles regarding the elements of Tibetan medicine and how they are integrated into biodynamic practice with the five winds of PR and the Nine Pulses of traditional Chinese medicine.

ELEMENTAL PRINCIPLES

The *first* principle is that the element of space must incarnate as origin, and it does so through the umbilical vein and future vena cava into the heart of the developing embryo. The quality of space is related to the perception of dynamic stillness that we are already know. Thus, the element of space is the most central structure of the heart via somites, wedge epithelia, and quiescent cells. Space, the dynamic stillness, thus resides in the structure and function of the heart and veins. The center of the heart is made of dynamically still (quiescent) cells. The practice is to sense the heartbeat synchronized with the stillness that extends in all directions toward the horizon. The element of space conducts the sound of creation such as the Om, but also the heartbeat itself is a divine sound that the entire universe makes.

The *second* principle is that the element of wind is mixed with space as the basic substrate of the incarnating consciousness. Wind incarnates second, although it is not a linear sequence. We know this as PR in its timeless dimension. When mixed with space, it gives an immediate sense of directionality and flow in the veins going toward the heart and then the arteries leaving the heart with the help of the water element (fluid body) comprising the majority (70 percent) of the fluid in the vein and artery. PR then takes up residence in the posterior heart fields and radiates from that location as the all-pervasive wind. Space and wind are the principal carriers of sacred sound, and thus the sense of hearing must open to listen to elements of space and wind. The upward-rising wind is connected to speech and thus the throat and vocal cords. Right speech is a function of PR in the upward-rising wind.

The *third* principle is that the physiological movement of the blood inside the veins is partially dependent on the proximity of its neighboring artery. In other words, the artery is smaller, with extra connective tissue, and thus stronger in its pulsation away from the heart while the vein is more open and relaxed in its slow tidal flow toward the heart. Veins have a system of one-way valves that do not allow blood to flow backward. However, the blood can back up and reverse flow in the artery as if stuttering in a limited way, which is not natural because of an inflammatory process affecting the endothelium. Thus, the pulse of the artery is one factor that helps propel the blood in the veins back toward the heart. Think about this directionality for some time, as it is under the control of PR.

A natural type of microbackflow more like a spiraling occurs in distinct locations in the vascular tree. This is where an artery bifurcates, such as the abdominal aorta into the two common iliac arteries or the popliteal artery into the anterior and posterior tibial arteries or the aorta into the subclavian and carotid arteries (among other small arteries coming off of the aorta, especially the coronary arteries). So even though the flow of the blood and PR is moving away from the heart in the artery via the life-sustaining wind, it assists the movement of the blood in the veins back to the heart. The life-sustaining wind of PR from the top of the head (Du 20) is enhanced in the vascular tree with the all-pervasive wind flowing throughout the interstitium of the body from the heart in the blood as well as subdivisions of the fluid body such as the lymph.

Biodynamic cardiovascular therapy is working with all the elements as they manifest in the cardiovascular system and in all directions of the five fulcrums of the wind element in the body. This is not limited to the life-sustaining and all-pervasive winds. There is fire in the blood coming from the gut, the structure of the artery is of the earth, and the fluid body is the water element in the blood itself. Once again, we must understand that biodynamics is a study of perception.

Thus, it is possible that PR can be perceived moving in both directions at once or in reciprocal phases—now the vein for a while and then the artery for a while. The perception is not a linear sequence; it is extrasensory. Therapists wait to enter the flow in either or both directions under the guidance of PR. It may seem as if one's fingers are merged in the flow of the artery or vein itself. This is a special invitation from PR and an extrasensory perception of the five elements.

The *fourth* principle relates to the dynamic stillness, the element of space.

This is experienced in the vein as a dynamic stillness in the center of a fluid body. The element of space in the vein encompasses all of space in the universe, or at least to the horizon. In shamanism, the therapist periodically extends their attention beyond the horizon to see the elements as they were in the beginning. It is a fundamental aspect of the biodynamic healing process. Sensing the wholeness of the embryo as we have learned in previous classes via PR and stillness in the present moment now includes sensing the origin of the universe as a necessary condition of healing the contemporary client. The natural world participates in the healing process as taught in all the courses and so does the entire cosmos. It starts with opening our senses, especially seeing and hearing the elements so that we may "be still and know."

The *fifth* principle involves the importance of settling and resting one's mind and interrupting our thoughts, especially while working to open one's hearing and vision in the dynamic stillness, the element of space. Restrain yourself from looking at objects and mentally labeling them, because this misses the point of looking at the element of space such as the sky. It is here where the other elements come into play and continually form, starting with space, then wind, then fire, then water, and finally earth.

In the same way, at the time of death this incarnating process of the elements reverses and becomes a continually dissolving process: earth dissolves to water dissolves to fire dissolves to wind dissolves to space. This process of forming and dissolving in the cosmos, body, and mind is happening constantly. Is this what automatic shifting means?

REVIEW

It is important when working with the veins and their elemental qualities that we also relate to the following facts:

1. The blood is 70 percent water, and water also makes the blood move and keeps it warm.
2. The venous system of the body acts as a radiator in dissipating core level heat/fire in the human body by bringing the veins closer to the surface of the skin.
3. The fine structure of both the artery and vein contains significant amounts of connective tissue (earth), although the artery has a bit more than the vein.

Thus, all the elements are at play in the cardiovascular system. You cannot have fire without wind. You cannot have a fluid body without water and earth. You cannot exist without space. This is the essence of Ignition and its perception in biodynamic practice.

34
Biodynamic Shamanism

Descent to the realm of the dead, home of disease spirits, speaks to the fundamental helplessness of humanity. Encountered in the depths are ravenous spirits that instruct as they destroy. The shaman's receptivity to the world of creatures opens after he or she has surrendered to death. . . . The shaman partakes of the raw nectar of the world of creatures. Raw death and a non-dualistic, amoral universe are revealed. There is no morality in the stare of the hawk; nor is there morality in death.

JOAN HALIFAX, *SHAMAN: THE WOUNDED HEALER*

We can contact a pulse through its specific artery or the capillary bed anywhere. We can feel the pulsing of the blood if we open our senses and experience the substrate of Primary Respiration underneath all of the elements. PR is an aspect of the wind element. Each of the five elements gain their power, so to speak, from the wind element. PR is considered the master control valve of all life. It makes everything move, even our thoughts. Without movement there is no life. This is a key principle in BCVT. When the artery and its pulse is sensed, attunement and synchronization with PR must happen to access the Health and the incorporation as a spiritual altruistic human being. This involves access to extrasensory perception guided by PR. Biodynamics becomes a shamanic procedure.

The life force, prana, or what we call PR are mixed with the air and oxygen that we breathe. As mentioned in the previous chapter, once it enters the body (or moves through the body or exits the body), it establishes and orients to five locations or fulcrums with which to guide the ordinary, subtle, and very subtle bodies. These five locations also have associations with the five elements and Tibetan medicine. These associations are derived from the ayurvedic tradition as it influences Tibetan medicine. There are many schools of Tibetan medicine, some more influenced by traditional Chinese medicine and Taoism.

I add the template of the five elements derived from ayurveda and expanded in Tibetan medicine within our exploration of biodynamic practice evolving spiritually into a shamanic practice. Western medicine is not working with the cause of disease, and older, Eastern traditions have the potential to help the contemporary client. The five elements lead into another order or level of organization of the three bodies called the channels and their nodal points called the chakras. I teach exploring the subtleties of flow and information through the veins and arteries as the principal expression of these channels, and thus the chakras are simply points where numerous channels come together to organize and integrate forms of sensory information. This means it is a natural way of looking at how the cardiovascular system is organized in conjunction with the autonomic nervous system, endocrine system, and immune system. This includes its relationship with the subtle and very subtle body as one continuous whole. This book is not expressly about the chakra system. Rather it is important to hold a larger vision of what the human body is, how it is made, and how it functions at a physical and at a subtle level.

The additional difference is that in Tibetan medicine, the formation of the incarnating consciousness that includes passion, aggression and ignorance, and the sense consciousnesses comes through the channels, veins, and arteries. It comes through the umbilicus and straight to the heart. Thus, biodynamic exploration includes the origin of the twin storms of cognition and emotion that frequently disrupt our sensibility and well-being as a function of blood flow and subtle energy flow in the meridians. I am contemplating PR and dynamic stillness throughout this book at the deeper levels of wind and space. This view expands the potential of biodynamic practice and the mystery of the Breath of Life given to us by Dr. Sutherland.

The deep well of biodynamic cardiovascular therapy includes knowledge and understanding of a model of healing called shamanism. Shamanism is the original health care system practiced for thousands of years on the planet and is still in existence in many traditional cultures. I use the term *shamanism* to mean extrasensory perception as it relates to infusing biodynamic practice with a sense of the sacred. It helps us understand how to organize this information about the elements and channels because it can provide a natural experience of spiritual incorporation as well as an integration with the natural world outside of the body. To do this we must keep all our senses open with the cycle of attunement. This is always our intention from the very beginning, to incorporate more fully, and so we just continue to deepen on this path.

We do not need to call ourselves a shaman because it is a metaphor for extrasensory perception. We simply need to know how extrasensory information embedded within PR and stillness is organized in order to be most effective in helping to relieve the pain and suffering of our client. I show stages of this process at the end of this chapter. Shamanism is the integration of the healing elements of the natural world waking up the wisdom knowledge of healing pre-existing on the inside of the body. This knowledge has always been linked to the elements inside and outside the body with the five senses. To facilitate this level of spiritual incorporation, I connect the five elements inside the body with the five elements outside the body through the pervasiveness of the cardiovascular system, PR, and dynamic stillness. Take a moment to review chapter 23 and the cosmology presented there as a basis of understanding the need for a shamanic approach (see figs. 23.1–3 on pages 245–47).

ELEMENTAL PERCEPTION

Biodynamics is a contemporary exploration of spiritual Health. Incorporation as a spiritual being encompasses both a cosmology and an embryology, as discussed in detail throughout this book. A symbolic return to origins through a well-bounded, ethical biodynamic ritual of healing requires safety. *The felt sense of safety is the gateway to being fully incorporated.* Safety is linked to the Neutral as defined in biodynamic theory. Everyone is bio-unique in terms of their ability to achieve a Neutral, which is the automatic shifting window of tolerance for change process in the autonomic nervous system. As Dr. Becker said, "The therapeutic process does not begin until the will of the patient yields to the will of Primary Respiration." The Neutral is the first of the three-step process of biodynamic practice being a rite of passage as mentioned in chapter 21. The Neutral is the first step to the portal or doorway to the other side of healing once the client feels safe. Then Ignition of the creative aspect of PR manifests its unerring potency; incorporation as a spiritual being comes through the manifestation of the potency of PR called the Health. Clients frequently express that they feel the meaning of the suffering they are experiencing.

The window of Neutral does not stay open for very long. Be wise and be cautious how you proceed while viewing through an open window. Waiting for the big game of dynamic stillness and PR is a lesson in transcendent patience!

First, you wait for the Neutral, then you wait for PR to reveal its priorities in the Neutral via Ignition of the heart and vascular system. And always, you must wait for those events to occur in their own timing. Waiting is practiced with calm abiding or zazen in which thoughts, concepts, and ideas about the healing process are allowed to fade to the background of perception. Not knowing and bearing witness are the attitudes of the therapist. There is only the dance of PR and stillness.

∞

Posture

Posture is a reference state for the mind and body to synchronize (repeat this sentence one hundred times). We start with the posture in the meditation practice of zazen. It is an asana practice with many nuances. It is what the Buddha taught. This is a shorter version of the instructions in chapter 22.

- Settle the posture: Gather your attention and settle into an upright posture that supports your practice.
- Cultivate an unselfish motivation: recall your intention to awaken in order to serve others. It is easy enough to say nonverbally: may I awake, may all awake.
- Stabilize attention on the breath in the abdomen to cultivate attentional balance and concentration (see below for more detail).
- As appropriate, notice the arising and passing of thoughts and sensations (impermanence), selflessness: insight.
- When concentration is very stable, the attentional field opens to nonreferential awareness: dynamic stillness.
- Dedication of merit: offer whatever good has arisen to others, may all awake.

When treating a client, know when your posture has automatically shifted and feel the degree of restriction with your respiratory diaphragm. Maximum comfort and freedom of breath in any assumed posture from the reference state is an incorporation practice. As therapists, we learn to shape-shift our bodies to accommodate the progression of hand placements in a session. In this way, biodynamic practice becomes like a vinyasa flow yoga class.

Know where home base is and return to it periodically in a session (and maybe also in life). I suppose you could call this mindfulness. "Be still and know . . . " from Psalm 46 is enough.

✂

Conscious Breathing:
Incorporating your own Pranayama from Chapter 22

- The first breathing practice is finding the inner breath up and down the central channel, referencing, for example, the descending and abdominal aorta or the spinal cord and brain.

- Second, practice embodying your inhalation into the lower dantian. This is the place between your umbilicus and pubic bone and between front and back. This begins balancing the lower warmer of the Triple Warmer and is vitally important for all three warmers.

- Third, practice embodying your exhalation as dissolving slowly into the gap between the exhalation and inhalation. Make your dying process easy and good to the last breath. There is no breath holding.

- Fourth, when the sitz bones are rocking forward, placing the pubic bone closer to the chair, and the chin is slightly retracted, the central channel is free to lengthen. The breath that fills the lower dantian becomes a river flowing up and down the central channel. When the sitz bones are rocked forward comfortably, the sacrum and spine are free to lift with the head. Differentiate the sitz bones from the sacrum.

✂

Heart Attunement Manifests a Neutral

- Listen to the heartbeat and periodically count 70 heartbeats.
- Feel the dorsal pericardium fulcrum for PR located in the back of the heart.
- Sense the heart field and the people in it, especially the client.
- Sense the heart spiraling in the pericardium. This ignites the flow of compassion in the Tide of PR from heart to heart.
- The heart spiral is linked to lengthening the arms for the hands to sense deeper into the client without added pressure. This takes practice in parts of the vinyasa flow.
- The heart spiral is continuous or reciprocal in the tempo of PR.

The elements arise sequentially at conception and dissolve sequentially in the reverse order while in the dying process. Clear knowing of the elements is a side effect of meditation. The knowing happens in the gaps between thoughts. Reduce thoughts and cognition and increase interoceptive awareness of all the viscera and their fasciae, especially the containers and contents of the peritoneum, pericardium, pleura, and dura.

The mind is the element of space. Stillness is the element of space. Just listen deeply to the silence for the sacred sound of the heartbeat. Other sacred sounds are also playing! *Thoughts are the elements of space and wind.* PR contains all the activities and levels of the wind element and consequently the chi. Becoming/dissolving of the elements is simultaneous. Conception–death is sequential and simultaneous metabolically. Knowing the elements includes knowing their different levels of function. An element is an entire domain of activity containing countless attributes and entities. Find the gap and visit creation and death simultaneously or sequentially! Your call.

Sky gazing is linked to meditation because it helps our nervous system access the void, the absolute ending of the previous universe. Cease naming the objects of perception. Gather your mind prior to sky gazing and always when you begin your meditation practice. First identify whether your mind is busy or spacey. Then notice if it contains numerous emotional storylines or disembodied self-documentaries. Observe this activity as if sitting watching traffic up and down a street outside a window. As is said: *all dharmas agree on one point, kill the neurosis.* But make friends with it first. Then kill it with kindness and allow it to retire in a gold-star long-term care facility.

Chi, wind, and PR are metaphors for one thing with three basic levels of structure and function. The sensing of such begins with one's incorporation of the subtle. In *The Light Inside the Dark,* John Tarrant said, "Spirit is not given in a session, it is uncovered by the quality of our attention." Attention moves with PR between self, client, and nature. This is called the cycle of attunement as detailed in chapter 24. Different types of chi flow between hands and feet reciprocally, hands to heart, and head to feet. At the same time these flows happen in the channels of the subtle body, their physical body locations are in the fasciae, the interstitium, the blood, the arteries, the veins, and the heart. These are the superficial flows. (We will learn the deeper flows in the next chapters.)

THE SIX EXTRASENSORY PERCEPTIONS

Extrasensory perception is a defining feature of shamanism. This is nothing new (PR requires extrasensory perception) but rather a focus on levels of biodynamic perception always being cultivated in life and in clinical practice. Perception in the treatment room continues outside the treatment room. The *first* extrasensory perception is *transparency*. In order to enter the stream of the all-pervasive wind from and to the heart, we place our fingers on specific locations in the vascular tree and immediately access a sense of transparency in the totality of our body such that PR is constantly moving back and forth through us. There is a quality of dissolving the various elements into their original substrate, which is PR.

The *second* extrasensory perception is to listen to the dynamic stillness and PR; we are listening for what is called the "sacred sound." In the Vedas this was the sound of the Om. This sound is already present and can be evoked by making a very low-level and brief humming sound in the base of the throat. It is simply about creating a vibration in the upward-rising wind of the throat. It is also the sound and sense of one's own heartbeat.

The *third* extrasensory perception we know as *dissipation*. Chapter 13 discusses this and provides a perceptual practice. Upon placing our hands onto the client, we become totally receptive by accessing our fluid body and allowing the client's fluid body to merge with ours and experience that through micromotion and finally settling. It is the same way with the nature of thoughts and emotions. We become totally receptive nonjudgmentally and allow mind and their objects to dissipate.

The *fourth* extrasensory perception is looking directly at the space of *stillness*. This is a variation on horizon therapy (sensing PR move between the horizon and the third ventricle of the brain). We simply allow our eyes to open to the horizon and the space immediately above the horizon. During practice, our vision has three focal points: the body of the client on the table in front of us, the horizon, and the space above the horizon (the void). Each of these three locations provides discrete information on the constitution of the five elements and how they are constantly coming together and dissolving. Wait until the elements begin to manifest this dance visually in the space in between your body and the object of perception, or as an internal visualization or as if the object of perception were a movie screen on which a magic show is being performed.

The *fifth* extrasensory perception is synchronizing one's heartbeat with the dynamic stillness of space as it extends through the vascular system and out to the horizon and beyond in all directions. The therapist, upon becoming aware of his or her heartbeat, immediately extends their perception and awareness gradually in all directions. This perception pauses at the horizon before going into the larger cosmos of our solar system, the Milky Way, and the universe in general. Sometimes the shaman needs to access the origin of the universe rather than the origin of the client's embryo for healing. PR will guide you, if necessary, beyond the horizon. Wait at the horizon for instructions from all the senses and all the elements with a calm mind of non-thinking.

The *sixth* extrasensory perception is *synchronizing* the breath of air with PR. This allows greater contact with how the five elements create the human body and uncreate the human body at the same time. PR is always the link to all the elements, including space.

A bridge to the deeper chi is in the literal heart. Practice the heart spiral when possible, as this engages the pericardium and middle burner in classical Chinese medicine for balance. Explore and differentiate more consciously the "gift" that you offer to clients. What is your gift? This will help you in your life practice.

THE WAY OF THE NATURAL WORLD

Throughout this book I am making a case for the spiritual in biodynamic practice. In the age that we live in we can begin healing the polarization rampant on the planet with a spirit of unification. The intention is to bring the unity of space forward as an offering to the contemporary client and their suffering. Shamanism itself is a metaphor for the most natural wisdom potential, the innate knowing in our mind and body of how to transform suffering to awakening. From this point of view, the biodynamic therapist can integrate the archaic skills of the past to invigorate the healing instinct already available in the present moment. It is based on attunement to the natural world outside and inside the body.

Initiation requires a near-death experience resulting in the direct experience and immediate accessibility of the extrasensory perception of such spiritual authority. By definition the experience of the COVID-19 pandemic was a shamanic initiation. The macabre images of bodies strewn about makeshift mortuaries, refrigerator trucks full of the dead, and constant daily reporting of the body count created a portal to the rich dimension of inner spiritual formation. The enormity of the fear gripping the planet became the object of concentration in this deadly meditation. In such initiations, being spiritually informed by prayer, transforming fear into a blessing, or just being lucky enough to have a sense of humor about it all continually manifests the power of initiation into compassion and service. This is the new spiritual authority, a spiritual ignition as biodynamic shamanism that permeates a laying-on-of-hands ministry so necessary in this moment in time.

Viruses, pathogens, drugs, and unrealistic views, not to mention processed food and added sugar, are some of the new elemental entities—so-called "negative energies"—along with the inner terror of death lurking around every corner that infect the consciousness of the contemporary client. Technically, no one gets out of this life alive anyway. Thus a contemporary exorcism, a blessing in disguise, is performed by the spiritual authority of such a "fully" initiated shaman.

Being spiritually informed means living by the vow to downregulate and reduce one's neurosis. Neurotic, compulsive thoughts and behaviors can drive the whole wheel of karma. The initiated jump ship and step off the wheel of concept, compulsivity, and emotional afflictions. We make a backward step into the inner terrain of stability and resilience, prayer and blessing, happiness and knowing the source of happiness unique to everyone's spiritual aptitude, of which there are thousands. The only way out is in, to a somatic reality of vitality and reverie, the instincts of sanity and unfettered exploration of the whole terrain of life without judgment. It is clearly easier said than done to cross through that portal into the fluid body of the natural world.

So I live my life in the warrior lineage as it is known in the major Eastern traditions, that regardless of what I face, I will never give up. Sacrifice is a necessary component of the healing journey to the freedom I am describing. You must sacrifice your neurosis. You never give up your honor and duty to protect your embodied spiritual formation and its continuity with the natural world of the planet earth. The biodynamic shaman is more of a poet, a Rumi, a Rilke, a Maya Angelou, an Amanda Gorman. It is the poetry of compassion and tough love from the Big Book of Alcoholics Anonymous, and the benevolence of the universe. No matter what state of mind you are in, the sun will always rise in the east and set in the west. The vast expanse of the universe mirrors our innate capacity for a spacious relaxed mind free of emotional afflictions, fixed inflexible opinions, judgments, and evaluations about which the sun and the moon couldn't care less. The Way of the Natural World is to connect with the intelligence of the natural world through the fluid body, the sun and moon, and the rhythm of slowness and stillness.

We must sacrifice our shared global neurosis now. Loss of mind, of body, and of the Holy Spirit is rampant. We are perpetually grieving. This is a critical extrasensory perception of the biodynamic shaman. Grieving is the deep repair righting the ship that has keeled over and stranded civilization on the rocks, in quarantine from the Way of the Natural World. We grieve our own losses, our own style of suffering that we share with all of humanity's unique style. This is now the extrasensory perception of sorrow, always available, always Prime and on-demand. Her brother is humility. You cannot figure out the world as it is. There is only the inner somatic geography to explore and seek answers from. It is the work of a lifetime. As Ikkyu said, "Only one koan matters, you." We bow to our inner spiritual formation. We bow to the client's inner spiritual formation.

35

Realignment of Heaven, Earth, and Human

All the rites of rebirth or resurrection, and the symbols that they imply, indicate that the novice has attained to another mode of existence, inaccessible to those who have not undergone the initiatory ordeals, who have not tasted death. We must note this characteristic of the archaic mentality: the belief that a state cannot be changed without first being annihilated (in the present instance, without the child's dying to childhood). It is impossible to exaggerate the importance of this obsession with beginnings, which, in sum, is the obsession with the absolute beginning, the cosmogony. For a thing to be well done, it must be done as it was done the first time.

MIRCEA ELIADE, *RITES AND SYMBOLS OF INITIATION: THE MYSTERIES OF BIRTH AND REBIRTH*

Eastern healing traditions prize an aesthetic for the position of a human being located between the earth and the heavens of the whole universe. In this chapter we will learn simple skills specifically related to acupuncture points and their corresponding arteries that invite the aesthetic of heaven, earth, and human to more fully manifest. There is a felt sense of this connection being an energetic and potent midline that literally extends from the core of the planet earth through the center of the human being and out the top of the head connecting to the centerpoint of the universe, thought to be a star in Ursa Major. What follows are a set of skills designed to bring a felt sense to the body and mind of this most sacred connection and relationship with the entire universe. It is subtle work because some of the arteries are small and it requires a quiet mind and patience for the manifestation of the connecting energy through the artery and acupuncture point. Be patient.

REALIGNMENT WITH THE COSMOS (SEE FIG. 35.1)

EARTH AREA OF SOMA

1. Metatarsalis dorsalis A. (Heaven). LIVER 3
2. Dorsalis pedis A. (Human). STOMACH 42
3. Posterior tibial A. (Earth). KIDNEY 3

HUMAN AREA OF SOMA

1. Radial A. (Heaven). LUNG 9
2. Ulnar A. (Human). Life essence artery. HEART 7
3. Metacarpal dorsalis A. (Earth). LARGE INTESTINE 4

HEAVEN AREA OF SOMA

1. Temporalis profundus anterior A. (Heaven). Tai yang point (close to GB 1)
2. Superficial temporalis A. (Human). TRIPLE WARMER 21
3. Facial–Angularis A. (Earth). STOMACH 3

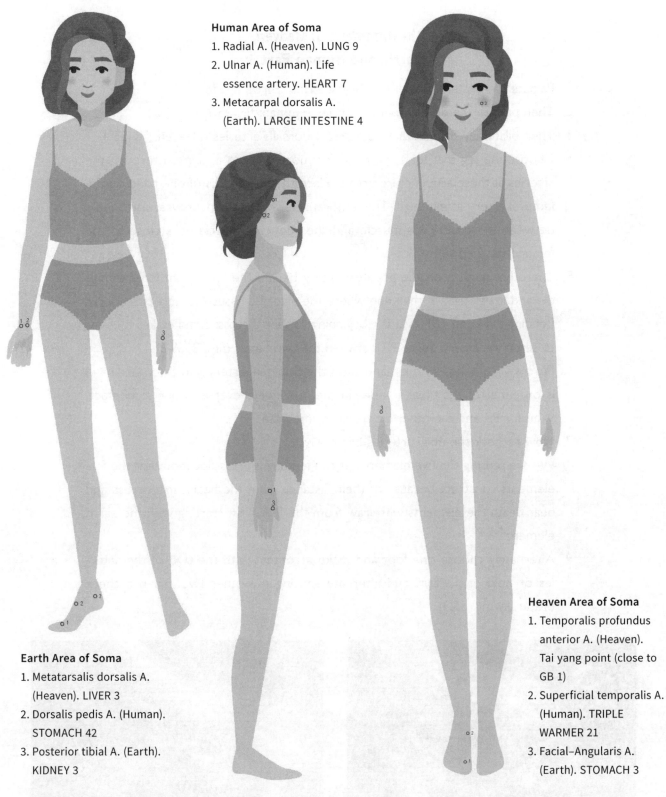

Human Area of Soma

1. Radial A. (Heaven). LUNG 9
2. Ulnar A. (Human). Life essence artery. HEART 7
3. Metacarpal dorsalis A. (Earth). LARGE INTESTINE 4

Earth Area of Soma

1. Metatarsalis dorsalis A. (Heaven). LIVER 3
2. Dorsalis pedis A. (Human). STOMACH 42
3. Posterior tibial A. (Earth). KIDNEY 3

Heaven Area of Soma

1. Temporalis profundus anterior A. (Heaven). Tai yang point (close to GB 1)
2. Superficial temporalis A. (Human). TRIPLE WARMER 21
3. Facial–Angularis A. (Earth). STOMACH 3

Fig. 35.1. Balancing the cosmos: Heaven–Earth–Human. These acupuncture points harmonize the body with the earth and the cosmos in the Taoist sense of being connected to the North Star in the constellation Ursa Major. In the very subtle body, the central channel extends to the center of the earth and upwardly to the North Star. It is a thread of chi that reestablishes our connection to the universe.

∝

Realignment of Heaven,
Earth, and Human Part I

1. Palpate the bilateral posterior tibial arteries (Earth; fig. 35.2).

2. Then palpate the dorsalis pedis arteries (Human; fig. 35.3).

3. Then bilaterally palpate the metatarsalis dorsalis arteries (Heaven; fig. 35.4).

4. Choose the leg that feels the need for more balance as sensed through the arteries at these acupuncture points. Place the finger pads of one hand on the femoral artery at midthigh. The femoral artery is in the neurovascular bundle between the quadriceps muscle and the adductor muscle. It is close to the femur (figs. 35.5–6).

5. The other hand is on the popliteal artery behind the knee. Aim for the middle and lower part of the knee where the artery crosses the tibia posteriorly. Bending the knee slightly at the beginning softens the tissue and makes it easier to sense the artery. Sense PR between the two hands (figs. 35.7–8).

6. Now switch hands so one hand is on the popliteal artery and the other hand is on either of the tibial arteries in the foot, whichever is easier to contact. Wait for PR and the other elements to integrate.

7. Now recheck the tibial arteries bilaterally.

8. We are sensing the five elements as the feet are the last location that the five elements construct because of their distance from the heart. In sickness and near death the elements withdraw from the feet first, starting with the earth element.

9. Alternately choose one foot and make a contact with the two of the arteries or hold one artery and alternate sensing the other two. Then recheck bilaterally (fig. 35.9).

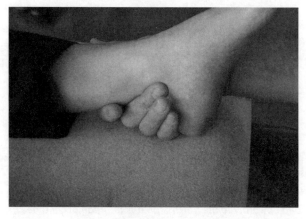

Fig. 35.2. Posterior tibial artery

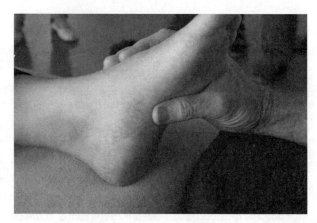

Fig. 35.3. Dorsalis pedis artery

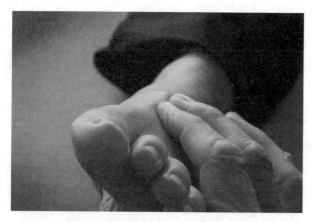

Fig. 35.4. Metatarsalis dorsalis artery

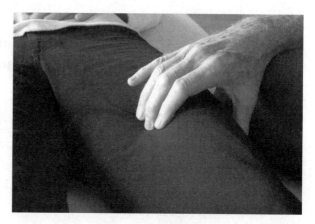

Fig. 35.5. Femoral artery 1

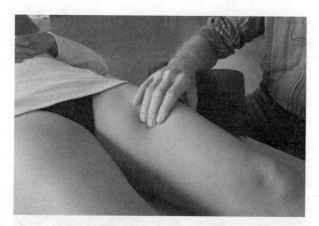

Fig. 35.6. Femoral artery 2

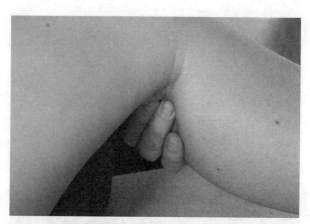

Fig. 35.7. Popliteal artery 1

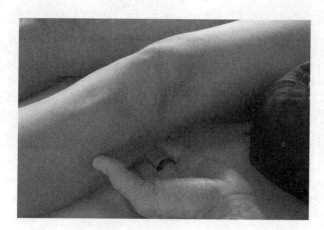

Fig. 35.8. Popliteal artery 2

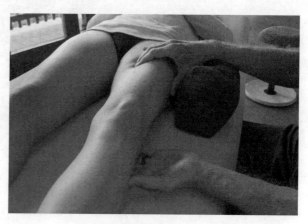

Fig. 35.9. Femoral–Popliteal arteries

☙

Realignment of Heaven, Earth, and Human Part 2

1. Palpate the radial artery (Heaven).

2. Then palpate the ulnar artery on one side (Human). The ulnar artery is called the life essence artery in Tibetan medicine. The client's arm is either palm up or palm down on the table by the side of their body.

3. Then palpate the metacarpal dorsalis artery on the medial side of the base of the index finger (Earth).

4. Now combine the metacarpal dorsalis contact with either the radial or ulnar artery or moving back and forth to see how the metacarpal dorsalis artery responds. Are the three arteries balanced?

5. Repeat on the other side of the client.

6. Sitting at the right side of the table, extend the client's arm palm up by the side of their body. Use one hand to palpate the ulnar artery. Then, with

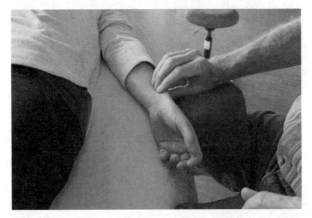

Fig. 35.10. Radial artery

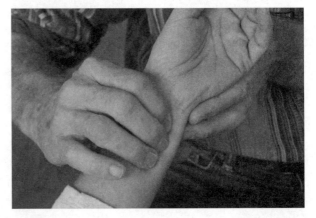

Fig. 35.11. Ulnar artery

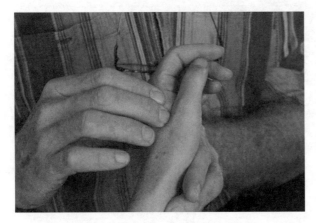

Fig. 35.12. Metacarpal dorsalis artery 1

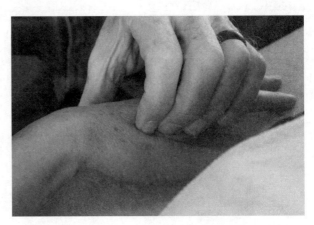

Fig. 35.13. Metacarpal dorsalis artery 2

the free hand, contact the heart center over the sternum either palm up or down. Sense the flow of PR as the life-sustaining wind from the heart to the ulnar artery at the wrist. Reverse hands if it is more comfortable and make sure the hands and arms are supported (figs. 35.15–18).

7. Finish with bilateral tibial arteries.

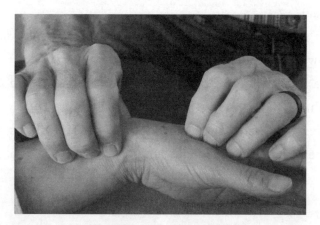

Fig. 35.14. Metacarpal radial arteries

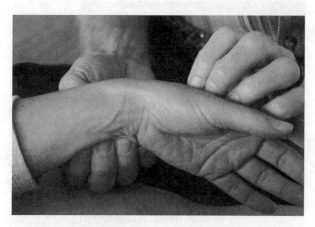

Fig. 35.15. Metacarpal–Ulnar arteries

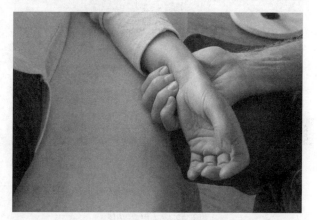

Fig. 35.16. Ulnar artery

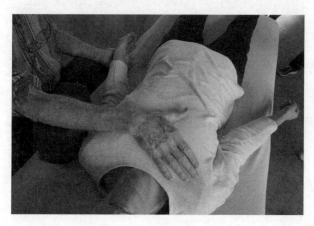

Fig. 35.17. Ulnar–Heart 1

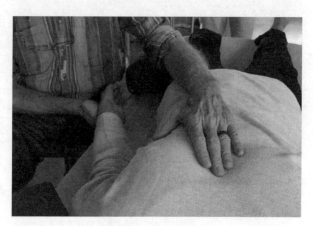

Fig. 35.18. Ulnar–Heart 2

✂

Realignment of Heaven,
Earth, and Human Part 3

1. Contact the client's shoulders bilaterally.

2. Palpate the superficial temporalis artery bilaterally between the ear canal and TMJ (Human).

3. Palpate the temporalis profundus anterior artery bilaterally directly over the greater wing of the sphenoid bone (Heaven).

4. Palpate the angularis artery bilaterally in the nasal labial fold adjacent to the nose (Earth).

5. Try palpating a different sequence with the three face pulses, but always finish with the temporalis profundus anterior artery in clinical practice.

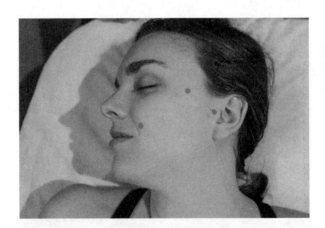

Fig. 35.19. Chi points

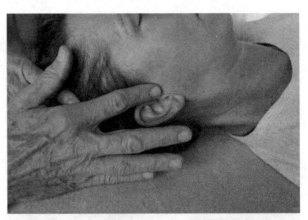

Fig. 35.20. Temporalis artery 1

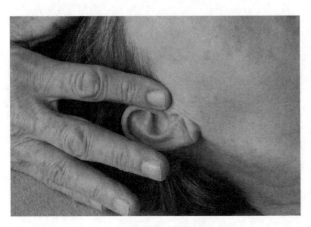

Fig. 35.21. Temporalis artery 2

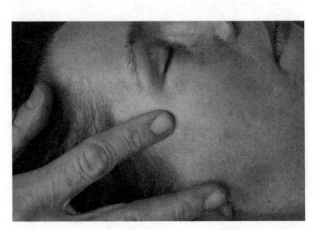

Fig. 35.22. Temporalis profundus anterior 1

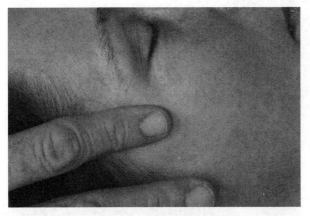

Fig. 35.23. Temporalis profundus anterior 2

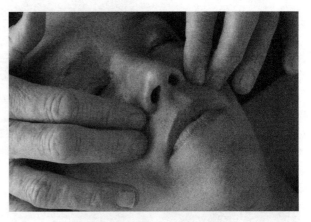

Fig. 35.24. Facial–Angularis Artery

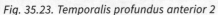

Realignment of Heaven, Earth, and Human Part 4

1. Contact and balance the client's three foot pulses. The femoral–popliteal sequence is optional.

2. Contact and balance the client's three hand pulses on both sides.

3. Contact and balance the client's three face pulses bilaterally.

4. Finish with either of the bilateral tibial arteries or the ulnar–heart sequence from above.

The Embryonic Channels to the Heart

1. Sitting at the right side of the table, gently place the index, middle, or ring finger of your right hand into the umbilicus of your partner.

2. Make a brief clockwise circular motion to come into relationship with the pulse of the abdominal aorta.

3. The inferior vena cava is immediately adjacent to the right of the abdominal aorta and close to the spine. Allow the finger to find the medial edge of the pulsation of the aorta, which is close to the IVC. It feels as if the fingers fall into an open space (the IVC). A slight awareness of the aorta remains as with the other hand positions in this whole sequence.

4. Remember that we do not want to lose the connection with the aorta or the artery, since it is intimately connected to the vein, especially with PR.

5. The other hand will be palm down over the costal arch approximating the surface geography of the IVC crossing through the respiratory diaphragm. Sense PR between

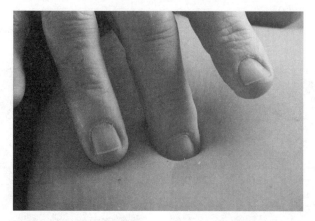

Fig. 35.25. Inferior vena cava–Umbilicus

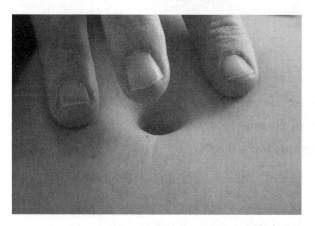

Fig. 35.26. Inferior vena cava above umbilicus

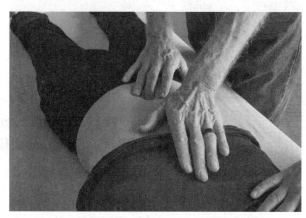

Fig. 35.27. Umbilicus–Inferior vena cava–Diaphragm

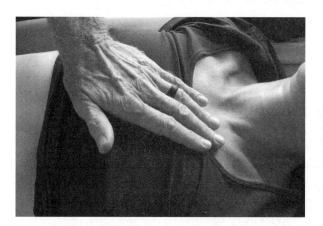

Fig. 35.28. Umbilicus–Inferior vena cava–Heart

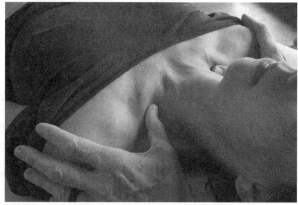

Fig. 35.29. Subclavian vein 1

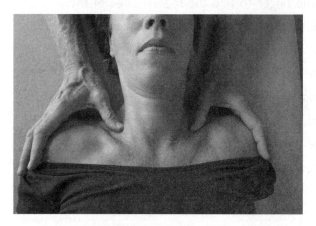

Fig. 35.30. Subclavian vein 2

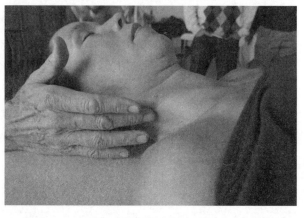

Fig. 35.31. Jugular vein

the two hands. The consciousness of the five senses is said to come through the umbilical veins, and we sense that through the IVC with stillness and PR.

6. Next move your hand from the costal arch directly over the heart and connect with PR at the level of where the IVC joins the superior vena cava (SVC). PR moves into the right atrium. Sense the space of stillness and wait for the movement of PR to reveal itself. It is the umbilical vein (IVC and SVC) that *brings the incarnating consciousness into form* through the umbilicus directly to the heart of the embryo.

7. Sitting at the head of the table, contact the shoulders of the client. Then contact the subclavian artery on the right. If the client is comfortable, then contact the left for bilateral contact. As with the palpation in the abdomen, very gently allow the fingers to move around and under the artery to contact the space of the subclavian vein. The right subclavian vein represents the inflow of what is called "Alaya," which is the *base consciousness of an ordinary, settled mind.* The left subclavian vein represents the *flow of the intellect moving* toward the heart. In Buddhism, the heart is said to be the location of the mind. Wait for PR to indicate its directional flow toward the heart associated with these two levels of discernment in Tibetan medicine.

8. Contact the middle of the length of the SCM muscle on the right side with the pad of one or two fingers. If this is comfortable then contact the left side for bilateral contact. Sense the carotid artery under the muscle. Once again, find the center of the pulse of the carotid artery and gently move your contact around the posterior edge of the SCM so that the dynamic open space of the vein can be sensed. The fingers are naturally attracted to the stillness of the veins. Again, wait until the flow of PR moves toward the heart. Sometimes it will feel as if the fingers are melting into the vein. Frequently, you will also sense the movement of PR in the vein toward the heart and then PR in the artery moving away from the heart. Sometimes this is experienced sequentially and sometimes simultaneously. In the right jugular vein, it is said that the mind of conflicting emotions moves to the heart. In the left jugular vein is the excellent mind conducive to enlightenment according to Tibetan medicine.

9. Finish this sequence with bilateral contact with either of the tibial arteries or a coccyx-diaphragm contact.

RECOMMENDED READING

A Manual of Acupuncture by Peter Deadman and Mazin Al-Khafaji (Journal of Chinese Medicine Publications, 2016).

Putting It All Together

A Biodynamic Rite of Passage

Throughout this book the view of a clinical session is that of a rite of passage and aligned with the Way of the Natural World, the fluid body in all its manifestations. It is a three-step process of perception and prayer. Integrating factors from medical and cultural anthropology into a contemporary state of mind, body, and spirit includes the following:

STEP ONE: THE NEUTRAL

The intention in the beginning of a session is to *stabilize the wind of water and earth elements* in the client. In the body, the water and earth elements are conjoined as biological water with dozens of different fluids that communicate with the whole through the interstitium, blood, and fascia. The fluid body is the *water-earth body*. In Tibetan medicine their combination has a neurological fulcrum (of several) in the brain and body called the autonomic nervous system. The wind moves the water just as stress physiology moves the autonomic nervous system. It is the same metaphor. We perceive our fluid body as demonstrated in part 2. The perfect fluid body is the Tide of Primary Respiration. When we meditate as described in parts 4 and 5, the perception and balancing of the earth element is enhanced by mindfulness of gravity and weightedness in the body. The posture of meditation itself is enlightenment as Suzuki Roshi said in *Zen Mind, Beginner's Mind*. The therapist brings a meditation posture to the treatment room.

We then attune to Primary Respiration. The client naturally attunes to our internal states (and we attune to their internal states) as we move our *fulcrum* of perception for Primary Respiration starting at the lower dantian and gradually between the third ventricle of our brain and the horizon following the initial exploration of a meditation posture and the fluid body. We are an interconnected two-person biology reciprocally establishing a felt sense of safety. We allow that fulcrum to automatically shift to the heart-to-heart connection with the client. When the wind and waves of stress physiology in the client begin to settle by attunement to the therapist's state of abiding in the calmness and serenity of not knowing how to help, a Neutral is perceived. This is a slowing down in the relational field and a stillpoint capable of expanding to the horizon. This is the wind of space opening the door to transformation determined by the intelligence of the elements. Such a stillpoint is clear and potent rather than inert and dissociated, which is the other end of the spectrum of the dorsal vagus being overstimulated and accessing an instinctual state of withdrawal. Remember, Dr. Jealous said to "wait, watch, and wonder."

STEP TWO: IGNITION

The perception of the wind of water, earth, and space generates an Ignition, a transition to the healing priorities of the elements. They move in a therapeutic direction assisted primarily by the diligence of the therapist maintaining a container of safety and open awareness. Ignition is about the *wind of fire*. The fire element needs to be contained and redirected in between the core of the body: the pleural, pericardial, and peritoneal cavities and the sleeve of the body consisting of the muscular skeletal system and skin. This is the Triple Warmer in classical Chinese medicine. The primary fulcrum of the fire element in the body is the superior mesenteric artery.

The superior mesenteric artery is the first artery in the abdomen and pelvis of the embryo to develop. It arises simultaneously with the mesentery, the anchor of the intestines on the posterior abdominal wall. It holds and nurtures the entire small intestine and two-thirds of the large intestine. It is the source of heat that digests our food from an elemental point of view. Just as there are five fulcrums of Primary Respiration, the fire element fulcrums include the liver, the heart, the eyes, and the skin. The constancy of physical contact skin to skin, a form of kangaroo mother care in a biodynamic session, conducts heat and can naturally settle the wind of the digestive fire. The therapist must learn to belly breathe and place the wind in the abdomen surrounding and filling the superior mesenteric artery. This is where your embryo is located in the lower dantian. This is achieved by concentrating on the focal point of the lower dantian for inhalation and exhalation. This type of breath is a gentle exploration of softening and opening the tensions held within the peritoneal cavity of abdomen and pelvis rather than a forceful mechanical pushing of the breath, which just creates more waves and hotter fire.

The wind of fire is the greatest modifier of temperature and the intensity of the lava flow of inflammation. Understanding the hot volcanic goddess Pele from Hawaiian legend helps us understand the alchemical transformation of food being digested when something melts to become a different shape or form from bile to feces, from blood to urine. The abdomen is now the *critical geography* of therapeutic input in the contemporary client. It must be contacted as frequently as is appropriate for a client. A map is not the territory. The exploration of the gut was detailed in previous chapters.

Ignition requires a strong container as the client has a foot in both worlds. There is a foot with its roots in the history and gestation of whatever condition or syndrome is presently arising. And at the same time because of the Neutral, the client now has a foot in the world of healing outside ordinary space and time. The client has access to the extraordinary space and time of the elements present from the beginning of the universe and coming to human form at conception. Thus, this phase in the biodynamic rite of passage must maintain an even stronger container for the client to navigate fearlessly between the seduction of one world to the other unknown world without interference such as excessive curiosity by the therapist or the client insisting on keeping their cell phone available during a session. The other world is simply the natural world. Ignition is the phase of bearing witness and building accurate therapeutic empathy for holding the client in their totality and uniqueness with loving kindness and humility. It is their process that must be honored and remain free of inappropriate interventions and the overly zealous desire to help. The client cannot be helped in a conventional sense, rather in the extraordinary sense.

STEP THREE: THE HEALTH

When Pele is satisfied and calmed by the cooling breeze of Primary Respiration, like a fountain of water springing from the lower dantian, the final stage of the biodynamic rite of passage can occur. The last stage is the *wind of space* deeply manifesting its grace and sacred sound located in the inner ear, vision in the eyes, the inner heart, and the entire rhythmic pulsation of the vascular system. This is the Health, a mind balanced by the wind of space in the heart and lower dantian. This is called potency in osteopathy. All such movement motivated by the wind as Primary Respiration is centered by the element of space, a self-knowing, nonthought awareness. Our perception periodically brings this awareness to the foreground and Primary Respiration fades automatically into the background. It is also known by its depth of stillness sometimes called the void. Thoughts become particles of space arising and dissipating by themselves, and the breath is discovered to be everything and nothing more than the wind of Primary Respiration moving the respiratory diaphragm. It is the flow of grace, nothing but the Tide. Unbiased and nonjudgmental choiceless awareness allows the physical body to synchronize with the subtle and very subtle bodies, and the flow of grace can be accessed when appropriate and necessary directly. This witness awareness comes forward, unbiased, nonthinking, and synchronized with posture, breath, and mind. The Health appears to the therapist with knowing and thinking hands synchronized with the potency of the Tide.

In this rite of passage to the Way of the Natural World, we are reclaiming dominion over our body. It is a politically active attitude of being pro soma. Each of us has authoritative knowledge regarding the care and nurturing of our bodies inside ourselves. Our bodies know what to accept and what to reject when given the opportunity at an elemental level. Our body can communicate the truth to us with interoceptive awareness. The care and nurturing of the body is the essence of the rite of passage that includes self-compassion and self-forgiveness for the ways in which we have harmed our body. We can wake up to engaging in self-safety and begin to avoid many of the noxious influences in the environment. We can establish a common somatic sensibility and restore the body's ability to heal itself and express its needs. This happens through an allegiance with conscious interoceptive awareness unpolluted by unwholesome external influences, concepts, and misperceptions of the external environment.

This biodynamic rite of passage is not a linear process in the treatment room or even in the natural world. Biodynamic practice is continuous practice. Sometimes we are lucky and steps in the process are skipped and sometimes they are prolonged in their phases. Each phase is a galaxy of potential, and the container that the therapist constructs builds alignment of the planets. Their orbits are eccentric, and they are centered by the sun radiating from our heart. Therefore we rest in our *beginner's heart* and relish the opportunity for not knowing, which is the dynamic stillness, a gap in discursive thinking without fear. Sometimes the void is accessed, the absolute end of the previous universe dissolving into the element of space. Death and birth are simultaneous and consequently do not exist at the deepest level of the element of space. It is there as a spontaneous potential and requires the continual maintenance of a strong perceptual container for renewal, regeneration, and incorporation as a spiritual human being endowed with common somatic sense.

Familiarity with death and dying must be known. Our work as biodynamic practitioners is palliative. The essence is in the experience of self-regulation, agency, and pro soma sovereignty. Never let anyone take your right to direct experience of your Health away from you. We all have a lot of work to do on ourselves to be of benefit to others. We learn how to serve rather than fix or give a treatment. Our treatments are an offering, a blessing. We serve the whole that is pre-existing rather than helping what is broken. The colors, the wisdoms, the elements, and the heart are the glue that binds the whole. "Be still and know . . ."

Real Food

Yummy Soups, Smoothies, and Breakfast Ideas

BY CATHY SHEA

CATHY SHEA has been a licensed massage and colon hydrotherapist in the state of Florida since 1992. She also holds full certification in Swiss Biological Medicine from Thomas Rau, M.D. Additionally, she is a certified instructor with the International Association of Colon Therapy and holds the highest credential in her profession as a nationally board certified colon hydrotherapy instructor. Her passion for health education is shared with her husband Michael J. Shea, Ph.D., as they have collaborated on teaching and writing since 1990. Cathy has personally instructed health care providers in thirty-four countries who share knowledge and experience as they continue to expand upon the value of gentle, routine cleansing practices and positive health outcomes.

YUMMY CLEANSING
LUNCH AND DINNER IDEAS

Simple veggie soups are the perfect way to cleanse and maintain stamina during days when we have colon hydrotherapy. Here are some of my favorites that are easy to prep if you chop the veggies ahead of time and freeze them (except the avocado). I start by sizzling the onions and garlic in a good oil to get them softened and slightly browned, then add the veggies and broth to simmer. These can be eaten either chunky with broth or pureed as you prefer.

- zucchini, yellow squash, onion, garlic; garnish with oregano
- asparagus, celery, onion; garnish with fresh tarragon
- cauliflower, onion, curry; garnish with toasted coconut or sesame seeds
- organic frozen veggie combo, garlic, onion, other savories
- butternut, carrot, onion, ginger; garnish with pumpkin seeds
- tomato, onion, garlic, peppers; garnish with fresh basil
- cucumber, garlic, avocado; garnish with green onion (this is a chilled soup)
- masa harina corn, onion, garlic, cumin/coriander
- green beans, onions, mushrooms, garlic; garnish with dill

Note that these recipes are using mild veggies vs. strong ones like broccoli and legumes that often cause too much gas. Consider adding either tofu, coconut milk/cream, avocado, or soaked cashews/almonds to thicken and provide good fat. Pouring soup over a bed of spinach or other greens will increase nutrient density. If you like, you may also add cooked grains or quinoa for density. ENJOY!

YUMMY SMOOTHIE IDEAS

You can make any of these combinations ahead and then freeze in mason jars that are just two-thirds full to allow for expansion. A good measurement is: 2 cups water, 1 cup veg, 1 cup fruit = almost 4 cups. If the lid is tight, it will keep refrigerated for 3 days maximum or frozen up to 3 months.

Red: beets and raspberries
Blue: blueberries and spinach
Orange: carrots and papaya
Green: kale and mango
Yellow: pineapple and yellow squash
Gold: mango and golden beet
Good garnishes: ginger in winter, mint in summer, other favorite herbs, plus lime, orange, or lemon juice

YUMMY BREAKFAST IDEAS

You may find it best to drink about sixteen to thirty-two ounces of warm water with a squeeze of lemon or lime in it first thing in the morning. This washes the digestive tract and helps create alkalinity. Also, it makes a nice herbal tea to warm the stomach. If you plan to take a walk, bike, or swim, eat a small portion of fruit. Remember to only eat one fruit at a time so it digests quickly and easily. After exercising, try one of these:

- Greens in the blender with fresh fruit or frozen. Add a few drops of stevia if you need it sweeter.
- Eggs are a great protein, either scrambled, fried, poached, or hard boiled.
- Gluten-free toast or waffles with nut butter/cinnamon on top. Sprinkle 1 tbsp. of flax seeds for that extra fiber boost.
- Squeeze fresh lemon or lime juice over pieces of avocado with papaya or mango slices; sprinkle toasted coconut flakes on top.
- It's okay to have chicken or fish or beans for breakfast; this is when we need our big protein.
- Veggie wrap with salsa or chopped tomatoes.
- Sweet potato mash with sprinkled cinnamon and chopped nuts.
- Gluten-free toast with tomato, lettuce/sprouts, and avocado.
- Whole grains: quinoa, rice, millet, buckwheat. Simmer gently with added nuts, seeds, cinnamon, and dairy-free milk.
- When I'm short on time, I eat cold cereal with warmed dairy-free milk and banana slices. It's quick and easy and YUMMY!!
- Garden burgers also make a super-fast, high-energy meal. Eat on bread or over a grain or salad.

Add the fiber from acacia, ground flax, or chia (or whole seeds soaked overnight and rinsed in the morning) or organic flax oil with lignans to any or all of the above. This increases the fiber content tremendously and adds EFA lubrication to the system and feeds beneficial microbes.

Bless it all and enjoy!

Glossary

Some of the terms defined below have a more universal usage in the fields of science, medicine, and/or spirituality. But many of the terms included here are defined specifically as used in biodynamic craniosacral/cardiovascular therapy and the Primary Respiration/Long Tide model.

autonomic nervous system (ANS): the part of the central nervous system that is coregulated by the hypothalamus in the brain and controls the physiology of bodily functions generally categorized as unconscious such as breathing, heartbeat, and digestion. However, those functions can be influenced consciously when awake. The ANS is made up of the sympathetic nervous system (SNS) and parasympathetic nervous system (PNS) (see these entries for more). The ANS is a dual reciprocal functioning system of the body not only associated with physiological but also metabolic regulation. The ANS functions at a metabolic level via its neurotransmitters and biochemistry for the regulation of anabolism and catabolism. This is particularly important in their flow within the ANS plexi built into and around the esophagus and organs of digestion and elimination, heart, aorta, descending aorta, abdominal aorta, and common iliac arteries.

awareness: directly experiencing the discovery of mindfulness and the willingness not to cling to the discoveries of mindfulness. Mindfulness is associated with precision of attention and recognizing when one's attention has been captured by the past or future. Awareness diffuses mindfulness into a larger container associated with the insight of no self, also called self-knowing awareness. It is associated with the deeper meanings of the element of space, the dharma teaching of emptiness, and dynamic stillness—called *shikantaza* in Zen. (See also "mindfulness.")

biodynamic: the growth of the whole organism and its perpetual differentiation of its wholeness over time in the context of the human embryonic morphology model of Erich Blechschmidt, M.D. This understanding became expanded by Jim Jealous, D.O., who included the whole to mean the natural world of the planet earth and its continuity with all sentient beings inside and out. His metaphor for such wholeness was the fluid body. Thus, biodynamic can mean the Way of the Natural World prior to cognition and conceptualization. (See also "fluid body" and "Way of the Natural World.")

biodynamic healing process: the timeless process of becoming fully human. Differentiated and manifesting over the life span before, during, and after sessions in unique and discrete ways for each person. It is not possible to know the client's healing trajectory, therefore the therapist maintains an attitude of not knowing, bearing witness, and self-compassionately engaging their own healing process. Biodynamics is an exploration of unconditioned phenomena inherent in the constant rhythmic interchange of the PR and the stillness for perhaps an hour in the larger context of the remainder of a client's lifestyle. Unconditioned states associated with healing within PR/stillness are innumerable and organized into three categories: gross, subtle, and very subtle. The therapist learns to serve the client heart to heart. (See also "Health" and "stillness.")

biodynamic therapeutic process: the direct experience of the rhythmic, balanced interchange of the PR and stillness in, through, and outside of the body during a single session. A self-directed and open-ended continuum of perceptual explorations of Health via the natural world bound by the time scheduled for the client. The therapist is an unbiased nonjudgmental observer in each session. (See also "Health.")

Breath of Life: a timeless state within PR. Sutherland described it variously as a flash of light, a spark, and Ignition. It is associated with spirituality and religion in the context of how Sutherland defined his perception of it based on the Book of Genesis in the Bible and his devotion to his Christian origins and that of his profession. It can be considered as the Wisdom Wind in Tibetan Medicine. (See also "Primary Respiration.")

cardiovascular system: a differentiated and interconnected vascular tree for biodynamic therapeutic exploration (the cardiovascular system as used in this book). It has ten components. First, the whole tree itself is moved by the wind of Primary Respiration. Second, the vascular tree has a center or core, which is the four chambered heart and coronary arteries. Third, a trunk called the life channel including the aorta, the descending aorta, the abdominal aorta, arteries differentiating from the abdominal aorta, and paired veins especially the portal vein and inferior and superior vena cava. Fourth, like a mangrove in the coastal waters of the tropics, it has a shallow root system above the ground of the legs consisting of the common and internal iliac arteries and all other pelvic floor arteries and veins. Fifth, it has a deep root system that continues below the pelvis when it transitions from the external iliac artery under the inguinal ligament and becomes the femoral artery and all other arteries and veins down to the tips of the toes. Sixth, the main branches of the vascular tree consist of the subclavian artery and veins including their extensions down through the arm, lungs, muscles of respiration, and breasts in general. In addition, the carotid and vertebral arteries are major branches that go through the neck into the face and cranium including the jugular vein. Seventh, the treetop is the Circle of Willis in the brain and all other cerebrovascular structures. Eighth, the leaves of the tree consist of the capillary beds. It is here in the capillary beds where a major interface with the interstitium and bone marrow, components of the fluid body, exist. Ninth, the blood is the sap of the tree with a spiritual essence coming from the heart flowing in the blood to and through every cell in the body. Tenth, the endothelium of the vascular tree is an endocrine-immune organ and coregulator of homeostasis in the body.

central nervous system (CNS): generally considered to be the brain and spinal cord. Many but not all metabolic process are coregulated by the central nervous system, which includes the endocrine and immune systems. Embryonically, the CNS arises from the third ventricle of the brain. This is important because Dr. Jealous moved the fulcrum of therapeutic concentration in the Cranial Concept from the fourth ventricle to the third ventricle of the brain because the third ventricle is the origin point for all embryonic differentiations of the central nervous system.

compassion: knowing our style of suffering and its depth, which is similar and thus shared with all other sentient beings. Everyone suffers on a scale of moderate to severe from emotional afflictions, unrealistic views, and cognitive obscurations. First, compassion is to know how these function in mind and body, which creates suffering in ourselves and others. Second, it is relating directly to personal suffering and engaging it skillfully—initially taught through mindfulness of the body-mind and gradually through complex visualizations and prayers. PR connects self with others reciprocally because it is the movement of compassion heart to heart. Self-compassion is the priority. Empathy forms a basis of compassion, the kindling that ignites compassion. (See also "empathy" and "mindfulness.")

empathy: to feel what another person is feeling. There are three types of empathy: First, somatic, originating in the core of the body through interoceptive awareness of one's visceral urges being sensed. Second, emotional through cardioception, which is awareness of one's heartbeat and its potency associated with the source of spiritual PR emanating from the back of the heart. Third, cognitive, the ability to put yourself in someone else's shoes, their mind of suffering from emotional afflictions and cognitive obscurations. (See also "compassion." and "mindfulness")

endocrine system: controls metabolism through the secretion of hormones. Some hormones have anabolic actions on the body; others have mainly catabolic actions. For example, testosterone is an anabolic hormone (build up), and synthetic steroids that produce the anabolic actions are known as anabolic steroids such as the widely prescribed drug called prednisone and many other forms used by athletes all over the world. On the other hand, cortisol (a steroid hormone produced by the adrenal gland) is a catabolic hormone (break down). The endocrine system (as well as the CNS) is influenced by the balance between the energy demands of the body and its energy stores, called glycogen and ketones processed in the liver and used by the mitochondria in all the cells of the body for metabolic energy.

fluid body: a metaphor for an experience of the natural world inside and outside the body. The fluid body is an instinctual intelligence that interconnects us to the natural world as one living, incorporated, spiritual being capable of giving and receiving love. PR exists both as a layer of experience within the fluid body as well as moving through it ("in the fluids not of the fluids," according to Dr. Sutherland). It is also considered the mixture of the elements water and earth in Eastern medicine. There is a perfect and an imperfect fluid body. An unhealthy metabolism generates an imperfect fluid body through the deposition of too many waste products in the lymphatic fluid, the interstitial fluid, the cytoplasm of the cell, the fascia, and the blood. The perfect fluid body is the Wisdom Wind of water. This is called the Tide. Primary Respiration breathes/moves the water element without any interference regardless of the amount of toxicity in the imperfect fluid body. (See also "Primary Respiration.")

four reminders: important contemplation of luck, life, death, and impermanence upon entering the Tantric Path. These four reminders are: First, I contemplate the preciousness of having a human body and being free from war and oppression, being well-favored with time and health, and having access to sacred teachings and an authentic teacher. Human birth is rare and difficult to gain, easy to lose; now I must do something meaningful for the benefit of all sentient beings. Second, the whole world and its inhabitants are impermanent. Whatever appears will disappear. I have the same nature. The life of all sentient beings is like a temporary bubble. Death comes without warning; this body will be a corpse. At that time, the dharma of pristine self-knowing awareness will be my only help; I must continually practice not-knowing and non-thinking with exertion 24/7 to overcome fear. Third, when death comes, I will be helpless to prevent it. Because I create karma, I must abandon compulsive ill-intentioned actions, and always devote my time to virtuous actions. Thinking this, every day I will examine the motivation and intention for all my mental, emotional and physical behavior. Fourth, the homes, friends, wealth, and the comforts of samsara are the constant torment of the three sufferings (old age-sickness-death, impermanence, and existentialism). Such comforts are like a feast before the executioner leads you to your death. I must cut desire and attachment and attain enlightenment through continuous meditation practice. The present moment is the supreme spiritual teacher.

fulcrum: a stillpoint in the embryo around which structure forms. It is called radial symmetry. Biodynamic practice includes three fulcrums for the perception of PR through the umbilicus/lower dantian, posterior heart/middle dantian, and third ventricle of the brain/upper dantian. Each is differentiated through the potency and direction of PR and the background of cellular quiescence (stillness). They are interconnected as the three dantians. Purposeful slowness (PR) and cellular and venous quiescence (stillness) are factors inducing growth and development that precede biochemistry. PR contains other numerous perceptual possibilities on a spectrum between form and formlessness because it is an aspect of the Wisdom Wind element. (See also "stillness.")

Health: embodied manifestation of Primary Respiration. It is used as a marker for session outcomes by Dr. Jealous and the biodynamic osteopathic community in general as the perception of PR's potency increasing, mutating, or transforming. For example, when someone is near death their Health becomes sweet and soft rather than depleted or missing. It is an intrinsic factor of PR but differentiated from its base rate of 6 CP–10 M and other subtle levels. The Health is one's felt sense of vitality, revery, and well-being and not limited to that. It is variable like the wattage and voltage of electricity and preexisting in the body. The fuse box for the Health is found in the rhythmic balanced interchange of Primary Respiration and the stillness. It is on a spectrum of variable perceptions, experiences, and metaphors such as grace, the Breath of Life, love, spiritual chi emanating from the heart, compassion, empathy, gratitude, and so forth. Such metaphors and others are representations of the Health. Each biodynamic therapist must have direct experience of their own fluctuating Health as a prerequisite for serving the Health of others. As a principle of interpersonal neurobiology, the client instinctually seeks contact with the Health of the therapist as the ground of safety in the therapeutic relationship and thus a reliable source to mimic. It is a basis of achieving a Neutral. (See also "Neutral" and "Primary Respiration.")

ketosis: the breakdown of fatty acids into ketones, the preferred source of energy for cells in most of the body especially the brain rather than sugar.

Long Tide: the original term coined by Dr. Sutherland that now means Primary Respiration. (See also "Primary Respiration.")

mandala: a symbolic representation of cosmic forces in a two- or three-dimensional form. It is a synthesis of an aspect of the cosmos used for one's individual spiritual formation through meditation and awakening to one's own unlimited ground of being.

macronutrients: consists of three categories of nutrition needed by the body for proper anabolism and catabolism: 1. proteins/types, 2. fats/types, 3. carbohydrates/types.

metabolism: the biochemical modification and exchange of molecules by the human body, especially through cells and their mitochondria. The term is often used to refer to the basal metabolic rate, the "set point" that each person has in breaking down food energy to fortify and maintain the mitochondria in providing energy to operate all functions in the body. Its meaning encompasses the overall ingestion of food, its transformation biochemically for the building and the growth of the body, and excretion of wastes from the mitochondria of each cell to the evacuation of the large intestine. Metabolism includes the chemical conversion of ingested items other than food, like drugs and poisons. Evolutionary factors influencing metabolism include feast/famine cycles, starvation studies, and paleo or ancestral nutrition. Evolutionary factors are bound by the relationship of epigenetics to mammalian instincts—especially survival, the oldest and most primitive human instinct.

metaphor: the terminology therapists and clients are expected to spontaneously develop to describe their own unique sensory experience (as a phenomenology of mind and body).

microbiome: a microbial community best described as the sum of all microbial life living in, on, or around the human body. These microbes are located in and on the tissue of the eyes, ears, nose, throat, digestive organs, reproductive organs, blood, and all vascular tissue. It is an entity that has wide-reaching metabolic, nutritional, psychological, and immunological effects on the body. The microbiome evolves within a flexible immune system host from conception to death, constantly fine-tuning itself to maintain a homeostatic balance with the body's immune system of which it coregulates. Continued evolution of the human microbiome after birth is governed by factors such as both the adaptive and innate immune system, as well as external factors such as diet, medication, toxin exposure, and illness. The microbiome begins its evolution in utero and extends across the life span, profoundly effecting both physical and mental well-being and has a role in the development of disease and neurological disorders.

micronutrients: a group of essential elements that feed the body throughout life and include water, vitamins, and minerals, micronutrients are one of the four pillars of essential human nutrition that include carbohydrates, protein, and fats.

midline: a metaphor for various interpretations of the experience of embodied order and organization in the manual therapeutic arts, also known as axial symmetry. Midline is the transitory organizing phenomena for the growth and development of the embryo, which leaves an imprint over the life span of the body.

The axial symmetry of the embryo is one such transitory phenomena. Midline is usually associated with some aspect of the anatomy of the spine in traditional craniosacral therapy. At a more subtle level the midline extends from the core of the planet earth through each person's neurological midline (or anterior to it) out the top of the head and connecting to a star in the constellation Ursa Major considered to be the center of the universe in Taoism. Thus, each person is connected through the universe via such a cosmological midline. The level of the spiritual formation midline is the stillness, the element of space, and the void as discussed in this book. (See also "fulcrum" and "stillness.")

mindfulness: the act and instinctual experience of noticing mental attention being captured by thoughts and concepts of the past, present, and future. Mindfulness is the art of returning over and over again to the direct experience of the present moment. It is the portal to self-knowing awareness and awakening. It is cultivated by meditation but is not meditation.

Neutral (holistic shift): when the autonomic nervous system senses safety and PR shifts from managing trauma to restoring harmony and balance. The Neutral is unique to everyone based on each client's discrete set point for overstimulation and trauma history. It is the first step in the biodynamic rite of passage unfolded in this book. Since it is frequently perceived as a stillpoint, the Neutral is one metaphor for numerous PR therapeutic and healing transition states. The Neutral begins with the therapist's neutral and then that of the client through attunement.

parasympathetic nervous system: the part of the autonomic nervous system generally responsible for relaxation, natural digestion, and elimination. It acts reciprocally with the sympathetic nervous system. Its principal component is the vagus nerve, which displays deeper physiological and metabolic regulation of the organism. (See also "autonomic nervous system," "polyvagal theory," and "sympathetic nervous system.")

pathology: a branch of medicine that explores and diagnoses diseases including metabolic syndrome, cardiovascular disease, diabetes, obesity, dementia/ Alzheimer's, and cancer.

pelvic floor: the structure of the human body that contains the reproductive and eliminative organs. This includes fascia/muscles, bladder, prostate, gonads, fallopian tubes, uterus, vagina, vulva (clitoris), and penis. Pelvic floor functions include defecation, urination, orgasm, and birthing.

polyvagal theory: describes a three-tiered group of ANS mechanisms through which physiological states communicate the experience of safety and contribute to a person's capacity either to feel safe and spontaneously engage cooperatively with others via the nucleus ambiguus-ventral vagus, to feel threatened and recruit defensive strategies through the SNS, or to become immobilized by feigning death or dissociating via the more ancient dorsal motor nucleus above the diaphragm. The polyvagal theory emphasizes the differential roles of two distinct vagal pathways identified in the mammalian ANS—the dorsal motor nucleus and the nucleus ambiguous—generally from the brain stem to the esophageal plexus on the respiratory diaphragm.

Primary Respiration (PR): the perception of a rhythmic gain and loss of the inherent completeness and equality of body-mind-natural world as "one drop." It is the starting point in a PR session. PR is a multilayered set of generative and spontaneously emerging phenomena associated with stillness and the element of wind in Eastern medicine. All PR states are viewed as intelligent session entry, mid, and end points. An important intention of the PR is to incorporate as a spiritual being: knowing what to accept and what to reject, claiming dominion with one's body, responding rather than reacting, being self-compassionate and empathetic, and expressing heartfelt love. Synonyms for PR include but are not limited to: the Tide, Breath of Life, Primary Respiratory Impulse, Long Tide, perfect fluid body, source chi, spiritual chi, and the Holy Spirit. (See also "spirituality.")

pro soma: embodied moral, metabolic, emotional, and social safety. Pro soma is the active separation from the body politic, the agency of mind-body spiritual authority, governing and intelligently manifesting the innate wisdom, and intentions of the Health in one's body. The definition is in concordance with the 1948 United Nations Universal Declaration of Human Rights. It is focused, committed self-compassion. (See also "compassion.")

Real Food: food that is eaten in its most natural state such as fruits, vegetables, whole grains, and water. Real Food is the opposite of "processed" food, which is chemically altered, highly processed, and packaged for convenience and longevity, causing metabolic syndrome.

six virtues: virtues perfected by a compassionate human being. They are generosity, discipline, patience, exertion, meditation, and wisdom.

somatic: the organism before thoughts and concepts. It is associated with the evolutionary intelligence and decision-making capacity of the fluid body.

spirituality: the timeless direct experience of PR and its intention. PR manifests at its deepest level as embodied love, compassion, and grace unfolding from inside, through, and around the whole body out to the edge of the universe and beyond. Spirituality is associated with reverence, respect, and reverie, considered essential attitudes of the therapist. Sorrow, empathy, and compassion are also essential spiritual attitudes of biodynamic practitioners. All healing is spiritual healing under the guidance of PR manifesting as the Holy Spirit in the guise of the Way of the Natural World. The spiritual authority of the therapist comes from a direct experience of PR and stillness, which transforms into a blessing offered to the client from the therapist's presence and manual contact. Each person has their own spiritual aptitude for direct experience of their own interconnected divinity with the cosmos and their own heart. Thus, each individual's spiritual formation is a lifelong learning, which may include atheism, agnosticism, and all other "isms" as part of the path of heart-mind awakening that has no beginning and no ending.

stillness: the differentiation of levels associated with accessing the Health as defined in this book. According to Dr. Jealous there are three levels. Level one stillness is the balance point between atmospheric pressure and the body fluids as a cellular metabolic quiescence—no breathing. Level two stillness is the stillness through which breathing relates to Zone B, the biosphere around the body. Breathing is regulated by Primary Respiration. Third level stillness emerges over time and is considered the dynamic stillness—no rate, only a direct perception of the element of space, panoramic awareness, and the void. (See also "Health" and "Primary Respiration.")

sympathetic nervous system (SNS): the branch of the autonomic nervous system that increases heart rate, blood pressure, and breathing rate when the body is under stress. Commonly known as the "fight or flight" branch. Metabolically, the SNS regulates vasodilation, which is the first function of the endothelium to fail in the inflammatory process. (See also "autonomic nervous system.")

trauma: overwhelming experience of the ANS resulting in suffering. In biodynamic therapy the therapist acknowledges trauma but does not orient to it unless PR does so. All such states are held with mindfulness, empathy, and compassion so PR can potentiate transformation and reconnection to a resourced state. PR—not the therapist—makes decisions about its therapeutic priorities. Trauma reactions governed by the ANS cannot be fixed, rather they become stabilized and recognized and resilience skills are built as valuable resources for riding the periodic ANS waves of being triggered. The therapist learns to serve the client by integrating the three tenets of not knowing, bearing witness, and appropriate compassionate exploration based on the therapist's own spiritual formation integrated with their personal trauma work.

Tide: See "Primary Respiration."

void: a direct experience of no beginning-no ending, no birth-no death without fear. Found in the present moment as the supreme spiritual teacher. (See also "stillness.")

Way of the Natural World: synonym for the fluid body. Inner spiritual formation includes direct experience of the whole of the natural world outside, biodynamic practice is thus the Way of the Natural World as conceived by Dr. Jealous. It is integrated into sessions because of its potential for igniting the healing process of sensing interconnection with the cosmological whole. The natural world participates in a biodynamic session and is capable of guiding each session and directing therapeutic outcomes. Consequently, the therapist moves their attention out to the horizon and back as an invitation for the natural world and all its beauty to help and support the session. This includes having visual access to the natural world by looking out a window for example and acute listening to the sounds of nature, especially the wind and bird song. The therapist manages the session interaction between the forces of nature outside the office with the forces of nature inside the therapist's body and that of the client. In the Way of the Natural World, the client cannot be fixed, only offered such an invitation for reconnection to the whole. (See also "fluid body," "Health," "Primary Respiration," and "stillness.")

Bibliography

Aird, William C. "Phenotypic Heterogeneity of the Endothelium: I. Structure, Function, and Mechanisms." *Circulation Research* 100, no. 2 (February 2007): 158–73.

———. "Phenotypic Heterogeneity of the Endothelium: II. Representative Vascular Beds." *Circulation Research* 100, no. 2 (February 2007): 174–90.

Alphonsus, Christella, and R. N. Rodseth. "The Endothelial Glycocalyx: A Review of the Vascular Barrier." *Anaesthesia* 69, no. 7 (July 2014): 777–84.

Asghar, Zeenat, Alysha Thompson, Maggie Chi, et al. "Maternal fructose drives placental uric acid production leading to adverse fetal outcomes." *Scientific Reports* (April 29, 2016): 625091.

Azad, Meghan B., Atul K. Sharma, Russell J. de Souza, et al. "Association between artificially sweetened beverage consumption during pregnancy and infant body mass index." *JAMA Pediatrics* published online July 1, 2016.

Bailey, Alice. *Esoteric Healing*. New York: Lucis Press, 1953.

Ball, Philip. "David Hare's Fiery Account of COVID-19." *Lancet* 396, no. 10255 (Sept 2020): 878–79.

Batra, Arvind, and Britta Siegmund. "The Role of Visceral Fat." *Digestive Diseases* 30, no. 1 (May 2012): 70–74.

Belančić, Andrej. "Gut Microbiome Dysbiosis and Endotoxemia—Additional Pathophysiological Explanation for Increased COVID-19 Severity in Obesity." *Obesity Medicine* 20 (December 1, 2020): 100302.

Bernard, Isabelle, Daniel Limonta, Lara K. Mahal, and Tom C. Hobman. "Endothelium Infection and Dysregulation by SARS-CoV-2: Evidence and Caveats in COVID-19." *Viruses* 13, no. 1 (December 26, 2020).

Bragg, Paul, and Patricia Bragg. *The Miracle of Fasting: Proven Throughout History for Physical, Mental, and Spiritual Rejuvenation*. Santa Barbara, Calif.: Bragg Health Sciences, 2004.

Briner, Barbara. *Esoteric Healing Part 1: Introduction to Esoteric Healing*. Okemos: National Association of Esoteric Healing, 1993.

Briner, Barbara. *Esoteric Healing Part 2: Integration*. Okemos: National Association of Esoteric Healing, 1993.

Briner, Barbara. *Esoteric Healing Part 3: The Bigger Picture*. Okemos: National Association of Esoteric Healing, 1993.

Carrington, Hereward. *Fasting for Health and Long Life*. Whitefish, Montana: Kessinger Publishing, 2006.

Centers for Disease Control and Prevention (website), "People with Certain Medical Conditions." Accessed May 2, 2021.

Chernyak, B. V., E. N. Popova, A. S. Prikhodko, O. A. Grebenchikov, L. A. Zinovkina, and R. A. Zinovkin. "COVID-19 and Oxidative Stress." *Biochemistry* (Moscow) 85, no. 12–13 (December 1, 2020): 1543–53.

Coelho, Marisa, Teresa Oliveira, and Ruben Fernandes. "Biochemistry of adipose tissue: An endocrine organ." *Archives of Medical Science* 9, no. 2 (April 20, 2013): 191–200.

Connelly, Dawn. "Everything You Need to Know about COVID-19 Vaccines." The Pharmaceutical Journal (website). Updated December 15, 2021.

Cuervo, Natalia Zamorano, and Nathalie Grandvaux. "ACE2: Evidence of Role as Entry Receptor for SARS-COV-2 and Implications in Comorbidities." *ELife* 9 (October 2020): 1–25.

Danese, Andrea, and Bruce S. McEwen. "Adverse childhood experiences, allostasis, allostatic load, and age-related disease." *Physiology and Behavior*, 106, no. 1 (April 16, 2012): 29–39.

Danese, Silvio, Elisabetta Dejana, and Claudio Fiocchi. "Immune Regulation by Microvascular Endothelial Cells: Directing Innate and Adaptive Immunity, Coagulation, and Inflammation." *The Journal of Immunology* 178, no. 10 (May 15, 2007): 6017–22.

Deanfield, John E., Julian P. Halcox, and Ton J. Rabelink. "Endothelial Function and Dysfunction: Testing and Clinical Relevance." *Circulation* 115, no. 10 (March 13, 2007): 1285–95.

Deputy, Nicholas P., Andrea J. Sharma, Shin Y. Kim, and Stefanie N. Hinkle. "Prevalence and Characteristics Associated with Gestational Weight Gain Adequacy." *Obstetrics & Gynecology* 125, no. 4 (April 2015): 773–81.

DeVries, Arnold Paul. *Therapeutic Fasting.* Los Angeles, Calif.: Chandler Book Company, 1963.

Dimitriadis, Kyriakos, Costas Tsioufis, Alexandros Kasiakogias, et al. "Waist circumference versus other obesity indices as determinants of coronary artery disease in essential hypertensive patients: A 6 year follow up study." *European Heart Journal* 33, Abstract Supplement (March 28, 2018): 494.

Din, Ahmad Ud, Maryam Mazhar, Muhammed Waseem, et al. "SARS-CoV-2 Microbiome Dysbiosis Linked Disorders and Possible Probiotics Role." *Biomedicine and Pharmacotherapy* 133 (January 2021): 110947.

Dogné, Sophie, Bruno Flamion, and Nathalie Caron. "Endothelial Glycocalyx as a Shield against Diabetic Vascular Complications: Involvement of Hyaluronan and Hyaluronidases." *Arteriosclerosis, Thrombosis, and Vascular Biology* 38, no. 7 (July 27, 2018): 1427–39.

Ehret, Arnold. *Rational Fasting.* (First published in 1910). New York: Ehret Literature Publishing, 2011.

———. *The Mucusless Diet Healing System* (Revised edition). Columbus, Ohio: Breathair Publishing, 2014.

Eliade, Mircea. *Rites and Symbols of Initiation: The Mysteries of Birth and Rebirth.* New York: Harper & Row, 1958.

Eliade, Mircea. *Myth and Reality.* New York: Harper & Row, 1963.

Eliade, Mircea. *Shamanism: Archaic Techniques of Ecstasy.* Princeton: Princeton University Press, 1964.

Epstein, Franklin H., John R. Vane, Erik E. Änggård, and Regina M. Botting. "Regulatory Functions of the Vascular Endothelium." *New England Journal of Medicine* 323, no. 1 (July 1990): 27–36.

Fildes, Alison, Judith Charlton, Caroline Rudisill, Peter Littlejohns, A. Toby Prevost, and Martin C. Gulliford. "Probability of an obese person attaining normal body weight: Cohort study using electronic health records." *American Journal of Public Health* 105, no. 9 (July 16, 2015): e54–9.

Fothergill, Erin, Juen Guo, Lilian Howard, et al. "Persistent metabolic adaptation 6 years after 'The Biggest Loser' competition." *Obesity* 24, no. 8 (August 2016).

Fowler, Sharon P. G., Ken Williams, and Helen P. Hazuda. "Diet Soda Intake Is Associated with Long-Term Increases in Waist Circumference in a Biethnic Cohort of Older Adults: the San Antonio Longitudinal Study of Aging." *Journal of the American Geriatrics Society* 63, no. 4 (April 2015): 708–15.

Fuhrman, Joel. *Fasting and Eating for Health: A Medical Doctor's Program for Conquering Disease*. New York: St. Martin's Griffin, 1995.

García, Luis F. "Immune Response, Inflammation, and the Clinical Spectrum of COVID-19." *Frontiers in Immunology* 11 (June 16, 2020): 1441.

Goni, Leticia, Marta Cuervo, Fermín I. Milagro, and J. Alfredo Martínez. "Future Perspectives of Personalized Weight Loss Interventions Based on Nutrigenetic, Epigenetic, and Metagenomic Data." *Journal of Nutrition* 146, no. 4 (April 1, 2015): 905S–12S.

Guo, Junyi, Zheng Huang, Li Lin, and Jiagao Lv. "Coronavirus Disease 2019 (COVID-19) and Cardiovascular Disease: A Viewpoint on the Potential Influence of Angiotensin-Converting Enzyme Inhibitors/Angiotensin Receptor Blockers on Onset and Severity of Severe Acute Respiratory Syndrome Coronavirus 2 Infection." *Journal of the American Heart Association* 9, no. 7 (April 7, 2020): e016219.

Hahn, Thich Nhat. *Interbeing: The 14 Mindfulness Trainings of Engaged Buddhism*. Berkeley, Calif.: Parallax Press, 2020.

Hamming, I., W. Timens, M. L. C. Bulthuis, A. T. Lely, G. J. Navis, and H. van Goor. "Tissue Distribution of ACE2 Protein, the Functional Receptor for SARS Coronavirus. A First Step in Understanding SARS Pathogenesis." *Journal of Pathology*, 203, no. 2 (June 2004): 631–37.

He, Li-Hong, Long-Fei Ren, Jun-Feng Li, Yong-Na Wu, Xun Li, and Lei Zhang. "Intestinal Flora as a Potential Strategy to Fight SARS-CoV-2 Infection." *Frontiers in Microbiology* 11 (June 9, 2020): 1388.

Horton, Richard. "Offline: COVID-19 Is Not a Pandemic." *The Lancet* 396, no. 10255 (September 26, 2020): 874.

Howie, G. J., D. M. Sloboda, T. Kamal, and M. H. Vickers. "Maternal nutritional history predicts obesity in adult offspring independent of postnatal diet." *Journal of Physiology* 587, part 4 (February 15, 2009): 905–15.

Ikkyū, *Crow with No Mouth*. Translated by Stephen Berg. Port Townsend, Wash.: Copper Canyon Press, 1989.

Jasti, Madhu, Krishna Nalleballe, Vasuki Dandu, and Sanjeeva Onteddu. "A Review of Pathophysiology and Neuropsychiatric Manifestations of COVID-19." *Journal of Neurology* 268, no. 6 (June 2021): 2007–12.

Jensen, B. *Dr. Jensen's Juicing Therapy: Nature's Way to Better Health and a Longer Life*. New York: McGraw-Hill Education, 2000.

Jialal, Ishwarlal, Sridevi Devaraj, Harmeet Kaur, Beverley Adams-Huet, and Andrew A. Bremer. "Increased Chemerin and Decreased Omentin-1 in Both Adipose Tissue and Plasma in

Nascent Metabolic Syndrome." *Journal of Clinical Endocrinology and Metabolism* 98, no. 3 (March 2013): E514–17.

Karachaliou, Marianna, Vaggelis Georgiou, Theano Roumeliotaki, et al. "Association of trimester-specific gestational weight gain with fetal growth, offspring obesity, and cardio-metabolic traits in early childhood." *American Journal of Obstetrics and Gynecology* 212, no. 4 (April 2015): 502.e1–14.

Khalil, Mohamad, Hala Khalifeh, Fatima Saad, et al. "Protective Effects of Extracts from Ephedra Foeminea Forssk Fruits against Oxidative Injury in Human Endothelial Cells." *Journal of Ethnopharmacology* 260 (May 16, 2020): 112976.

Khansari, Nemat, Yadollah Shakiba, and Mahdi Mahmoudi. "Chronic Inflammation and Oxidative Stress as a Major Cause of Age-Related Diseases and Cancer." *Recent Patents on Inflammation & Allergy Drug Discovery* 3, no. 1 (January 2009): 73–80.

Khomina, Anna. "The Doctrine of Discovery: On This Day, 1493." The Gilder Lehrman Institute of American History (website), May 4, 2017.

Kolacz, Jacek, and Steven W. Porges. "Chronic Diffuse Pain and Functional Gastrointestinal Disorders After Traumatic Stress: Pathophysiology Through a Polyvagal Perspective." *Frontiers in Medicine* 5, no. 145 (May 2018).

Kompaniyets, Lyudmyla, Alyson B. Goodman, Brook Belay, et al. "Body Mass Index and Risk for COVID-19–Related Hospitalization, Intensive Care Unit Admission, Invasive Mechanical Ventilation, and Death—United States, March–December 2020." *Morbidity and Mortality Weekly Report* 70, no. 10, Centers for Disease Control and Prevention (CDC) (March 12, 2021): 355–61.

Larson, Joni. "Back to Basics: The First Law of Healing." *LIFESTREAM* 10, no. 2 (2020): 16–20.

Leddy, Meaghan A., Michael L. Power, and Jay Schulkin. "The Impact of Maternal Obesity on Maternal and Fetal Health." *Reviews in Obstetrics and Gynecology* 1, no. 4 (2008): 170–78.

Lee, Wen Shi, Adam K. Wheatley, Stephen J. Kent, and Brandon J. DeKosky. "Antibody-Dependent Enhancement and SARS-CoV-2 Vaccines and Therapies." *Nature Microbiology* 5, no. 10 (October 2020): 1185–91.

Li, Yanwei, Wei Zhou, Li Yang, and Ran You. "Physiological and Pathological Regulation of ACE2, the SARS-CoV-2 Receptor." *Pharmacological Research* 157 (July 2020): 104833.

Libby, Peter, and Thomas Lüscher. "COVID-19 Is, in the End, an Endothelial Disease." *European Heart Journal* 41, no. 32 (September 2020): 3038–44.

Lowen, Alexander. *Bioenergetics*. New York: Penguin/Arkana, 1994.

Ludwig, David. *Always Hungry? Conquer Cravings, Retrain Your Fat Cells, and Lose Weight Permanently*. New York: Grand Central Life & Style Publishing, 2016.

Lustig, Robert H. *The Hacking of the American Mind: The Science Behind the Corporate Takeover of Our Bodies and Brains*. New York: Avery, 2018.

———. *Metabolical, The Lure and the Lies of Processed Food, Nutrition, and Modern Medicine*. New York: Harper Collins, 2021.

Lustig, R. H., K. Mulligan, S. M. Noworolski, V. W. Tai, M. J. Wen, A. Erkin-Cakmak, A. Gugliucci, and J. Schwarz. (2016). "Isocaloric fructose restriction and metabolic improvement in children with obesity and metabolic syndrome." *Obesity* 24 (2016): 453–60

Lupien, Sonia J., Bruce S. McEwen, Megan R. Gunnar, and Christine Heim. "Effects of stress throughout the lifespan on the brain, behavior and cognition." *Nature Reviews Neuroscience* 10, no. 6 (June 2009): 434–45.

Mohammad, Sameer, Rafia Aziz, Saeed Al Mahri, et al. "Obesity and COVID-19: What Makes Obese Host so Vulnerable?" *Immunity and Ageing* 18, no. 1 (January 4, 2021): 1–10.

Monk, C., J. Spicer, and F. A. Champagne. "Linking Prenatal Maternal Adversity to Developmental Outcomes in Infants: The Role of Epigenetic Pathways." *Developmental Psychopathology*, 24 no. 4 (2012): 1361–76.

Mudd, Austin T., Lindsey Alexander, Rosaline Waworuntu, Brian Berg, Sharon M. Donovan, and Ryan N. Dilger. "What Is in Milk? How Nutrition Influences the Developing Brain." *Frontiers for Young Minds* 5, no. 16 (May 2017).

Myatt, L. "Placental Adaptive Responses and Fetal Programming." *Journal of Physiology* 572 no. 1 (2006): 25-30.

Nakao, Wendy Egyoku. "Hold to the Center." Tricycle (online), Summer 2017.

Nalbandian, Ani, Kartik Sehgal, Aakriti Gupta, et al. "Post-Acute COVID-19 Syndrome." *Nature Medicine* 27, no. 4 (April 2021): 601–15.

National Institute for Health and Care Excellence (NICE) (website). "Clinical Knowledge Summaries." Accessed May 2, 2021.

National Institute for Health Research. "Living with Covid19—Second Review." March 16, 2021.

National Institutes of Health (NIH). COVID-19 Treatment Guidelines, "Therapeutic Management of Hospitalized Adults With COVID-19." Last updated December 16, 2021.

Neumann, Erich. *The Great Mother.* Princeton, N.J.: Princeton University Press, 1963.

Norwitz, Nicholas G., and Uma Naidoo. "Nutrition as Metabolic Treatment for Anxiety." *Frontiers in Psychiatry* 12 (February 12, 2021): 598119.

Oken, Emily, Elsie M. Taveras, Ken P. Kleinman, Janet W. Rich-Edwards, and Matthew W. Gillman. "Gestational weight gain and child adiposity at age 3 years." *American Journal of Obstetrics and Gynecology* 196, no. 4 (April 2007): 322.e1–8.

Osuchowski, Marcin F., Martin S. Winkler, Tomasz Skirecki, et al. "The COVID-19 Puzzle: Deciphering Pathophysiology and Phenotypes of a New Disease Entity." *The Lancet Respiratory Medicine* 9, no. 6 (June 2021): 622–42.

Padwal, Raj, William D. Leslie, Lisa M. Lix, and Sumit R. Majumdar. "Relationship Among Body Fat Percentage, Body Mass Index, and All-Cause Mortality: A Cohort Study." *Annals of Internal Medicine* 164, no. 8 (April 19, 2016): 532–41.

Phillips, Catherine M. "Metabolically healthy obesity across the life course: epidemiology, determinants, and implications." *Annals of The New York Academy of Sciences.* The Year in Diabetes and Obesity (2016): 1–16.

Porges, Stephen W. *The Polyvagal Theory: Neurophysiological Foundations of Emotions, Attachment, Communication, and Self-Regulation.* New York: W. W. Norton, 2011.

———. *The Pocket Guide to the Polyvagal Theory: The Transformative Power of Feeling Safe.* New York: W. W. Norton, 2017.

Pries, A. R., and W. M. Kuebler. "Normal Endothelium." *Handbook of Experimental Pharmacology* 176, part 1 (2006): 1–40.

Pruimboom, Leo. "Methylation Pathways and SARS-CoV-2 Lung Infiltration and Cell Membrane-Virus Fusion Are Both Subject to Epigenetics." *Frontiers in Cellular and Infection Microbiology* 10 (May 26, 2020): 290.

Puchalski C., B. Ferrell, R. Virani, S. Otis-Green, P. Baird, J. Bull, H. Chochinov, G. Handzo, H. Nelson-Becker, M. Prince-Paul, K. Pugliese, and D. Sulmasy. "Improving the Quality of Spiritual Care as a Dimension of Palliative Care: The Report of the Consensus Conference. *J Palliat Med.* 12 no. 10 (October 2009): 885–904.

Ramcharan, Khedar S., Gregory Y. H. Lip, Paul S. Stonelake, and Andrew D. Blann. "The Endotheliome: A New Concept in Vascular Biology." *Thrombosis Research* 128, no. 1 (July 2011): 1–7.

Reich, Wilhelm. *The Mass Psychology of Fascism.* 3rd ed. New York: Farrar, Straus, and Giroux, 1980.

Reich, Wilhelm. *The Function of the Orgasm: Sex-Education Problems of Biological Energy.* New York: Farrar, Straus, and Giroux, 1986.

Reich, Wilhelm. *Character Analysis.* 3rd ed. New York: Farrar, Straus, and Giroux, 2000.

Ronti, Tiziana, Graziana Lupattelli, and Elmo Mannarino. "The Endocrine Function of Adipose Tissue: An Update." *Clinical Endocrinology* 64, no. 4 (April 2006): 355–65.

Saad, Antonio F., Joshua Dickerson, Talar B. Kechichian, et al. "High-fructose diet in pregnancy leads to fetal programming of hypertension, insulin resistance, and obesity in adult offspring." *American Journal of Obstetrics and Gynecology* 214, no. 1 (January 2016): Supplement, S48.

Saben, Jessica L., Anna L. Boudoures, Zeenat Asghar, et al. "Maternal Metabolic Syndrome Programs Mitochondrial Dysfunction via Germline Changes across Three Generations." *Cell Reports* 16, no. 1 (June 28, 2016): 1–8.

Sahakyan, Karine R., Virend K. Somers, Juan P. Rodriguez-Escudero, et al. "Normal-weight central obesity: implications for total and cardiovascular mortality." *Annals of Internal Medicine* 163, no. 11 (Dec 2015): 827–35.

Sandman, Curt A., and Elysia Poggi Davis. "Neurobehavioral risk is associated with gestational exposure to stress hormones." *Expert Review of Endocrinology and Metabolism* 7, no. 4 (July 2012): 445–59.

Scaer, Robert C. *The body bears the burden: Trauma, dissociation and disease.* 2nd ed. New York: The Haworth Medical Press, 2007.

———. *8 Keys to Brain-Body Balance.* New York: W. W. Norton & Company, 2012.

Schmiegelow, M., C. Andersson, L. Kober, et al. "Body mass index is a strong predictor of myocardial infarction and stroke in fertile women, a nationwide study." *European Heart Journal,* 33 (2012): Abstract Supplement, 493.

Schore, Allan N. "Back to Basics: Attachment, Affect, Regulation and the Developing Right Brain: Linking Developmental Neuroscience to Pediatrics." *Pediatrics in Review* 26, no. 6 (June 2005): 204–18.

Segerstrom, Suzanne C., and Gregory E. Miller. "Psychological Stress and the Human Immune System: A Meta-Analytic Study of 30 Years of Inquiry." *Psychological Bulletin* 130, no. 4 (July 2004): 601–30.

Seng, J. S., L. K. Low, M. Sperlich, D. L. Ronis, and I. Liberzon. "Post-traumatic stress disorder, child abuse history, birthweight and gestational age: A prospective cohort study." *BJOG: An International Journal of Obstetrics and Gynaecology* 118, no. 11 (October 18, 2011): 1329–39.

Sheldon, William H. *Atlas of Men: A Guide for Somatotyping the Adult Male of All Ages.* New York: MacMillan Publishing Company, 1970.

Shelton, Herbert M. *Fasting Can Save Your Life*. New York: American Natural Hygiene Society Press, 1978.

Shonkoff, Jack P., W. Thomas Boyce, and Bruce S. McEwen. "Neuroscience, Molecular Biology, and the Childhood Roots of Health Disparities Building a New Framework for Health Promotion and Disease Prevention." *JAMA* 301, no. 21 (June 3, 2009): 2252–59.

Simionescu, M., and F. Antohe. "Functional Ultrastructure of the Vascular Endothelium: Changes in Various Pathologies." *Handbook of Experimental Pharmacology* 176, part 1, (2006): 41–69.

Skinner, Asheley Cockrell, Eliana M. Perrin, and Joseph A. Skelton. "Prevalence of Obesity and Severe Obesity in US Children, 1999–2014." *Obesity* 24, no. 5 (May 24, 2016): 1116–23.

Sovio, Ulla, Helen R, Murphy, and Gordon C. S. Smith. "Accelerated Fetal Growth Prior to Diagnosis of Gestational Diabetes Mellitus: A Prospective Cohort Study of Nulliparous Women." *Diabetes Care* 39, no. 6 (June 2016): 982–87.

Steyers, Curtis M., and Francis J. Miller. "Endothelial Dysfunction in Chronic Inflammatory Diseases." *International Journal of Molecular Sciences* 15, no. 7 (June 25, 2014): 11324–49.

Still, Andrew Taylor. *Philosophy of Osteopathy*. Kirksville, Mo.: Published by the author, 1899.

———. *Autobiography of Andrew Taylor Still* (rev. ed.). Kirksville, Mo.: Published by the author, 1908.

Sudre, Carole H., Benjamin Murray, Thomas Varsavsky, et al. "Attributes and Predictors of Long COVID." *Nature Medicine* 27, no. 4 (April 2021): 626–31.

Sun, Hai Jian, et al. "Role of Endothelial Dysfunction in Cardiovascular Diseases: The Link between Inflammation and Hydrogen Sulfide." *Frontiers in Pharmacology* 10 (January 21, 2020): 1568.

Sutherland, Adah Strand, and Anne L. Wales (eds). *Collected Writings of William Garner Sutherland, D.O., D.Sc. (Hon.) Pertaining to the Art and Science of Osteopathy: Covering the Years 1914–1954*. Ford, Ky.: Sutherland Cranial Teaching Foundation, 1967.

Suzuki, Shunryu. *Zen Mind, Beginner's Mind*. Boston: Shambhala, 2006.

Tarrant, John. *The Light Inside the Dark: Zen, Soul, and the Spiritual Life*. New York: HarperPerennial, 1998.

Van den Bergh, B., E. Mulder, M. Mennes, and V. Glover, "Antenatal maternal anxiety and stress and the neurobehavioral development of the fetus and child: Links and possible mechanisms. A review." *Neuroscience and Biobehavioral Reviews* 29 (April 2005): 237–58.

Varga, Zsuzsanna, Andreas J. Flammer, Peter Steiger, et al. "Endothelial Cell Infection and Endotheliitis in COVID-19." *The Lancet* 395, no. 10234 (May 2, 2020): 1417–18.

Villapol, Sonia. "Gastrointestinal Symptoms Associated with COVID-19: Impact on the Gut Microbiome." *Translational Research: The Journal of Laboratory and Clinical Medicine* 226 (December 2020): 57–69.

Vimaleswaran, Karani S., Nita G. Forouhi, and Kamlesh Khunti. "Vitamin D and Covid-19." *The BMJ* 372, no. 544 (March 4, 2021).

Wadhwa, Pathik D. "Psychoneuroendocrine processes in human pregnancy influence fetal development and health." *Psychoneuroendocrinology* 30, no. 8 (September 2005): 724–43.

Wadhwa, Pathik D., Laura Glynn, Calvin J. Hobel, et al. "Behavioral perinatology: Biobehavioral processes in human fetal development." *Regulatory Peptides* 108, no. 2–3 (October 15, 2002): 149–57.

Wadhwa, Pathik D., Sonja Entringer, Caludia Buss, and Michael C. Lu. "The contribution of maternal stress to preterm birth: Issues and considerations." *Clinics in Perinatology* 38, no. 3 (September 2011): 351–84.

Walker, N. W. *Fresh Vegetable and Fruit Juices: What's Missing in Your Body?* Prescott, Ariz.: Walker Press, 1978.

Wann, Marilyn. *FAT!SO?: Because you don't have to apologize for your size.* Berkeley, Calif.: Ten Speed Press, 1998.

Warren, Rick, Daniel Amen, and Mark Hyman. *The Daniel Plan: 40 Days to a Healthier Life.* Grand Rapids, Mich.: Zondervan, 2013.

Wolfson, Julia A., Sarah E. Gollust, Jeff Niederdeppe, and Colleen L. Barry. "The Role of Parents in Public Views of Strategies to Address Childhood Obesity in the United States." *The Milbank Quarterly* 93, no. 1 (March 2015): 73–111.

World Health Organization. WHO Coronavirus (COVID-19) Dashboard | WHO Coronavirus (COVID-19) Dashboard With Vaccination Data. Accessed April 28, 2021.

World Obesity Federation. "Obesity and COVID-19: Policy Statement." Accessed May 4, 2021.

Yang, Lin, and Graham A. Colditz. "Prevalence of Overweight and Obesity in the United States, 2007–2012." *JAMA Internal Medicine* 175, no. 8 (August 2015): 1412–13.

Yehuda, Rachel, Stephanie Mulherin Engel, Sarah R. Brand, Jonathan Seckl, Sue M. Marcus, and Gertrud S. Berkowitz. "Transgenerational effects of posttraumatic stress disorder in babies of mothers exposed to the World Trade Center attacks during pregnancy." *Journal of Clinical Endocrinology and Metabolism* 90, no. 7 (July 2005): 4115–18.

Younossi, Z. M., A. B. Koenig, D. Abdelatif, Y. Fazel, L. Henry, and M. Wymer. "Global epidemiology of nonalcoholic fatty liver disease—Meta-analytic assessment of prevalence, incidence, and outcomes." *Hepatology* 64, no. 1 (July 2016): 73–84.

Zhang, Ying-Xiu, Zhao-Xia Wang, Jin-Shan Zhao, and Zun-Hua Chu. "Trends in overweight and obesity among rural children and adolescents from 1985 to 2014 in Shandong, China." *European Journal of Preventive Cardiology* 23, no. 12 (August 2016): 1314–20.

Resources

HOW TO REACH THE SHEAS

You may reach Michael Shea, Ph.D., at his website: **SheaHeart.com**.

You may reach out to Cathy Shea directly for guidance and coaching via her website, **www.cathysheaschool.com**. She also offers National Board Certification for professionals wanting to practice the trademark SheaWay^{SM} Colon Hydrotherapy, including the gentle SloFil^{SM} Method.

RESEARCHERS/ORGANIZATIONS

Center for Compassion and Altruistic Research and Education (CCARE) at Stanford University

Center for Healthy Minds at University of Wisconsin

Greater Good Science Center at the University of California, Berkeley

Naropa University

Real Food at Robert Lustig's website

Weston Price Foundation—authoritative knowledge on ancestral nutrition for the past ninety years

PRACTITIONERS

Thomas Rau, M.D., Swiss Biological Medicine, treats patients at his clinic in Switzerland

Zach Bush, M.D., has a website, Farmer's Footprint, with many resources, including an award-winning documentary about the impact of chemical farming

Sheila Shea, MA, LMT, is a GAPS (gut and psychology syndrome) certified instructor for healing leaky gut; an expert on metabolic syndrome, colon hydrotherapy, and eating disorders; she can be found on her website of the same name

Robert Lustig, M.D., is an international authority on the danger of sugar and founder of the Real Food movement starting with children; he is a pediatric neuroendocrinologist at the University of California San Francisco and best-selling author

Nina Teicholz, Ph.D., is an international authority on ketogenic diet and the politics of nutrition and a best-selling author

Catherine Shanahan, M.D., is an international authority on nutrition and human metabolism and a best-selling author

Jason Fung, M.D., is an international authority on intermittent fasting, obesity, and low carb diets and a best-selling author

Frank Lipman, M.D., is an international authority on nutrition and human metabolism

Aseem Malhotra, M.D., is an international authority on low carb diets and the politics of nutrition in Great Britain and Europe and a best-selling author

Tim Noakes, M.D., is an international authority on low carb diets and athletic performance

OTHER RESOURCES

International Council of Thirteen Indigenous Grandmothers, all of whom come from different tribes—these are wise, healer women who have nurtured and nourished many with their knowledge of home remedies and natural healing ways. You can find more information about them at their website.

Emotional Freedom Technique at Tapping.com

Index

Page numbers in *italics* refer to illustrations.

BOOKS OF RELATED INTEREST

Handbook of Chinese Medicine and Ayurveda
An Integrated Practice of Ancient Healing Traditions
by Bridgette Shea, L.Ac., MAcOM

The Encyclopedia of Ailments and Diseases
How to Heal the Conflicted Feelings, Emotions, and Thoughts at the Root of Illness
by Jacques Martel

Holistic Medicine and the Extracellular Matrix
The Science of Healing at the Cellular Level
by Matthew Wood
Foreword by Stephen Harrod Buhner

Healing from the Inside Out
Overcome Chronic Disease and Radically Change Your Life
by Nauman Naeem, M.D.
Foreword by Bernie S. Siegel

Anything Can Be Healed
The Body Mirror System of Healing with Chakras
by Martin Brofman
Foreword by Anna Parkinson

Healing the Thyroid with Ayurveda
Natural Treatments for Hashimoto's, Hypothyroidism, and Hyperthyroidism
by Marianne Teitelbaum, D.C.
Foreword by Anjali Grover, M.D.

Energetic Cellular Healing and Cancer
Treating the Emotional Imbalances at the Root of Disease
by Tjitze de Jong
Foreword by Robert Holden, Ph.D.

The Body Clock in Traditional Chinese Medicine
Understanding Our Energy Cycles for Health and Healing
by Lothar Ursinus

INNER TRADITIONS • BEAR & COMPANY
P.O. Box 388
Rochester, VT 05767
1-800-246-8648
www.InnerTraditions.com

Or contact your local bookseller